Gender-Based Violence

Yanyi K. Djamba • Sitawa R. Kimuna
Editors

Gender-Based Violence

Perspectives from Africa, the Middle East, and India

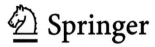 Springer

Editors
Yanyi K. Djamba
Department of Sociology, Anthropology
  and Geography
Auburn University at Montgomery
Montgomery, AL, USA

Sitawa R. Kimuna
Department of Sociology
East Carolina University
Greenville, NC, USA

ISBN 978-3-319-38319-4   ISBN 978-3-319-16670-4   (eBook)
DOI 10.1007/978-3-319-16670-4

Springer Cham Heidelberg New York Dordrecht London

Printed on acid-free paper

Springer International Publishing AG Switzerland is part of Springer Science+Business Media
(www.springer.com)

Contents

About the Editors

Yanyi K. Djamba is Professor of Sociology at Auburn University at Montgomery. He received his M.A. and Ph.D. degrees in Sociology from Louisiana State University and was a postdoctoral fellow at the Population Research Center, University of Texas at Austin. Dr. Djamba has previously worked at Brown University and Southeastern Louisiana University, where his last position was Associate Professor and Graduate Program Coordinator. He has received many professional awards and grants from different sources and has served as a consultant to a variety of organizations, as well as the United Nations. Dr. Djamba is the author and coauthors of many publications including *Sexual Health of Young People in the U.S. South* (2012), *Sexual Behavior of Adolescents in Contemporary Sub-Saharan Africa* (2004), and numerous peer-reviewed articles and newspaper columns on population-related topics.

Sitawa R. Kimuna is Associate Professor of Sociology at East Carolina University. Her research is interdisciplinary and covers substantive areas from gender-based violence, social demography, population dynamics, and immigration to sexual behavior and HIV in Sub-Saharan Africa and socioeconomic support of older people. Dr. Kimuna's Ph.D. degree in Sociology is from Kansas State University. She was a Population Reference Bureau Communications fellow and a Rockefeller Foundation fellow. She has served as a consultant to United Nations Population Fund Humanitarian Response Unit. Dr. Kimuna has publications in peer-reviewed journals and co-edited a book, *Women in African Development: The Challenge of Globalization and Liberalization in the Twenty-First Century.*

Contributors

Pranita Achyut International Center for Research on Women, New Delhi, India

Mosisa G. Aga Auburn University at Montgomery, Montgomery, AL, USA

Nandita Bhatla International Center for Research on Women, New Delhi, India

Dima Dandachi American University of Beirut, Family Medicine Department, Beirut, Lebanon

Yanyi K. Djamba Auburn University at Montgomery, Montgomery, AL, USA

Ruchi Jain National Council for Applied Economic Research, New Delhi, India

Alice Jacqueline Azebaze Kagou MINEPAT, Yaoundé, Cameroon

Hélène Kamdem Kamgno IFORD, Yaoundé, Cameroon

Marwan Khawaja UN-ESCWA, Beirut, Lebanon

Sitawa R. Kimuna East Carolina University, Greenville, NC, USA

Sunita Kishor The DHS Program, ICF International, Rockville, MD, USA

Kerry L.D. MacQuarrie The DHS Program, Avenir Health, Glastonbury, CT, USA

Amelia Reese Masterson American University of Beirut, Family Medicine Department, Beirut, Lebanon

Sarah Memmi CEPED—Paris Descartes Sorbonne University, Paris, France

Aparna Mukherjee Department of Population Policies and Programmes, International Institute for Population Sciences, Mumbai, India

Ajay Kumar Singh John Snow Research and Training Institute (JSI), New Delhi, India

Rabindra Kumar Sinha Independent Consultant, Mumbai, India

Mylene Tewtel Qatar Biomedical Research Institute, Qatar Foundation, Doha, Qatar

Jinan Usta American University of Beirut, Family Medicine Department, Beirut, Lebanon

Ravi Verma International Center for Research on Women, New Delhi, India

Nicole De Wet Demography and Population Studies, University of the Witwatersrand, Johannesburg, South Africa

Rebecca Winter The DHS Program, ICF International, Rockville, MD, USA

Introduction

Gender-Based Violence: A Call to Action

Gender-based violence is probably the most pervasive yet least recognized human rights violation of our time. Although both males and females are often victims of this type of violence, its prevalence remains higher for women and girls. As the UNFPA Executive Director, Dr. Babatunde Osotimehin said in his November 25, 2014 call to action for ending violence and discrimination against women, "today there is no country, not one, where women and girls live free from violence" (UNFPA 2014). According to some estimates, about one in three women have experienced physical or sexual abuse (UNFPA 2010). The situation is even more alarming in less developed regions where poverty is positively associated with gender-based violence, especially intimate partner violence (Duvvury 2009).

This book presents new perspectives on gender-based violence in Africa, the Middle East, and India, regions where the subject has been taboo in everyday discourse, due in part to their strong patriarchal cultural norms that limit women's autonomy. The book contains ten chapters of empirical research written by 22 scholars, who not only discuss the levels and the sociodemographic determinants of domestic violence but also examine topics that range from men's attitudes toward wife beating, domestic violence-related adolescent deaths, to women's reproductive tract infections and HIV due to sexual and physical abuse. The majority of the work in this book is based on papers presented at the 27th International Population Conference of the International Union for the Scientific Study of Population (IUSSP) held in South Korea in 2013 and the 2013 Annual Meeting of the Southern Demographic Association held in the United States.

In this introduction, we discuss the definitions of gender-based violence as well as the state of research on gender-based violence in non-Western world. This is followed by the presentation of the core conceptual framework within which fall all studies presented in this book. The subsequent part of the introduction provides a summary of the contents of each chapter. The last section gives a succinct conclusion of the book, including its contributions and suggestions for further research.

Defining Gender-Based Violence

Gender-based violence is not a new phenomenon. Through human history, the relations between males and females have involved various forms of discrimination based on gender, including cases where male genocides have been used in post-conflict environments (Carpenter 2006). However, the term gender-based violence has been well defined only in the last few decades as activists and advocates of gender equality fight to reduce discrimination and harmful practices against women. One major achievement in this regard was the 1993 United Nations Declaration on the Elimination of Violence against Women, which offered the first official definition of gender-based violence: "Any act of gender-based violence that results in, physical, sexual or psychological harm or suffering to women, including threats of such acts, coercion or arbitrary deprivations of liberty, whether occurring in public or in private life" (Health and Human Rights Info 2014).

While it is true that much of gender-based violence acts are directed toward women, there is evidence that men also have been victims of such abuse (Christian et al. 2011). As a result, we adopt the following definition in this book: "Gender based violence is any act of threat of harm inflicted on a person because of their gender" (Duvvury 2009). This definition incorporates all forms of abuse, including sexual, physical, emotional, and psychological harms. More specifically, the above definition encompasses all forms of violence discussed in this book, from physical abuse (e.g., wife beating in Chap. 1 and female death in Chap. 3) to the consequences of sexual violence (e.g., reproductive health issues in Chap. 8 and HIV risk in Chap. 4), as well as coercive marriage (e.g., Chap. 5).

The State of Research on Gender-Based Violence in Non-Western World

Research on gender-based violence in non-Western countries is still very limited, due to the lack of adequate data and limited methodological development. Nonetheless, there have been some promising developments in some non-Western parts of the world in recent years. However, the majority of such studies have been limited in both depth and quality of data, as well as geographic coverage.

For example, a 2011 publication by European Union (2011) based on the national situation analyses provides some basic information on the prevalence of gender based in nine countries: Algeria, Egypt, Israel, Jordan, Lebanon, Morocco, the Occupied Palestinian Territory, Syria, and Tunisia. Limited to these nine countries of the southern part of the European Union territory, that study does not offer a broader view of the gender-based violence in non-Western world. Moreover, its use of situation analysis as the primary data source does not allow the kind of empirical analyses needed to compare findings across regions.

Between 2000 and 2003, the World Health Organization (WHO) conducted the WHO Multi-country Study on Women's Health and Domestic Violence against Women (World Health Organization 2005). This study was carried out in ten countries across the globe. Because of its focus on health and domestic violence, the WHO study does not offer information on some of the current issues that increase women's vulnerability to gender abuse. For example, no substantial discussion is provided on the impact of war and political unrest on women's risk of spousal violence. Moreover, Sub-Saharan African countries were only marginally represented in the WHO study.

A more comprehensive study on gender-based violence in non-Western world published by ORC Macro used data from the Demographic and Health Surveys (DHS) in nine developing countries: Cambodia, Colombia, Dominican Republic, Egypt, Haiti, India, Nicaragua, Peru, and Zambia (Kishor and Johnson 2004). The results from these surveys, conducted mostly after 1998, show the percentages of women who said an intimate partner had ever abused them ranged from 48 % in Zambia and 44 % in Colombia to 18 % in Cambodia and 19 % in India. Additional findings show that more than one in six married women in each country reported being pushed, shaken, slapped, or targeted with a thrown object by their male partners.

While the ORC Macro study provides interesting comparative data on the levels and determinants of domestic spousal violence in nine countries, its regional coverage is very limited. For example, it includes only one country from the Sub-Saharan African region. The present study extends current knowledge on gender-based violence in non-Western world by examining data from three regions that have been historically excluded from previous research. In addition, this study employs different data sources and an ecological framework to determine the impact of various sociocultural factors on women's risks and consequences of spousal violence.

Conceptual Framework

Until the end of 1980s, much of the work on gender-based violence has been primarily influenced by different disciplines such as psychology, sociology, criminology, and feminism. Although such approaches have helped understand factors of gender abuse, their contributions have been limited due to their emphases on single or limited factors. The first attempts to conceptualizing gender-based violence begun in 1998 with Lori L. Heise's etiological framework (Heise 1998). The particular framework was built on the works of Belsky (1980) and Edleson and Tolman (1992).

Heise's conceptual framework, which focuses on violence against women, is composed of four categories. The first category includes personal history factors such as witnessing marital violence as a child, being abused as a child, and living without a father or with a rejected father. The second category contains microsystem factors such as male dominance in the family, male control of wealth in the family, alcohol use, and marital conflict. The third category comprises exosystem variables related to employment and socioeconomic status, isolation of women and family, and delinquent peer association. The fourth category includes macrosystem factors or variables related to social structures. This category contains variables such as male entitlement or male's perception of ownership of women, masculinity linked to aggression and dominance, rigid gender norms, acceptance of interpersonal violence, and acceptance of physical chastisement of women (Heise 1998: 265).

This book uses one of the most recent versions of that framework published by the World Bank (2009). Like Heise's framework, the World Bank conceptual model is an ecological framework based on four types of factors that have been empirically shown to explain gender-based violence. Such factors are divided into the following categories: (1) societal, (2) community, (3) relationship, and (4) individual levels. The model is presented below.

While this model encompasses the empirical analyses presented in this book, it is not used in the same way across chapters. For example, societal data on conflict and refugee camps are used mainly in Chaps. 6 and 7, whereas some relational variables such as intergenerational violence and parental conflict involving violence are examined in Chaps. 2 and 10. Nonetheless, as a whole, the chapters in this volume address various factors represented in the conceptual framework below. By doing so, we provide the first comprehensive analysis of gender-based violence across Africa, the Middle East, and India.

Ecological model of gender-based violence

Societal	Community	Relationship	Individual
Broad factors that reduce inhibitions against violence	Neighborhood, schools, and workplaces	With family, intimate partners, and friends	Personal factors that influence individual behavior
• Poverty	• High unemployment	• Family dysfunction	• Gender, age, and education
• Economic, social, and gender inequalities	• High population density	• Intergenerational violence and poor parenting practices	• A family history of violence
• Poor social security	• Social isolation of females and family	• Parental conflict involving violence	• Witnessing GBV
• Masculinity linked to aggression and dominance	• Lack of information	• Association with friends who engage in violence or delinquent behavior	• Victim of child abuse or neglect
• Weak legal and criminal justice system	• Inadequate victim care	• Low socioeconomic status, socioeconomic stress	• Lack of sufficient livelihood and personal income
• Perpetrators not prosecuted	• Schools and workplaces not addressing GBV	• Friction over women's empowerment	• Unemployment
• No legal rights for victims	• Weak community sanctions against GBV	• Family honor more important than female health and safety	• Mental health and behavioral problems

Societal	Community	Relationship	Individual
Broad factors that reduce inhibitions against violence	Neighborhood, schools, and workplaces	With family, intimate partners, and friends	Personal factors that influence individual behavior
• Social and cultural norms support violence	• Poor safety in public spaces		• Alcohol and substance abuse
• Small fire arms	• Challenging traditional gender roles		• Prostitution
• Conflict or post-conflict	• Blaming the victim		• Refugee internally displaced
• Internal displacement and refugee camps	• Violation of victim confidentiality		• Disabilities
			• Small fire arms ownership

Source: World Bank (2009)

Note: Reprinted with permission granted by the World Bank on September 22, 2014

Organization of the Book

This book contains ten chapters divided into three parts. The first part comprises four chapters on gender-based violence in Africa. The second part includes three chapters on gender-based violence in the Middle East; and the third has three chapters on gender-based violence in India. The contents of these chapters are summarized below.

Part I: Gender-Based Violence: Perspectives from Africa

The first chapter examines men's attitudes toward wife beating in Ethiopia. Analyzing the 2011 Ethiopia Demographic and Health Survey data in logistic regression models, Djamba, Kimuna, and Aga found that unmarried men were significantly more likely than married men to agree with the statements that the husband is justified to beating his wife if she refuses to have sex with her husband and if she burns food. The authors also uncovered important regional differences in men's attitudes toward wife beating, with residents of the national capital city, Addis Ababa, being the least likely to agree with such behavior. The effects of other sociodemographic variables are also discussed, along with policy implications and predictions for men's attitudinal change in Ethiopia.

In the second chapter, Kagou and Kamgno explore the relationship between fertility and physical violence, net of the effect of other sociodemographic variables. Using the 2011 Cameroon Demographic and Health Survey data, the authors found that six in ten (59.1 %) women in marital unions have been victims of physical marital violence. Results from the proportional hazards model indicate that fertility has a detrimental impact on marital relations. Such findings suggest that reducing fertility can help lower the occurrence of intimate physical violence against women in Cameroon. The authors also found significant positive associations between intimate physical violence and a number of other variables.

The third chapter by Nicole De Wet looks at the causes of higher female mortality due to assault in South Africa during the period 1997–2009. The author used data from the 2010 Victims of Crime Survey and the information from the Death Notification Form to analyze the association between assault and mortality. She found more reports of physical than sexual assaults in the country, with higher reports of both types of assaults among females with secondary education. Results from multivariate models show that females were significantly more likely to die from assaults than males. The author proposes some practical measures for reducing female abuse and resulting mortality among young women in South Africa.

The fourth chapter by MacQuarrie, Winter, and Kishor analyzes the linkage between spousal violence and HIV in five Sub-Saharan African countries (Kenya, Malawi, Rwanda, Zambia, and Zimbabwe). Using Demographic and Health Survey data from the five countries, the authors applied a couple-based approach in which a woman's experience of spousal violence and her HIV status are mediated by her husband's and her own behavioral and situational HIV risk factors. Despite the high prevalence of sexual violence in these countries (12–17 %), sexual violence is not associated with women's HIV status. In contrast, physical violence is significantly associated with women's HIV status in Kenya and Zimbabwe. These results show the importance of country-specific policies and programs that use prevailing local gender role norms.

Part II: Gender-Based Violence: Perspectives from the Middle East

In Chap. 5, Usta, Khawaja, Dandachi, and Tewtel question whether the risk of intimate partner violence is higher in consanguineous marriages. To answer the question, the authors analyzed Demographic and Health Survey data from Egypt (2005) and Jordan (2007). Their analysis focused on physical, emotional, and sexual violence that occurred within the 12 months prior to the survey. The results show that physical violence is higher in Egypt (18 %) than in Jordan (12 %), emotional violence is similar in both countries (10 %), and sexual violence is higher in Jordan (6 %) than in Egypt (4 %). The prevalence of consanguineous marriage is higher in Jordan (39 %) than in Egypt (33 %). Findings from multivariate models show significant association between consanguinity and experience of emotional, but not physical or sexual violence in both countries.

Chapter 6 offers an important analysis of the impact of refugee status on women's reproductive health. Written by Usta and Masterson, this chapter is based on interviews conducted in 2012 among 452 Syrian women who have been living in Lebanon for an average of 5.1 months. Additional data came from three focus group discussions with 29 women. The results show high reports of preterm deliveries (27 %) as well as several pregnancy-related problems such as anemia, abdominal pain, and bleeding. Menstrual irregularity, dysmenorrhea, and symptoms of reproductive tract infections were also common among these displaced women. These women justified intimate partner violence primarily as a result of stress and tension in the home, frustration among unemployed or emasculated men, and general worry or anger about the situation back home in Syria. In addition to spousal violence, several cases of sexual violence were reported, all allegedly perpetrated by armed people in Syria. The present findings are consistent with previous research, which showed increases in domestic violence in post-conflict settings (Loue 2001).

Chapter 7 examines the link between political unrest and domestic violence in Palestine. In this chapter, Sarah Memmi argues that political conflict can lead to the "normalization" of violence and may also increase domestic violence against women. Using data from the 2006 Palestinian Family Health Survey, this author shows the extent to which patriarchy and Israeli occupation are associated with domestic violence. More specifically, Memmi found that the probability of accepting violent behavior is significantly associated with domestic violence experience. Moreover, women who live in the areas most affected by political violence and mobility restrictions are more likely to report having experienced violence and to accept it. As such, Mimi's findings confirm the assumption that political insecurity leads to acceptance and increases domestic violence against women.

Chapter 8 by Singh, Sinha, and Jain focuses on the association between nonconsensual sex and sexual health among young married women in India. Using cross-sectional data of 300 married women age 15–29 interviewed in Delhi during the years 2007–2008, the authors found that more than two-thirds of women reported ever experiencing coercive sex by husband in their life time. The results from multivariate analyses show a significant negative association between domestic violence experience and sexual health. Among respondents who ever experienced sexual violence, nearly half had at least one STD symptom during the last 6 months compared to one-third who did not experience such violence. The authors present a number of obstacles that inhibit young married women from protecting themselves from nonconsensual sexual relations and from taking action against their partners or withdrawing from a coercive relationship. They also call for the creation of supportive environments in which trusted adults and peers can provide sexual health counseling to young women. Such programs will help young women learn how to prevent and confront a potentially threatening situation. Another suggestion in Chap. 8 is to make marital rape an offence under the Indian Penal Code.

Chapter 9, by Achyut, Bhatla, and Verma, reports on the results of an experimental program designed to reduce risky sexual behaviors among adolescents.

The underlying assumption is that positive socialization at younger age leads to better decisions regarding sexual and reproductive behaviors. Achyut, Bhatla, and Verma analyzed data from the Gender Equity Movement in Schools (GEMS) collected in Mumbai schools among early adolescent girls and boys ages 12–14 years in 2008–2010. The results show that girls and boys exposed to the interventions showed much greater improvement in self-reported measures of sexual and reproductive health than those with no interventions. These findings underscore the importance of gender-focus initiatives at early ages as a means for improving sexual and reproductive knowledge and behaviors.

Chapter 10 by Aparna Mukherjee attempts to find the levels and determinants of intergenerational transmission of spousal violence against women in India. The data came from the National Family Health Survey-3, 2005–2006, the first ever nationally representative survey that collected data on the dynamics of domestic violence in India. The results from multivariate analysis that controls for gender show that a woman's exposure to childhood violence has more devastating effect on developing her understanding toward her gender norms than on men. Based on the significant and positive effect of education on gender equity shown in this chapter, the author recommends that students be taught to avoid violence and adopt peaceful ways of conflict resolutions. In addition, there is a need for legislative policies and laws to make spousal violence or violence of any type against women a crime.

Conclusion

This book is the first of its kind to analyze and bring to the forefront of policy making the linkages that exist between gender-based violence, inequality, sociocultural norms, and socioeconomic development in Africa, the Middle East, and India. It is also the first publication to use a variety of data sources and to cover a wide range of gender-based violence topics in the same volume. With its ten chapters written by 22 researchers from different countries, this book places an emphasis not only on levels and determinants of gender-based violence but also on practical solutions for decision-makers in local, government, and international agencies. As such, it serves as a reference document for researchers, decision-makers, and organizations that are searching for ways to reduce gender-based domestic violence in less developed regions.

Nonetheless, further research is needed to enhance our understanding of the correlates of gender-based violence. As Marleen Temmerman argues, until now much of the current data on gender-based violence are based on cross-sectional studies (Temmerman 2014). Therefore, the results presented in this book represent only the associations between gender-based violence, as a dependent variable, and its correlates. To establish causal relationships, we need longitudinal studies, especially in the developing regions covered in this book.

Montgomery, AL, USA   Yanyi K. Djamba
Greenville, NC, USA   Sitawa R. Kimuna

References

Belsky, J. (1980). Child maltreatment: An ecological integration. *American Psychologist, 35*, 320–335.

Carpenter, R. C. (2006). Recognizing gender-based violence against civilian men and boys in conflict situations. *Security Dialogue, 37*(1), 83–103. doi: 10.1177/0967010606064139.

Christian, M., Safari, O., Ramazani, P., Burnham, G., & Glass, N. (2011). Sexual and gender based violence against men in the Democratic Republic of Congo: Effects on survivors, their families and the community. *Medicine, Conflict, and Survival, 27*(4), 227–246.

Duvvury, N. (2009). Keeping gender on the agenda: Gender based violence, poverty and development. An Issues Paper from the Irish Joint Consortium on Gender Based Violence. http://www.realizingrights.org/pdf/Keeping_Gender_on_the_Agenda.pdf. Accessed 17 Dec 2014.

Edleson, J., & Tolman, R. M. (1992). *Intervention for men who batter: An ecological approach.* Newbury Park, CA: Sage.

European Union. (2011). *State of play: Gender-based violence in southern Mediterranean countries.* Brussels, Belgium: European Union.

Health and Human Rights Info. (2014). Selected links on gender based violence. http://www.hhri.org/thematic/gender_based_violence.html. Accessed 10 Dec 2014.

Heise, L. L. (1998). Violence against women: An integrated, ecological framework. *Violence Against Women, 4*(3), 262–290.

Kishor, S., & Johnson, K. (2004). *Profiling domestic violence: A multi-country study.* Columbia, MD: ORC Macro.

Loue, S. (2001). *Intimate partner violence: Societal, medical, legal and individual responses.* New York: Kluwer Academic/Plenum Publishers.

Temmerman, M. (2014). Research priorities to address violence against women and girls. *The Lancet*, doi: http://dx.doi.org/10.1016/S0140-6736(14)61840-7. Accessed 21 Nov 2014.

UNFPA. (2014). Ending violence and discrimination against women: A call to action. http://www.unfpa.org/news/ending-violence-and-discrimination-against-women-call-action. Accessed 17 Dec 2014.

UNFPA. (2010). *Gender-based violence: A global toolkit for action.* New York: UNPFA. http://www.unfpa.org/sites/default/files/pub-pdf/cap-6.pdf. Accessed 17 Dec 2014.

World Health Organization (2005). *WHO Multi-country study on women's health and domestic violence against women. Country findings: Ethiopia.* Geneva: World Health Organization.

World Bank. (2009). *Gender-based violence, health and the role of health sector at a glance. Sweden: The World Bank.*

Part I
Gender-Based Violence:
Perspectives from Africa

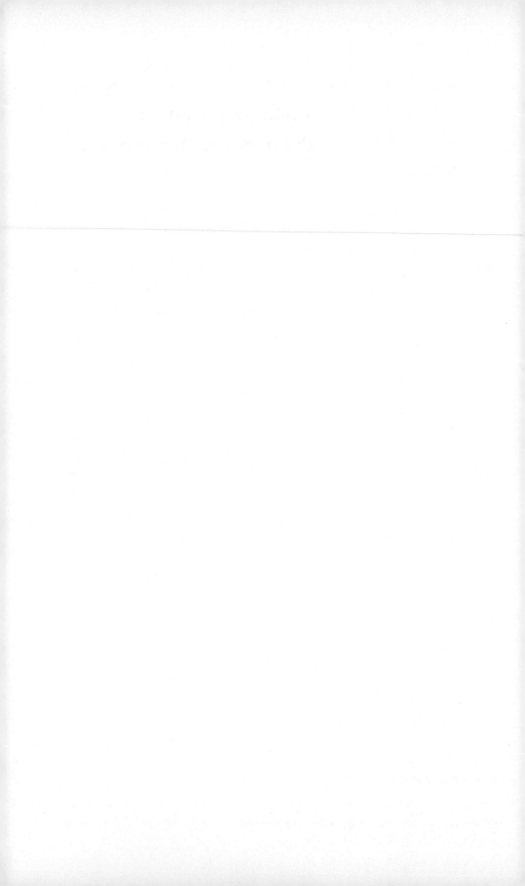

Chapter 1
Socio-demographic Factors Associated with Men's Attitudes Toward Wife Beating in Ethiopia

Yanyi K. Djamba, Sitawa R. Kimuna, and Mosisa G. Aga

Abstract Violence against women, especially intimate physical violence, is widely recognized as a public health and a human rights issue. However, most studies on this subject have focused on women's reports. This chapter examines men's attitudes toward wife beating using the 2011 Ethiopia Demographic and Health Survey, and compares never-married and currently married men's responses to a five-scenario question for which men believe that wife beating would be justified. The results from bivariate analysis show that married men were more likely than never-married men to agree with the statements that wife beating is justified if the "wife goes out without telling her husband," "neglects the children," "argues with husband," "refuses to have sex with the husband," and "burns food." However, these differences were statistically significant in logistic regression models only for refusal to have sex with the husband and burning food, for which married men appeared less likely to agree with wife beating than never-married men. Important regional differences are found with residents of Addis Ababa being the least likely to agree with wife beating followed by those in the Oromia region, whereas Somali and S.N.N.P. residents were significantly more likely to agree with wife beating statements. The effects of other socio-demographic variables are also discussed, including the policy implications and predictions for men's attitudinal change in Ethiopia.

Keywords Men • Attitudes toward wife beating • Socio-demographic factors • Ethiopia

Y.K. Djamba (✉) • M.G. Aga
Auburn University at Montgomery, Montgomery, AL, USA
e-mail: ydjamba@aum.edu; maga@aum.edu

S.R. Kimuna
East Carolina University, Greenville, NC, USA
e-mail: kimunas@ecu.edu

Background

According to the 2013 Population Reference Bureau (PRB) report, Ethiopia is the second most populous country in Africa, with 89.2 million inhabitants (PRB 2013). It is a multinational (multilingual) society with about 80 ethno-national groups; the main four groups are Oromo (34.5 %), Amhara (26.9 %), Somali (6.2 %), and Tigray (6.1 %) (CIA 2008). Consequently, Ethiopia is a multicultural society with diverse languages, customs, and religions. Its 11 federal regions are mainly based on the ethno-national groups inhabiting them: Oromia region (home of Oromos), Amhara regions (home of Amharas), Somali region (home of Somalis), and so on. It is also a multireligious society; the main three are Orthodox Christian (43.5 %), Islam (33.9 %), and Protestant (18.6 %) (CIA 2008).

A common denominator to this diverse cultural, linguistic, and religious composition of Ethiopia is that gender relations are not all equitable and many women suffer from various forms of partner violence in all settings. In a March 27, 2013, blog, Emnet Assefa wrote, "Everyone knows the presence of domestic abuse against women in Ethiopia; unfortunately no one knows how bad it is" (Assefa 2013). The Multi-country Study on Women's Health and Domestic Violence against Women, sponsored by the World Health Organization and conducted between 2000 and 2003, showed that nearly half (49 %) of ever-partnered women in Ethiopia have experienced physical violence by a partner at some point in their lives; 59 % reported sexual violence and 71 % reported having experienced either one or both of these two types of abuse (World Health Organization 2005).

Further, qualitative studies conducted in Ethiopia found evidence of intimate partner violence. For example, a study in Northwest Ethiopia based on data from focus groups among women showed that "[t]he normative expectation that conflicts are inevitable in marriage makes it difficult for society to reject violence" (Yigzaw et al. 2010: 39). More recently, researchers have considered both men's and women's views of intimate partner violence in some parts of Ethiopia. A 2012 qualitative study in West Ethiopia in which 55 men and 60 women participated in focus group discussions revealed that most subjects perceived intimate partner violence to be widely accepted in the community, particularly in the case of infidelity (Abeya et al. 2012).

Quantitative research on men's attitudes and the socio-demographic factors of their gendered behaviors toward women is very limited. One important work in this regard is the 2004 article published in the African Journal of Reproductive Health. In this comparative study of seven African countries based on Demographic and Health Survey data collected between 1999 and 2001, Rani and colleagues found that Ethiopian men were more likely to justify wife beating than their counterparts in five other countries with comparable data (Rani et al. 2004). Yet, because of its focus on comparative perspectives, no in-depth analysis of cultural norms embedded in regional differences of gender roles was examined.

In this chapter, we examine men's attitudes toward wife beating, a physical abuse that is usually associated with greater harms. Studies conducted elsewhere show that spousal violence adversely affects the health and well-being of women. A study in urban slums in Bangladesh revealed that more than three-quarters of physically violated women suffered injuries; more than 80 % of sexually violated women complained of pelvic pain and more than 50 % had reproductive tract infections (Salam et al. 2006). Similar results were found in Egypt, where ever-beaten women were more likely to report health problems necessitating medical attention (Diop-Sidibe et al. 2006).

In this study, we provide national estimates of Ethiopian men's views of wife beating using the most recent Ethiopia Demographic and Health Survey (2011 EDHS). Previous research in Africa has identified certain socio-demographic variables that increase or otherwise decrease men's acceptance of wife beating. Among these, education has been associated with reduced likelihood of acceptance of wife beating in Ethiopia, as well as in Benin, Mali, Rwanda, and Uganda (Rani et al. 2004). Men who have higher educational attainment are more amenable to negotiation when it comes to marital conflicts and spousal relations. Therefore, we expect educated men to be less inclined to approving of wife beating in contemporary Ethiopia.

Age was also found to be negatively linked to men's acceptance of wife beating in an earlier study in Ethiopia (Rani et al. 2004). It seems like older men are more tolerant to wife beating than younger men. Thus, we expect similar findings in the present study. Nonetheless, our study goes beyond previous research by including both the type of place of residence (rural/urban) and the region of residence in the analysis to capture differences in local gender norms. Due to exposure to various cultures in cities, we expect urban residents to be less supportive of wife beating than their rural counterparts. In the same way, we expect men who listen to radio, watch TV, and read newspapers to be less inclined to agreeing with statements that wife beating is justifiable.

In some parts of Ethiopia, including the capital, Addis Ababa, the Orthodox Church is the main religious denomination. In that church, Mary, mother of Jesus, is considered as one of the main messengers of God (Jesus). Followers of the Ethiopian Orthodox believe that Saint Mary has a supernatural power to convince Jesus. They call her "*amalaj*" which means negotiator (with Jesus) in Amharic language. Her picture exists in nearly every Orthodox believer's home and most of them pray mainly to her (not to Jesus). As such, we expect members of the Ethiopian Orthodox church to be less supportive of wife beating than their counterparts in other religious denominations, including those without religion.

Methods

Data

This study is based on the 2011 EDHS. The survey was carried out over a 5-month period from December 27, 2010, to June 3, 2011, by the Ethiopia Central Statistical Agency (CSA) under the auspices of the Ministry of Health. The 2011 EDHS was a nationally representative survey with a sample of 17,018 occupied households of which 16,702 were interviewed, representing a household response rate of 98.1 %. All women aged 15–49 and all men aged 15–59 in these households were selected

Table 1.1 Percent of men 15–59 who agree that a husband is justified to beating his wife for specific reasons, Ethiopia, 2011 EDHS

Husband is justified to beating his wife if she:	Percent
Goes out without telling the husband	25.8
Neglects the children	30.1
Argues with the husband	25.6
Refuses to have sex with the husband	21.2
Burns food	21.0
At least one of the above reasons	43.0

for interview. A total of 15,908 men were selected and 14,110 were interviewed, representing a response rate of 88.7 % (Central Statistical Agency [Ethiopia] and ICF International 2012: 11–12). This study is limited to the 13,192 men who were married or never married at the time of the survey.

Dependent Variables

In addition to regular demographic and health questions, the 2011 EDHS included a module measuring the number of situations in which the respondent considers wife beating justifiable. More specifically, survey participants were asked to say whether they agree or not that a husband is justified in beating his wife in the following circumstances: if the wife (1) goes out without telling the husband; (2) neglects the children; (3) argues with the husband; (4) refuses to have sex with the husband; and (5) burns food. The valid response options were yes (1) or no (0). Table 1.1 below shows the percent of men who agreed with each of the above statements about wife beating.

We consider each of the five scenarios as a dependent variable. In addition, a new variable representing men who agreed with wife beating in at least one of the situations was created. Therefore, there are six dependent variables.

Independent Variables

There are three sets of independent variables. The first set contains sociodemographic characteristics. This set includes marital status, age, education, and wealth index. Marital status has two categories: never married and (currently) married. We excluded divorced and other forms of unions because they may be directly or indirectly associated with domestic violence. For example, some men may have lost their wives through divorce or death; therefore, their answers to wife beating questions could be problematic. Age was regrouped into three categories: 15–24, 25–34, and 35+. Wealth index is a measure of level of wealth that is consistent with expenditure and income (Rutstein 1999). It is expressed in wealth quintiles: poorest, poor, middle, richer, and richest.

The second set of variables contains three sociocultural factors: type of place of residence (urban/rural), region of residence, and religion. The latter is very important in Ethiopia, where nearly half of the inhabitants are members of the Orthodox Church. Members of this religious denomination see women in the image of "Holly Mary" or "Saint Mary." Therefore, we expect Orthodox men to be less likely to condone wife beating practices.

The third set of variables contains media exposure information. Respondents were asked about how often they read newspapers or magazines, listen to the radio, and watch television. Response categories for each of these three questions were the following: not at all, less than once a week, and at least once a week. Because they expose men to new ideas and the world, these variables are expected to be negatively associated with acceptance of wife beating.

Results

In this study, results show that a significant number of Ethiopian men agree with each of the statements about wife beating. About 3 in 10 men (30.1 %) agree that a husband is justified to beating his wife if she neglects the children; one-fourth (25.8 %) in case she goes out without telling the husband; and about the same percent (25.6 %) if she argues with him (see Table 1.1). Wife beating received lower approval in cases of refusal to have sex with the husband (21.2 %) and burning food (21.0). Apparently, Ethiopian men rank the safety and well-being of children very high. Nearly half of the men (43.0 %) agreed that wife beating is justified in at least one of the situations considered in this study.

The results of the binary analysis between each of the independent variables and the dependent variables are given in Table 1.2. The information in that table shows that married men agree more with wife beating than unmarried ones. Nonetheless, there were no significant differences between the two groups in terms of refusal to have sex with the husband and burning food. Age is significantly associated with all dependent variables, except one—going out without telling the husband. Overall, younger men seem to agree more that the husband is justified to beating his wife than do older men.

Education is negatively associated with agreement of wife beating in all circumstances considered in this study. In the same way, wealth index has a negative association with wife beating. Men who lived in poorer households were more likely to agree with each and all of the statements justifying wife beating than those men who lived in better-off households.

Each of the sociocultural factors examined here is statistically significantly associated with each of the dependent variables. Urban residents were less likely to agree with wife beating than their rural counterparts. In addition, there are important regional differences. For example, men in the S.N.N.P. region were the most likely to agree with four of the five wife beating statements than men in other regions: going out without telling the husband (37.6 %); neglecting the children

Table 1.2 Men's attitudes toward wife beating by selected socio-demographic characteristics, Ethiopia, 2011 EDHS

Variables		Percent of men who said wife beating is justified if the wife:					
		Goes out without telling husband	Neglects the children	Argues with husband	Refuses to have sex with the husband	Burns food	At least one of the five reasons
Demographic characteristics							
Marital status	Never married	23.3***	29.3+	24.1***	20.9	20.7	41.5**
	Married	27.7	30.7	26.7	21.4	21.2	44.1
Age group	15–24	25.8	33.1***	27.2**	23.5***	23.3***	46.1***
	25–34	25.1	28.8	24.4	19.8	19.6	41.1
	35+	26.4	27.9	24.7	19.8	19.6	41.2
Education	No education	37.9***	39.9***	36.5***	30.9***	30.7***	56.8***
	Primary	25.5	31.7	26.4	21.7	21.8	44.9
	Secondary	11.2	15.3	9.8	7.6	6.9	23.6
	Higher	5.5	8.1	5.1	3.6	2.7	12.4
Wealth index	Poorest	37.3***	40.4***	37.4***	33.6***	33.1***	56.2***
	Poor	34.9	40.1	34.6	29.5	29.4	54.9
	Middle	32.2	36.8	32.4	24.8	26.4	53.9
	Richer	26.1	32.5	26.3	21.0	22.2	46.3
	Richest	10.9	14.1	9.9	7.6	6.0	21.9
Sociocultural factors							
Place of residence	Urban	10.5***	13.8***	9.3***	7.0***	5.8***	21.6***
	Rural	32.1	36.8	32.3	27.1	27.3	51.9

Region	Tigray	28.2***	35.8***	27.1***	19.7***	24.0***	46.2***
	Affar	35.3	34.1	34.3	32.0	27.8	47.6
	Amhara	30.4	34.6	27.5	21.0	22.8	50.7
	Oromia	19.8	24.4	23.7	21.7	19.1	38.9
	Somali	34.0	39.1	36.3	38.4	20.6	58.1
	Benishangul-Gumuz	32.8	38.5	28.5	21.2	24.9	50.5
	S.N.N.P.	37.6	42.4	34.9	29.1	34.2	57.3
	Gambela	25.0	30.8	26.5	21.4	25.2	44.9
	Harari	19.6	25.2	21.1	17.5	12.8	37.3
	Addis Ababa	3.9	5.8	3.4	2.1	1.7	9.5
	Dire Dawa	17.7	19.2	20.3	14.4	12.7	31.0
Religion	Orthodox	21.9***	26.2***	19.9***	15.1***	17.7***	37.2***
	Catholic	20.5	30.2	24.4	14.2	25.2	43.7
	Protestant	30.1	35.2	30.8	25.4	28.4	48.5
	Muslim	28.2	32.1	29.4	25.8	20.6	46.4
	Traditional	27.6	39.1	31.0	41.4	42.5	52.9
	Other	35.8	34.3	36.0	30.5	39.0	58.1
Media exposure indicators							
Read newspaper or magazine	Not at all	33.2***	37.0***	32.7***	27.6***	27.8***	52.6***
	Less than once a week	17.4	23.2	17.5	14.0	13.0	33.4
	At least once a week	10.5	14.1	10.4	7.9	7.6	20.7
Listen to radio	Not at all	34.2***	38.1***	33.1***	27.2***	29.3***	54.1***
	Less than once a week	29.0	34.4	29.7	25.5	24.4	48.3
	At least once a week	18.0	21.7	17.6	14.0	13.1	31.8
Watch TV	Not at all	33.9***	37.8***	34.5***	29.2***	29.2***	54.4***
	Less than once a week	27.3	32.3	26.8	22.1	22.5	45.3
	At least once a week	13.9	17.7	12.8	10.1	8.9	26.0

$***P \leq 0.001, **P \leq 0.01, *P \leq 0.05, ^{+}P \leq 0.10$

(42.4 %); arguing with the husband (34.9 %); and burning food (34.2 %). Somali men topped the list for agreeing with wife beating in case of refusing to have sex with the husband (38.4 %). For each of the scenarios of wife beating, inhabitants of the capital city, Addis Ababa, reported the lowest level of agreements (from 1.7 % in the case of burning food to 5.8 % in the case of neglecting the children, and 9.5 % for at least one of the five reasons).

As for religion, the data in Table 1.2 show that compared to other men, men who are members of the Orthodox Church were significantly less likely to agree with three of the five causes of wife beating: neglecting the children (26.2 %); arguing with the husband (19.9 %); and burning food (17.7 %). They were second in disagreement of wife beating behind those men who belong to the Catholic Church on two wife beating statements: going out without telling the husband (20.5 % for Catholic and 21.9 % for Orthodox) and refusal to have sex with the husband (14.2 % for Catholic and 15.1 % for Orthodox). Overall, men who belong to Ethiopia Orthodox Church were significantly less likely to agree with at least one of the five statements of wife abuse as compared to men in other religious denominations.

Binary results on media exposure indicators are all consistent. Men who read newspapers and/or magazines, those who listen to radio, and those who watch television were more likely to disagree with each of the five statements of wife beating than their counterparts who had no or little exposure to these media. Are these differences still significant once the effects of other factors are held constant? To answer this question, we now turn to the multivariate analysis in the form of logistic regression models. The results are shown in Table 1.3, where we discuss these results along with the three sets of variables.

The Importance of Demographic Characteristics

The results of demographic characteristics in Table 1.3 show that the two categories of marital status considered in this study are not statistically different when all other variables are taken into account regarding wife beating for the following causes: going out without telling the husband, neglecting the children, and arguing with husband. In other words, Ethiopian men, whether married or not, share the same view on those situations. They do, however, hold different views regarding refusal to having sex with the husband and burning food. In these two situations, married men are significantly more tolerant than never-married men. No significant difference was found in the last model for agreeing with at least one reason for wife beating.

Age, education, and wealth index were significantly associated with lower acceptance of wife beating in all circumstances examined in this study. Such findings are consistent with the results from previous research in Ethiopia, especially that of Rani and associates (2004). In terms of age, our findings suggest that maturity leads to more understanding of gender relations. The negative association between the acceptance of wife beating and education shows that formal schooling seems to improve men's view of women and thus reduces the use of force to correct

Variables		Percent of men who said wife beating is justified if the wife:					
		Goes out without telling husband	Neglects the children	Argues with husband	Refuses to have sex with the husband	Burns food	At least one of the five reasons
Demographic characteristics							
Marital status	Never married (ref)	1.000	1.000	1.000	1.000	1.000	1.000
	Married	0.959	1.007	0.950	0.808**	0.826*	0.919
Age group	15–24 (ref)	1.000	1.000	1.000	1.000	1.000	1.000
	25–34	0.918	0.774***	0.814**	0.797**	0.807**	0.797***
	35+	0.771***	0.588***	0.654***	0.660***	0.640***	0.613***
Education	No education (ref)	1.000	1.000	1.000	1.000	1.000	1.000
	Primary	0.668***	0.742***	0.716***	0.688***	0.684***	0.682***
	Secondary	0.423***	0.477***	0.387***	0.362***	0.346***	0.436***
	Higher	0.230***	0.280***	0.234***	0.216***	0.173***	0.236***
Wealth index	Poorest (ref)	1.000	1.000	1.000	1.000	1.000	1.000
	Poor	0.991	1.039	0.975	0.958	0.890+	1.016
	Middle	0.919	0.934	0.923	0.785***	0.806**	1.023
	Richer	0.768***	0.844**	0.769***	0.696***	0.727***	0.839**
	Richest	0.577***	0.582***	0.552***	0.518***	0.412***	0.568***
Sociocultural factors							
Place of residence	Urban (ref)	1.000	1.000	1.000	1.000	1.000	1.000
	Rural	1.281*	1.210*	1.462***	1.567***	1.405**	1.142
Region	Tigray	3.315***	3.445***	3.052***	2.984***	3.729***	3.050***
	Affar	3.393***	2.333***	2.809***	3.595***	3.699***	2.231***
	Amhara	2.958***	2.664***	2.411***	2.587***	2.712***	2.832***
	Oromia	1.936***	1.755***	2.093***	2.853***	2.700***	1.962***
	Somali	3.491***	3.158***	3.399***	5.630***	2.736***	3.841***
	Benishangul-Gumuz	3.362***	3.082***	2.328***	2.358***	3.196***	2.734***
	S.N.N.P.	4.739***	4.092***	3.335***	3.933***	5.115***	4.142***
	Gambela	3.163***	2.945***	2.893***	3.348***	4.276***	3.094***
	Harari	3.460***	3.251***	3.708***	4.467***	4.040***	3.514***
	Addis Ababa (ref)	1.000	1.000	1.000	1.000	1.000	1.000
	Dire Dawa	2.478***	1.931***	2.793***	2.761***	3.089***	2.146***

(continued)

Table 1.3 (continued)

Variables		Percent of men who said wife beating is justified if the wife:					At least one of the five reasons
		Goes out without telling husband	Neglects the children	Argues with husband	Refuses to have sex with the husband	Burns food	
Religion	Orthodox (ref)	1.000	1.000	1.000	1.000	1.000	1.000
	Catholic	0.739	1.047	1.115	0.736	1.148	1.067
	Protestant	1.220*	1.246**	1.520***	1.495***	1.327***	1.263***
	Muslim	1.167*	1.244***	1.336***	1.393***	0.959	1.255***
	Traditional	0.722	1.123	1.040	2.227***	1.667*	1.064
	Other	1.055	0.838	1.357+	1.382+	1.456*	1.339+
Media exposure indicators							
Read newspaper or magazine	Not at all (ref)	1.000	1.000	1.000	1.000	1.000	1.000
	Less than once a week	0.749***	0.833***	0.772***	0.760***	0.695***	0.798***
	At least once a week	0.701***	0.750***	0.720***	0.683***	0.738**	0.683***
Listen to radio	Not at all (ref)	1.000	1.000	1.000	1.000	1.000	1.000
	Less than once a week	1.009	1.026	1.090	1.196**	1.020	1.027
	At least once a week	0.841**	0.818***	0.848**	0.864*	0.800***	0.806***
Watch TV	Not at all (ref)	1.000	1.000	1.000	1.000	1.000	1.000
	Less than once a week	0.992	1.009	0.915+	0.933	0.924	0.938
	At least once a week	1.114	1.096	0.966	1.028	0.899	1.018

Note: ref reference category

*** $P \leq 0.001$, ** $P \leq 0.01$, * $P \leq 0.05$, + $P \leq 0.10$

what are considered bad behaviors within the Ethiopian context. As for wealth index, men who live in richer households are significantly less likely to approve of wife beating than those in poorer households. This is consistent for all scenarios, indicating that poverty may be a contributing factor of wife abuse in Ethiopia.

The Role of Culture

All three measures of cultural norms used in this study are statistically significantly correlated with attitudes toward wife beating. As we hypothesized, residents of urban places are less likely to agree that wife beating can be justified in any of the five circumstances, except in the last model in which we examined the case of men who agreed with at least one of the scenarios. The effect of the type of place of residence remained significant even when the region variable was excluded from the logistic regression equation (results not shown), proving that urbanization does play an important role in melting cultures and thus reducing the influence of traditional gender role views.

Region of residence is another very important variable of men's attitudes toward wife beating in Ethiopia. Compared to Addis Ababa residents, men in all other regions are more likely to agree with each of the five scenarios that are the cause of wife beating. Nonetheless, there are significant differences across regions. For example, men from the S.N.N.P. region top the list in terms of agreeing with wife beating in cases of going out without telling the husband (odd ratio=4.739), neglecting the children (odd ratio=4.092), burning food (odd ratio=5.115), and at least one of the five scenarios (odd ratio=4.142). Somali men (men in Somali regional state) lead for justifying wife beating in cases of arguing with the husband (odd ratio=3.399), and refusal to having sex with the husband (odd ratio=5.630). Another interesting pattern is that of the Oromo men (men in Oromia regional state), who rank second after Addis Ababa in five of the six models in Table 1.3.

The third variable in this set is religion. Interestingly, belonging to Orthodox or Catholic does not statistically significantly affect men's views on wife beating in all the six regression models. In contrast, compared to men in the Orthodox churches, those in the Protestant denomination were significantly more likely to agree with each of the scenarios of wife beating. The same was observed for Muslim men, except for burning food for which they were not significantly different from Orthodox and Catholic men.

The Impact of Media Exposure

Two of the media exposure variables are significantly associated with each of the six dependent variables in the multivariate models in Table 1.3. Those who read newspapers and/or magazines are significantly more likely to reject the views that wife beating can be justified in any of the scenarios proposed to them during the survey. More important, the relationship is even stronger for regular readers.

Although significant, the relationship between radio listening and men's attitudes toward wife beating is not all linear. While it is true that weekly exposure to radio is associated with significant reduction of support to each of the six situations presented in Table 1.3, limited exposure is found to even increase support for wife beating, particularly in the case of refusing to have sex with the husband, which the association was statistically significant.

Discussion and Conclusion

The purpose of this chapter was to examine men's attitudes toward wife beating in Ethiopia in order to provide a national profile of the situation, as well as determine socio-demographic factors associated with such views. The results show that nearly half of the men (43.0 %) agree with at least one of the five statements describing situations in which the husband is justified to beating his wife. However, there are some variations in men's agreement across the scenarios: for example, whereas most men (30.1 %) agree with wife beating in case the wife neglects children, only 21 % agree that the husband is justified to beating his wife for burning food. Such a range of disagreement is largely due to the influence of men's demographic characteristics, the cultural environment in which they live, and media influences to which they are exposed. The analysis of these variables in multivariate equations shows important results and confirms our presumption that men's views on wife beating are rooted in their background characteristics and the socio-cultural space.

In terms of demographic variables, the hypothesis that marriage influences men's attitudes toward wife beating was not fully supported in this study. Instead, we found that married men are more lenient than never-married men in terms of wife beating in cases of refusing to have sex with the husband and burning food. The lack of significant differences between married and never-married men's attitudes toward wife beating for other scenarios shows that those are high-ranking behaviors that most men condemn in Ethiopia. This is true considering the high percent of agreement accounted for those cases in descriptive and bivariate analysis sections of this chapter.

We also found that age, education, and wealth are important negative correlates of aspects of wife beating. Older men, those with higher education, and men in wealthier households are significantly less likely to agree with wife beating in any circumstance. This educational effect, which was also echoed in previous research (Rani et al. 2004), is an important policy variable. In the same way as scholars advocate for women's schooling as a significant female empowerment and sexual health variable (Roudi-Fahimi and Moghadam 2003), increasing men's educational attainment can significantly reduce wife abuse in Ethiopia. In addition, delaying marriage can also help, as older men show less support for wife beating. Naturally, wealth is a useful ingredient of marital harmony and gender relation, but its use in population policy is a daunting task.

This study also uncovered the key role of sociocultural factors in determining men's attitudes toward wife beating in Ethiopia. As we hypothesized, rural men hold more conservative views on wife abuse, even after controlling for the effects of all other variables. For a country that remains essentially rural, urbanization is not an immediate policy variable for improving gender relations. Only 14.2 % of Ethiopians live in urban areas according to estimates by Schmidt and Kedir (2009).

Results on regional variations suggest that some parts of the country are more apt to condone wife beating than others. For example, given their high levels of agreement with wife beating justification statements, S.N.N.P. and Somali regions should be the target areas for any large-scale campaigns for reducing wife beating in Ethiopia. Our findings show that men in the Somali region of Ethiopia take wife submission very seriously and they support wife beating as a corrective action tool. Those in the S.N.N.P. region seem to use wife beating primarily for family cohesion rather than pure submission to the husband. Hence, unlike Somali men who are ranked number one for support of wife beating for refusing to have sex with the husband and arguing with the husband, S.N.N.P. men are number one in agreeing that the husband is justified to beating his wife if she goes out without telling him, neglecting the children, and burning food.

Religion, especially the Ethiopian Orthodox and Catholic religions, is deterrent to wife beating in Ethiopia. Men of the Orthodox Church and those in the Catholic Church were significantly less likely to justify wife beating, regardless of the woman's behavior. In contrast, members of the Protestant denomination were significantly more likely to agree with all aspects of wife beating. Unlike Orthodox Church in which a woman is seen in the image of "Saint Mary," the Protestant religion teachings encourage the woman to be submissive to her husband. This may explain why Protestant men are in support of wife beating more than men in other religious denominations.

Exposure to mass media has a negative association with wife beating. We found that men who read newspapers and/or magazines and those who listen to radio are significantly less likely to approve of wife beating than their counterparts who do not use these types of media. Because such media are linked to educational attainment, improving men's education is again an important tool for combating domestic violence in Ethiopia. Therefore, as the country's educational level rises (Kabuchu 2013), along with age at marriage (Save the Children 2011), we expect some improvement in gender relations, including a reduction in support for wife beating.

This study contributes to literature on intimate partner violence in two main ways. First, it covers the entire country and uses quantitative data to examine men's attitudes toward wife beating. Previous studies were mostly qualitative works conducted in small areas (Abeya et al. 2012; Yigzaw et al. 2010). Second, this study explores the connection between socio-demographic variables and each of the scenarios in which husbands often use force as a mechanism for correcting their wives' behaviors. By doing so, we were able to find key sociocultural factors of gender relations and propose practical ways to reducing men's support for wife beating in Ethiopia.

Acknowledgements Earlier results of this study were presented at the 2013 Annual Meeting of the Southern Demographic Association held in Montgomery, Alabama, on October 23–25. The authors thank the conference participants for their comments and suggestions that helped improve the quality of this chapter.

References

Abeya, S., Afework, M., & Yalew, A. (2012). Intimate partner violence against women in west Ethiopia: A qualitative study on attitudes, woman's response, and suggested measures as perceived by community members. *Reproductive Health, 9*, 14. doi:10.1186/1742-4755-9-14.

Assefa, E. (2013). Domestic abuse against women in Ethiopia: The price of not knowing her pain. *Addis Standard.* http://addisstandard.com/domestic-abuse-against-women-in-ethiopia-the-price-of-not-knowing-her-pain/. Accessed 26 Aug 2014.

Central Intelligence Agency (CIA). (2008). *World factbook.* Ethiopia. https://www.cia.gov/library/publications/the-world-factbook/geos/et.html. Accessed 26 Aug 2014.

Central Statistical Agency [Ethiopia] and ICF International. (2012). *Ethiopia demographic and health survey 2011.* Addis Ababa, Ethiopia and Calverton, MD, USA: Central Statistical Agency and ICF International.

Diop-Sidibe, N., Campbell, J., & Becker, S. (2006). Domestic violence against women in Egypt-wife beating and health outcomes. *Social Science and Medicine, 62*(5), 1260–1277.

Kabuchu, H. (2013). *MGDF gender: Ethiopia LNWB final evaluation report.* Addis Ababa, Ethiopia: UN Joint Programme on Leave No Woman Behind (LNWB). http://www.mdgfund.org/sites/default/files/Ethiopia%20-%20Gender%20-%20Final%20Evaluation%20Report.pdf. Accessed 7 June 2014.

Population Reference Bureau. (2013). *2013 World population data sheet.* Washington, DC: Population Reference Bureau. http://www.prb.org/pdf13/2013-population-data-sheet_eng.pdf. Accessed 7 June 2014.

Rani, M., Bonu, S., & Diop-Sidibé, N. (2004). An empirical investigation of attitudes towards wife-beating among men and women in seven sub-Saharan African countries. *African Journal of Reproductive Health, 8*(3), 116–136.

Roudi-Fahimi, F., & Moghadam, V. M. (2003). *Empowering women, developing society: Female education in the Middle East and North Africa.* Washington, DC: The Population Reference Bureau. http://www.prb.org/pdf/EmpoweringWomeninMENA.pdf. Accessed 7 June 2014.

Rutstein, S. (1999). *Wealth versus expenditure: Comparison between the DHS wealth index and household expenditures in four departments of Guatemala.* Calverton, MD: ORC Macro.

Salam, A., Alim, A., & Noguchi, T. (2006). Spousal abuse against women and its consequences on reproductive health: A study in the urban slums in Bangladesh. *Maternal Child Health Journal, 10*(1), 83–94.

Save the Children. (2011). *Child marriage in North Gondar Zone of Amhara Regional State, Ethiopia.* Addis Ababa, Ethiopia: Save the Children Norway.

Schmidt, E., & Kedir, M. (2009). Urbanization and spatial connectivity in Ethiopia: Urban growth analysis using GIS. *ESSP2 Discussion Paper 003.* http://www.ifpri.org/sites/default/files/publications/esspdp03.pdf. Accessed 5 June 2014.

World Health Organization. (2005). *WHO Multi-country study on women's health and domestic violence against women. Country findings: Ethiopia.* Geneva: World Health Organization.

Yigzaw, T., Berhane, Y., Deyessa, N., & Kaba, M. (2010). Perceptions and attitude towards violence against women by their spouses: A qualitative study in Northwest Ethiopia. *Ethiopia Journal of Health Development, 1*, 39–45.

Chapter 2
First Intimate Physical Violence and Fertility in Cameroon

Alice Jacqueline Azebaze Kagou and Hélène Kamdem Kamgno

Abstract Despite the social importance attached to childbearing in Africa, fertility in relation to intimate partner violence has not received considerable attention in research and policy. This chapter examines the association between the number of children and the occurrence of the first intimate physical violence, net of the effect of other socio-demographic variables. The analysis is based on the 2011 Cameroon Demographic and Health Survey. The results show that 59.1 % of women in marital unions have been victims of physical marital violence. Results from the proportional hazards model (Cox regression) indicate that while fertility remains an important social factor in the Cameroonian society, it has a detrimental impact on marital relations: women who have children are significantly more likely to experience the first intimate physical violence in the hands of their husbands or male partners than their counterparts who have no children. Such results suggest that reducing fertility can help lower the occurrence of intimate physical violence against women in Cameroon. Other key contributing factors that are positively associated with intimate physical violence are: woman's education (when higher than that of her husband/partner), witnessed parental spousal violence, and having a husband or male partner who drinks alcohol.

Keywords Fertility • Intimate physical violence • Women • Cameroon

Introduction

Male domination is often seen through the ways men use physical violence against their female partners or wives. This kind of intimate partner violence (IPV) is observed around the world, including Africa. Worldwide, at least one-third of

A.J.A. Kagou (✉)
MINEPAT, Yaoundé, Cameroon
e-mail: al.azebaze@gmail.com

H.K. Kamgno
IFORD, Yaoundé, Cameroon
e-mail: hekamgno@yahoo.fr

© Springer International Publishing Switzerland 2015   17
Y.K. Djamba, S.R. Kimuna (eds.), *Gender-Based Violence*,
DOI 10.1007/978-3-319-16670-4_2

women have ever been physically abused by their intimate male partners (UNFPA 2000). According to the 2011 Cameroon Demographic and Health Survey [Enquête Démographique et de Santé (EDSC-VI)], 59.1 % of women in marital unions have been victims of intimate partner abuse (see also the report by Institut National de la Statistique (INS) et ICF International 2012:328). Such violence may have serious consequences on physical, sexual, and mental health of women. Therefore, efforts should be made to reduce its prevalence. Following the recommendations of various international organizations, such as the International Conference on Population and Development (ICPD) Programme of Action (UNFPA 1995) and the Beijing Declaration and Platform for Action (UNWOMEN 2014), the Government of Cameroon has made the elimination of violence against women one of its priorities. Despite this effort, the prevalence of gender-based violence remains high.

The causes of violence against women have been the subject of several studies, most of which looked at socio-demographic factors such as female education, age difference between spouses, and household wealth (Rani et al. 2004; Djamba and Kimuna 2008). However, only few studies have examined the potential impact of fertility on IPV, with the majority of them resulting in contradictory findings. These studies are discussed below.

Some researchers have found a positive relation between the number of children a woman has and her risk of being a victim of IPV. Martin and colleagues, for example, found that women who had multiple children were more likely to be physically abused by their male partners than their counterparts who had one or no children (Martin et al. 1999). In contrast, a more recent study in Uganda revealed that women who had six or more children had significantly lower risks of violence than those with 0–1 child (Koenig et al. 2003). Such contradictory findings indicate a need for further investigation, especially in Africa, where childbearing is highly revered and women are still socially valued primarily as mothers and wives, whereas men are generally considered the heads and decision makers of the household.

Another factor to consider is the current changes in women's conditions in many African countries. The most significant change has been female education. For example, despite persistent gender inequality, female school enrollment rate has significantly increased in Cameroon (UNICEF 2003). As women gain more education, they also improve their overall status in society because education opens a range of opportunities; from paid jobs to a better understanding of how society works. In addition, female education has been evidently linked to lower fertility (Population Reference Bureau 2011) and female empowerment. In male-dominated countries, such as Cameroon, changes in fertility can affect gender relations, particularly in marriage. Therefore, the key research question is the following: Does the presence of children increase or otherwise decrease the probability of physical violence in marriage in Cameroon?

Before answering this question, we should recognize the possibility that the relationship between fertility and female physical abuse can go both ways. That is, physical abuse in marriage can affect women's childbearing. Previous studies conducted in the USA have shown that domestic violence has serious health consequences, including trauma and other psychological problems that can affect childbearing capability and outcomes (Mezey et al. 2005; Sharps et al. 2007). In such cases, physical abuse can lead to lower fertility. On the other hand, women can be subjected to more violence as a result of their childbearing outcomes in two ways. First, if higher fertility is valued in a society, women who do not have many children can be subjected to domestic violence as their husbands/partners expect to have larger families. Second, larger families can bring more challenges to women, especially in poor households.

This study aims to advance our understanding of the association between childbearing and physical violence against women. More specifically, we examine the timing of the first occurrence of intimate physical violence in relation to the number of children a woman has at the time of the initial event. From a policy perspective, understanding the interplay between physical abuse and fertility can provide insights on practical ways to reduce domestic violence in Cameroon as well as in other countries with similar demographic characteristics and cultural norms.

Theoretical Framework

Several theoretical perspectives have been used to explain physical violence against women. In general, such explanations are based on the premise that domestic violence against women results from the type of interactions that happen between male and female partners, within a specific sociocultural environment (Bouchon 2009: 20). A closer review of those interactions suggests that much of the domestic violence against women can be explained by individual, gender, economic and institutional, and cultural conceptual frameworks.

Individual and Gender Explanations

One of the individual explanations of domestic violence comes from the European Psychoanalyst Sigmund Freud. According to Freud, men are biologically wired to be more aggressive than women (Freud 1933). Broadly put, the Freudian explanation posits that men are physically and morally stronger than women. As such, men who abuse women must be mentally ill (Laughrea et al. 1996). In their review of theory-driven explanations of male violence against women, Cunningham and colleagues state that "woman abuse is seen as a 'mate retention tactic' […] used […] when a man senses his wife could attract and keep a better partner" (Cunningham et al. 1998: 5). However, the authors recognize the challenge associated with that biological explanation of male jalousie.

Others have argued that relationships between men and women, or most specifically, between sex partners vary from one society to the next and are the products of socioeconomic and cultural systems. Under that framework, gender theory offers a way to analyze the relationships between men and women taking into account their differences and similarities, and how such connections affect and are affected by social and cultural factors (Hamza 2006: 18). In recent decades, the gender explanation has also included the feminist theory, which argues that women abuse is rooted in the patriarchal system of male dominance (Tracy 2007).

Economic and Institutional Explanations

According to some scholars, domestic violence is due to stress resulting from unemployment, bad work conditions, alcohol abuse, and poverty (Steinmetz 1977). In general, there is some evidence that economic conditions are also causes and effects of violence. A study in India found strong associations between domestic violence and low household income, low educational level of husband, consumption of alcohol and drugs, and witnessing domestic violence during childhood, and also an inverse relationship between a woman's educational attainment and domestic violence (Chandrasekaran et al. 2007; Kimuna et al. 2013). Several decades ago, Goode (1971) argued that violence occurs when economic resources are lacking, or when individuals feel that they have low prestige, are not respected in the society, or perceive to not being loved. However, for most women, access to resources happens generally within marital unions, especially when wives are devoted to their husbands and their children's well-being.

Domestic violence can also be associated with social organizations, namely institutional circumstances, such as written laws and unwritten rules and regulations that give men more power over women. From the beginning of time, patriarchal norms and other social practices have subjected women to lower status in many societies. As such, women tend to have limited resources of their own. This lack of resources leads to limited decision making because the value of the resources one brings into the family is positively associated with power and greater autonomy (Kabeer 1997). In short, proponents of the economic and institutional theories of gender see the economic inequality between men and women as rooted in the patriarchal structure of society, which gives males advantages over females. But, if that argument were true, then we would expect women who earn income to be less likely to experience domestic violence than unemployed women; yet, empirical data show a very complex picture (Renzetti 2011).

Cultural Explanations

According to the cultural theories of gender, the use of violence is the result of normative values individuals learn through socialization. Therefore, both the perpetrators and the victims find abusive behaviors as acceptable practices. Moreover, the victims may feel shame to talk about the abusive acts they have experienced, especially in societies where wife beating is common and socially accepted. A multi-country study by the World Health Organization reveals that "it is particularly difficult to respond effectively to [this] violence because many women accept such violence as 'normal'" (WHO 2005: vii).

Many women may also refrain from reporting domestic abuse in fear of repercussions for more abuse, if their male partners find out that their wives (or female partners) accused them. In some circumstances, speaking about husband's abusive behavior can lead to divorce, something many women avoid at all cost because they do not want to leave their children through divorce or separation (Wolfang and Ferracuti 1967); in most African countries husbands have custody of children in case of divorce.

Other research has indicated that a woman's childbearing experience can affect her relationship with her husband (Kamdem 2006; Andro 2001). Nonetheless, that relationship is complex. For example, some studies found a positive association between the number of children a woman has and her risk of IPV (Kishor and Kiersten 2006; Brown and Jaspard 2004). In Peru, only 22 % of women without children reported being victims of partner violence, compared to 38 % among those with 1–2 children; 45 % for women with 3–4 children; and 53 % among those with 5 or more children (Kishor and Kiersten 2006). The argument is that larger families tend to have lower per capita income, which may increase the stress for the head of the household (usually the man) who then uses violence as a corrective weapon.

In contrast, in Mozambique, the risk of IPV against women is higher among childless women and women with five children and more (Mc Closkey et al. 2005). Similar results were found in Cameroon, where women with more than five children were at higher risk of physical violence as compared to their counterparts who had no children (Azebaze Kagou 2012). In all those studies, both the fertility and IPV were reported without determining the timeline of the events. As a result, it is difficult to determine the direction of the association between the two variables. In other words, lower and/or higher fertility can trigger stress and other problems that may lead to IPV. Likewise, violence against women can negatively affect childbearing by increasing the risk of sexually transmitted diseases, preterm labor, and low birth weight (Sharps et al. 2007).

This study contributes to the literature on the association between fertility and intimate partner abuse by determining the sequence of events in order to assess the causal effects between the two phenomena. More specifically, we use an event history approach to measure the timing of the first act of intimate physical violence against women, in relation to the number of children, controlling for other sociodemographic variables in the West African country of Cameroon.

Methodology

Data

This study is based on the 2011 Cameroon Demographic and Health Survey [Enquête Démographique et de Santé (EDSC-VI)]. EDSC-VI was carried out by the Cameroon National Institute of Statistics (*Institut National de la Statistique*) in collaboration with the Ministry of Public Health. EDSC-IV used a nationally representative sample of household members. A total of 15,050 households were selected using a multistage stratified sampling design. All women of 15–49 years who were present in the selected households the night before the survey were eligible for interview. In addition, a subsample of households (half of all selected households) was used to select all men aged 15–59 as survey participants.

Out of the 15,852 women selected, 15,426 were successfully interviewed, representing a response rate of 97.3 %. Among men, 7,525 were selected but only 7,191 were successfully interviewed, producing a response rate of 95.6 %. The data collection was carried out from January to August 2011 (Institut National de la Statistique (INS) et ICF International 2012). Since the focus of this study is on the association between fertility and IPV, we only used data from the women sample.

Variables

EDSC-VI included detailed questions on intimate physical violence experienced by women, as well as that of their own mothers. The dependent variable of interest is the occurrence of the first physical violence against the woman in marital union. We call that variable "first intimate physical violence," (FIPV in short). A woman is said to have experienced FIPV if she answered yes to at least one of the following statements about her current (or last) husband/partner. The questions were framed as follows. Did your (last) husband/partner ever:

1. Push you, shake you, or throw something at you?
2. Slap you?
3. Twist your arm or pull your hair?
4. Punch you with his fist or with something that could hurt you?
5. Kick you or drag you?
6. Try to choke you or burn you on purpose?
7. Threaten or attack you with a knife, gun, or any other weapon?
8. Physically force you to have sexual intercourse with him when you did not want to?
9. Physically force you to perform any other sexual acts you did not want to?

Answers to these questions were compared to the woman's number of children in order to determine the temporal association between FIPV and fertility. Since we do not have the exact dates of the events, we divided women in terms of their number of children. Hence, using the total fertility rate of Cameroon, which is 5.1 children per woman (Institut National de la Statistique (INS) et ICF International 2012: 73), respondents were divided into three categories based on their current number of children:

1. Low—women who have no children.
2. Moderate—women who have 1–4 children.
3. High—women who have five or more children.

To measure the net effect of fertility on physical violence against women, several control variables were included in the analyses. They are (1) religion, (2) couple's education—measured as the difference between husband and wife educational attainment, (3) healthcare decision making—determining whether one spouse or the couple decides on healthcare matters, (4) household wealth index, (5) mother's spousal violence experience, (6) husband's alcohol drinking, and (7) year or cohort of marriage.

Analytical Approaches and Research Hypotheses

This study follows an event history approach in which the dependent variable is measured in terms of the actual time before the woman experiences intimate physical violence in marital union, commonly called time to event (TTE) in statistical analysis (Fike 2014). The time frame is between 0 and 40 years. Hence, the dependent variable will take a value of 1 if the woman experienced physical violence in the hands of her husband/partner, or 0 if she did not have such experience. This event history approach leads to censoring of certain respondents based on the occurrence or nonoccurrence of the event (right censoring) within the time frame of reference.

Data were then prepared in the form of person-year observations. In that file, the first year of observation is the first year of marital union for women who were in their first marital unions and who were interviewed about domestic violence. The analysis is based on the Kaplan-Meier method (Kaplan and Meier 1958), a nonparametric technique used to estimate the probability of survival within a given time frame. Therefore, we calculated the probability of experiencing the first physical violence in marital union within the time interval considered in this study (0–40 years), and then obtained a curve of survival rate for women who have not yet experienced such violence (Bocquier 1996).

The method for calculating these probabilities is as follows:

- d(ti) is the number of events—intimate physical violence—that occurred in time ti.
- N(ti) is the number of women who have not experienced intimate physical violence.
- ti = t1, t2, t3, … years in which women experienced intimate physical violence.

Therefore, the probability of occurrence of intimate physical violence in years (ti), also known as the instantaneous hazard rate h(ti), is

$$h(\text{ti}) = \frac{d(\text{ti})}{N(\text{ti})}$$

And the proportion of women who have not experienced intimate physical violence (survival distribution S(ti)) will be

$$S_{(\text{ti})} = \prod_{j \le i}\left(1 - h_{(\text{tj})}\right)$$

The probability curves obtained via the Kaplan-Meier method were compared using log-rank test results (Bland and Aluman 2004) in order to verify the validity of the following main research hypothesis: fertility is positively associated with intimate physical violence against women. That is, the more children a woman has, the higher her risk of being physically abused by her husband or male partner. In addition, we expect other independent variables to influence the likelihood of intimate physical violence directly or indirectly as hypothesized below.

As found in other countries (Djamba and Kimuna 2008; O'Farrell et al. 1999), we expect that man's alcohol drinking will increase the likelihood of IPV against women in Cameroon. Further, women who have been married in recent years are expected to have been exposed to individualistic values and knowledge of human rights more than women who were married 20 years or more before the survey. As such, recently married women may resist some gender norms of male dominance. By doing so, they might infuriate their husbands and therefore increase their risk of physical abuse.

These hypotheses are tested in Cox regression models. Whereas the Kaplan-Meier method with log-rank test is useful for comparing survival curves in two or more groups, Cox regression (or proportional hazards regression) is more appropriate in multivariate analysis where the effect of several independent variables is examined. In our case, the Cox regression equation is used to show that the risk of IPV against women is proportionally associated with a woman's socio-demographic factors, mainly her number of children. The results of both descriptive and multivariate analyses are presented in the next section.

Results

Findings from Descriptive Analysis

The descriptive analysis focused on determining the association between the occurrence of the first physical violence against women in marital union and number of children controlling for each of the following variables: (1) duration of marriage, (2) religion, and (3) timing (cohort) of marriage. The results are presented in graphic forms.

The results in Fig. 2.1 show that the occurrence of the first physical violence against women is significantly associated with the number of children (log-rank test). When the duration of marriage is taken into account, the data in Fig. 2.1 show that during the first 10 years of marriage, women who had 1–4 children were more likely to experience physical violence in the hands of their husbands/partners than other women. More specifically, 50 % of women with 1–4 children experienced physical violence within the first 5 years of marriage and 75 % within the first 10 years of marriage. In contrast, physical violence was rare among women who had no children; only less than 25 % of them experienced physical violence during all their exposure time (0–40 years of marriage).

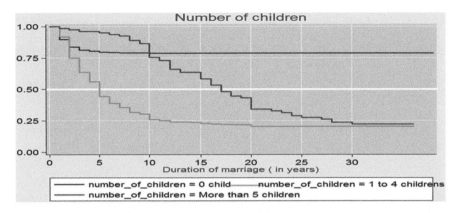

Fig. 2.1 Probability of not experiencing first intimate physical violence by duration of marriage and number of children, Cameroon, 2011 CDHS-VI

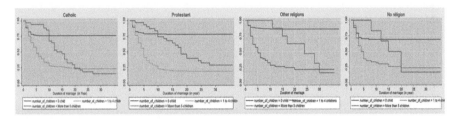

Fig. 2.2 Probability of not experiencing first intimate physical violence by duration of marriage and number of children and religion, Cameroon, 2011 CDHS-VI

Regardless of a woman's religious affiliation, the relation between number of children and first marital physical violence was statistically significant ($P \leq 0.01$; log-rank test). For all four religious categories considered here, data in Fig. 2.2 show that women who have 1–4 children were significantly more likely to experience physical violence sooner than other women. More than 75 % of women with 1–4 children experienced physical violence within the 10 years of marriage among Catholics and Protestants, and within 12 years of marriage for Muslims. Here again, physical violence was significantly lower among women who had no children.

Figure 2.3 shows the results of bivariate analyses between first physical marital violence and number of children, controlling for the cohort of marriage. The results show that the association between the first intimate physical violence and number of children was statistically significant among women who were married between 1990 and 2011 ($P \leq 0.01$; log-rank test). Among those recently married women (the 1990–2011 cohort), those who had an average number of children (1–4 children) experienced physical violence earlier in marriage than their counterparts with no children. No significant differences were found between the number of children and first physical violence among women who were married during the period of 1961–1989.

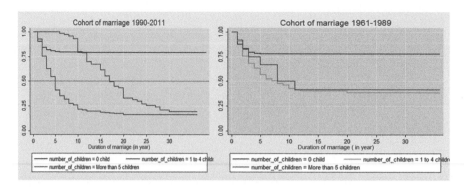

Fig. 2.3 Probability of not experiencing first intimate physical violence by duration of marriage and number of children, by Cohort of Marriage, Cameroon, 2011 CDHS-VI

We also analyzed the association between number of children and first physical violence, controlling for household wealth, couple's education, parent's experience of IPV, couple's decision-making style, and husband's alcohol drinking. The results are similar to those presented above. In brief, the findings from the descriptive analysis show that women who have 1–4 children are more likely to experience intimate physical violence sooner in their marital unions than their counterparts with fewer or more children (Table 2.1).

Findings from Multivariate Analysis

The results of multivariate analysis are presented in Table 2.2. We discuss only variables that were significantly associated with the occurrence of first intimate physical violence against women at the level of significance of 0.05 or lower. Those variables are number of children, religion (woman's), spouse's relative educational level, couple's decision-making style on health matters, parent's experience of intimate partner violence, husband's alcohol drinking, and timing (cohort) of marriage.

Data in Table 2.2 show that the number of children is a significant factor of first intimate physical violence in Cameroon. The risk of physical violence was higher among women with 1–4 children (hazard ratio of 4.255) followed by those with five children or more (hazard ratio of 2.561), as compared to women with no children. In other words, first physical violence happens sooner in marriage among women who have 1–4 children. Religion is only statistically significant for Muslim women. Compared to Catholics, Muslim women are about 30 % less likely to experience physical violence in the hands of their husbands/partners. These results may be due to the differences in the level of cohabitation. Such illegitimate unions are more frequent among Christian women than Muslim women. Therefore, the present results are consistent with previous research which showed that physical abuses are more common in cohabitating relationships than in legal marital unions (Kenney and McLanah 2006).

Table 2.1 Selected characteristics of the sample, Cameroon, 2011 CDHS-VI

Variables	Distribution of the sample	
	N	%
Religion		
Catholic	2,423	35.5
Protestant	2,342	34.3
Muslim	1,587	23.2
Other	482	7.1
Spouses' relative educational level		
Same level low	2,646	38.01
Same level high	1,455	20.90
Husband higher than wife	2,154	30.94
Wife higher than husband	706	10.14
Who decides about health matter?		
Wife alone	874	14.69
Wife and husband together	1,645	27.65
Husband alone	3,429	57.65
Level of household wealth		
Low	2,733	39.26
Average	1,448	20.80
High	2,780	39.94
Mother ever battered by her husband?		
Yes	1,909	29.85
No	4,487	70.15
Does respondent's husband drink alcohol?		
Yes	4,026	57.87
No	2,931	42.13
Year of marriage		
1990–2011	5,801	83.34
1961–1989	1,160	16.66
Total	6,961	100.0

Notes: Due to missing values some totals for some variables may be lower than the number reported in the last row. Also, percent for some variables may not add to 100 due to rounding

In terms of education, our findings show that intimate physical violence is more likely to occur in households where wives are more educated than their husbands. These results suggest that while female education is often perceived as a factor of women empowerment, its effects on gender relations can lead to unintended consequences, including physical violence in the hands of less educated men. Another interesting finding is that joint decision making reduces the likelihood of intimate physical violence in Cameroon. Compared to couples where the husband/partner alone makes decisions about health matters, in relationships where couples jointly make those decisions, women are significantly less likely to experience physical violence.

Being the daughter of a woman who has experienced domestic violence significantly increases the respondent's risk of intimate physical violence. Hence, women

Table 2.2 Results from Cox proportional hazards regression of first marital physical violence against women, Cameroon, 2011 CDHS-VI

Variables	Hazard ratios
Number of children	
No children (ref)	1.000
Between 1 and 4	4.255***
5 or more	2.561***
Religion	
Catholic (ref)	1.000
Protestant	1.020
Muslim	0.676***
Other	1.132
Spouses' relative educational level	
Same level low (ref)	1.000
Same level high	0.906
Husband higher than wife	1.076
Wife higher than husband	1.200*
Who decides about health matter?	
Wife alone	0.941
Wife and husband together	0.815*
Husband alone (ref)	1.000
Level of household wealth	
Low (ref)	1.000
Average	1.029
High	0.964
Mother ever battered by her husband?	
Yes	1.264**
No (ref)	1.000
Does respondent's husband drink alcohol?	
Yes	1.465***
No	1.000
Year of marriage	
1990–2011 (ref)	1.000
1961–1989	0.839**

Note: *ref* reference category
***$P \leq 0.001$, **$P \leq 0.01$, *$P \leq 0.05$

whose mothers have been physically abused by their husbands/partners are 1.264 times more likely to experience intimate physical violence during the period considered in this study. This result is consistent with previous research, which shows that women who lived in abusive families have a higher risk of experiencing intimate violence in their lives (Black et al. 2010).

Similar to previous studies (O'Farrell et al. 1999; Quigley and Leonard 2000), women whose husbands/partners drink alcohol are also significantly more likely to experience physical violence than those living with non-alcohol drinkers (hazard ratios of 1.465 vs. 1.000). Evidently, alcohol impairs judgment and may thus lead to physical confrontation.

There are significant cohort effects; women who were married during the period of 1961–1989 were significantly less likely to experience physical violence in their marital unions (hazard ratio of 0.839) than their counterparts who were married during the period of 1990–2011. In other words, physical violence happened sooner in marital unions for women who got married during the period of 1990–2011. It is possible that these recently married women encounter many conflicts in their relationships because of their exposure to new ideas currently available in the mass media and on the Internet. In a society that remains largely patriarchal, any attempt to challenge male domination could lead to female abuse.

Conclusion

Physical violence against women is one of the key issues for decision makers and the entire community today in many countries, including the Republic of Cameroon. This study examined the impact of fertility on the occurrence of the first act of physical violence against women in marital unions. In addition, other socio-demographic variables that have been associated with intimate partner violence in previous studies were included in the regression model to determine the net effect of fertility on physical violence.

The main research hypothesis that fertility is positively associated with IPV against women was confirmed. Nonetheless, the relationship was not all linear. Women who had 1–4 children were more than four times likely to experience physical violence than their counterparts who had no children, net of the effects of other socio-demographic variables. Those who had five children or more were about three times more likely to experience intimate physical violence.

Other significant correlates of physical violence were religion, spouses' differences in educational attainment, spouses' decision making in health matters, parent's experience of physical violence, husband's (male partner's) alcohol drinking, and timing/cohort of marriage. We also found that Muslim women were significantly less likely to experience physical violence earlier in their marriages/unions than Catholic women; but, there was no significant difference between Catholics and Protestants. We attributed the difference between Muslims and Christians to their differences in marital status. In Cameroon, Christians are more likely to be in consensual unions. Yet, such unions have been found to be more physically violent than traditional/legal marriages (Kenney and McLanah 2006). Therefore, the higher probability of physical abuse among Christians can be explained by their higher prevalence of cohabiting unions.

Consistent with findings of earlier studies (O'Farrell et al. 1999; Quigley and Leonard 2000), this study showed that the husband's alcohol drinking was significantly and positively associated with early onset of physical abuse. This result confirms our hypothesis that alcohol consumption may lead to conflicts in marriage, which can trigger physical abuse against women. The hypothesis of cohort effect was also confirmed in this study: women who have been married in recent years were more likely to experience physical violence, suggesting that their exposure to today's individualistic values and aspirations to personal freedom may appear conflictual to their male partners' vision of gender relations. Men who continue to believe in gender inequality probably use physical violence to force their female partners to submit to the norms of the patriarchal society. Under such circumstances, women who are aware of their human rights may refuse to submit to traditional patriarchal norms, which would then lead to physical violence against women. This may explain why women who were married within the last 20 years of the survey were significantly more likely to experience physical violence than their counterparts of previous cohorts.

Another interesting finding is that intimate physical violence was significantly more likely to occur in couples where the wife was more educated than her husband/partner. This result suggests that less educated men may feel frightened by highly educated women and use force to impose themselves as dominant in the marriage. We also found that women in unions where both spouses make joint decisions about health matters were significantly less likely to experience physical abuse than women whose husbands/partners made such decisions alone. Finally, our analysis showed that women whose mothers experienced physical abuse were more likely to be victims of the same type of violence in their own lives. This result is consistent with previous studies (Black et al. 2010).

We must point out some potential limitations of our study. For example, because the data used here come from a cross-sectional survey, detailed information on gender relations is lacking. Knowing how wives and husbands interact in marital unions can enhance our understanding of conflict. In addition, this study assumes that only men use violence against women. Such an assumption excludes the fact that a woman can physically or emotionally abuse her husband/partner, a situation that can lead a man to use physical violence against his female partner. Despite such potential limitations, this study contributes to the literature on gender relations by showing the impact of fertility on the risk of physical violence against women.

References

Andro A. (2001). Fertily's projet in west africa, in LOCOH Therese (dir): Gender and society in africa. p 373–391, INED, 432p.

Azebaze Kagou, A. J. (2012). *Fécondité, durée de marriage et premieres violences conjugales physiques faites aux femmes: le cas du Cameroun. Thèse de maitrise en démographie*. Institut de Formation et de Recherche Démographiques (IFORD), Yaoundé, Cameroun. http://www.ceped.org/ireda/inventaire/ressources/azebaze_2012-F.pdf. Accessed 28 Aug 2014.

Black, D. S., Sussman, S., & Unger, J. B. (2010). A further look at the intergenerational transmission of violence: Witnessing interparental violence in emerging adulthood. *Journal of Interpersonal Violence, 25*(6), 1022–1042. doi:10.1177/0886260509340539.

Bland, J. M., & Aluman, D. G. (2004). Statistics notes: The Logrank test. *British Medical Journal, 328*(7453), 1412.

Bocquier, P. (1996). *Analysis of biographic's surveys. Documents and manuals of CEPED no 4, July 1996*. Paris: CEPED. 202p.

Bouchon, M. (2009). *Violences faites aux femmes: Genre, culture et sociétés*. Médecins du Monde. http://issuu.com/medecinsdumonde/docs/guidevff_fr.pdf. Accessed 28 Aug 2014.

Brown, E., & Jaspard, M. (2004). La place de l'enfant dans les conflits et les violences conjugales. *Recherches et Previsions, 78*, 5–19.

Chandrasekaran, V., Krupp, K., George, R., & Madhivanan, P. (2007). Determinants of domestic violence among women attending an human immunodeficiency virus voluntary counseling and testing center in Bangalore, India. *Indian Journal of Medical Sciences, 61*(5), 253–262.

Cunningham, A., Jaffe, P. G., Baker, L., Dick, T., Malla, S., Mazaheri, N., & Poisson, S. (1998). Theory-derived explanations of male violence against female partners: Literature update and related implications for treatment and evaluation. http://www.lfcc.on.ca/maleviolence.pdf. Accessed 27 Aug 2014.

Djamba, Y., & Kimuna, S. (2008). Intimate partner violence among married women in Kenya. *Journal of Asian and African Studies, 43*(4), 457–469. doi:10.1177/0021909608091976.

Fike, L. (2014). How to set up censored data for event history? http://www.theanalysisfactor.com/how-to-set-up-censored-data-for-event-history-analysis/. Accessed 3 Aug 2014.

Freud, S. (1933). New introductory lectures on psychoanalysis. Lecture 33: Femininity. *Standard Edition, 22*, 136–157. http://www.haverford.edu/psych/ddavis/p109g/freudfem.html. Accessed 27 Aug 2014.

Goode, W. (1971). Force and violence in the family. *Journal of Marriage and the Family, 33*, 624–636.

Hamza, N. (2006). Gender based violences. Training manual for the attention of the national network listens to center for women victims of violences. 110p.

Institut National de la Statistique (INS) et ICF International. (2012). *Enquête démographique et de santé et à indicateurs multiples du Cameroun 2011.* Calverton, MD, USA: INS et ICF International.

Kabeer, N. (1997). Women, wages and inter-household power relations in urban Bangladesh. *Development and Change, 28*, 261–302.

Kamdem Kamgno, H. (2006). Gender and fertility in Cameroon. A comparative studies between Bamiléké and, Doctorate in Démographie, University of Yaoundé II, IFORD, 258 p.

Kaplan, E. L., & Meier, P. (1958). Nonparametric estimation from incomplete observations. *Journal of the American Statistical Association, 53*, 457–481.

Kenney, C. T., & McLanah, S. S. (2006). Why are cohabiting relations more violent than marriage? *Demography, 43*(1), 127–140.

Kimuna, S. R., Djamba, Y. K., Ciciurkaite, G., & Cherukuri, S. (2013). Domestic violence in India: Insights from the 2005–2006 National Family Health Survey. *Journal of Interpersonal Violence, 28*(4), 773–807.

Kishor, S., & Kiersten, J. (2006). Domestic's violences: A study in several countries, Calverton Maryland: Macro International Inc. 104p.

Koenig, M. A., Lutalo, T., Zhao, F., Nalugoda, F., Wabwire-Mangen, F., Kiwanuka, N., Wagman, S. D., Wawer, M., & Gray, R. (2003). Domestic violence in rural Uganda: Evidence from a community-based study. *Bulletin of WHO, 81*, 53–60.

Laughrea, K., Bélanger, C., & Wright, J. (1996). Existe-t-il un consensus social pour definer et comprendre la problématique de la violence conjugale? *Santé Mentale au Québec, XXI*(2), 95–116.

Martin, S. L., Tsui, A. O., Maitra, K., & Marinshaw, R. (1999). Domestic violence in Northern India. *American Journal of Epidemiology, 150*(4), 417–426.

Mc Closkey, L., Williams, C., & Larsen, U. (2005). Gender inequality and intimate partner violence among women in Moshi, Tanzania. *International Family Planning Perspectives, 31*(3), 124–130.

Mezey, G., Bacchus, L., Bewley, S., & White, S. (2005). Domestic violence, lifetime trauma and psychological health of childbearing women. *BJOG, 112*, 197–204.

O'Farrell, T. J., Van Hutton, V., & Murphy, C. M. (1999). Domestic violence before and after alcoholism treatment: A two-year longitudinal study. *Journal of Studies on Alcohol, 60*, 317–321.

Population Reference Bureau. (2011). The effect of girls' education on health outcomes: Fact sheet. http://www.prb.org/Publications/Media-Guides/2011/girls-education-fact-sheet.aspx. Accessed 27 Aug 2014.

Quigley, B. M., & Leonard, K. E. (2000). Alcohol and the continuation of early marital aggression. *Alcoholism: Clinical and Experimental Research, 24*(7), 1003–1010.

Rani, M., Bonu, S., & Diop-Sidibé, N. (2004). An empirical investigation of attitudes towards wife-beating among men and women in seven sub-Saharan African countries. *African Journal of Reproductive Health, 8*(3), 116–136.

Renzetti, C. M. (2011). *Economic stress and domestic violence.* Harrisburg, PA: National Resource Center on Domestic Violence/Pennsylvania Coalition Against Domestic Violence. http://www.vawnet.org/applied-research-papers/print-document.php?doc_id=2187. Accessed 1 Aug 2024.

Sharps, P., Laughon, K., & Giangrande, S. (2007). Intimate partner violence and the childbearing year: Maternal and infant health consequences. *Trauma Violence and Abuse, 8*(2), 105–116.

Steinmetz, S. K. (1977). *The cycle of violence: Assertive, aggressive and abusive family interaction.* New York, NY: Praeger Publishers.

Tracy, S. R. (2007). Patriarchy and domestic violence: Challenging common misconceptions. *Journal of the Evangelical Theological Society, 50*(3), 573–594.

UNFPA. (1995). *Report of the International Conference on Population and Development.* New York: Unites Nations. https://www.unfpa.org/public/global/publications/pid/1973. Accessed 1 Aug 2014.

UNFPA. (2000). Ending violences against girls and women: a priority in the rigth and health field, world's population state, Chapter 3, 6 p.

UNICEF. (2003). *Girls' education in Cameroon.* New York: UNICEF. www.unicef.org/girlseducation /index.html. Accessed 1 Aug 2014.

UNWOMEN. (2014). *Beijing declaration and platform for action.* New York: United Nations. http://www.un.org/womenwatch/daw/beijing/platform/. Accessed 1 Aug 2014.

WHO. (2005). *WHO multi-country study on women's health and domestic violence against women: Summary report of initial results on prevalence, health outcomes and women's responses.* Geneva: World Health Organization. http://www.who.int/gender/violence/who_ multicountry_study/summary_report/chapter1/en/index1.html. Accessed 3 Aug 2014.

Wolfang, M. E., & Ferracuti, F. (1967). *The subculture of violence. Towards an integrated theory in criminology* (p. 140). London: Tavistock Publications.

Chapter 3
Violence Against Young Females in South Africa: An Analysis of the Current Prevalence and Previous Levels of Youth Mortality, 1997–2009

Nicole De Wet

Abstract Violence against females, in its many forms, is a recognized social and public health concern. In South Africa, studies have examined the consequences (HIV transmission) and social causes (patriarchal practices) of violence against females. This study contributes to this body of knowledge by examining the national prevalence of violence as reported by females and the national mortality rates of females due to assault—which is an aggressive act perpetrated by another person. The analysis is based on the nationally representative Victims of Crime Survey (2010) and Death Notification Form data. Rates, proportions, and logistic regression producing odds ratios are generated. The results show that more physical than sexual assaults are reported by young females in the country. Both types of assault are reportedly higher among females with a secondary education. Female mortality due to assault increased between 1997 and 2009, and the odds of a female dying from assault are higher than that of a male. Some practical measures are proposed to reduce the prevalence of female abuse and resulting mortality among young South African females.

Keywords Female mortality rates • Physical and sexual assaults • South Africa

Introduction

Violence against females is a global problem. Recent results on physical violence have estimated that between 13 and 61 % of females had experienced physical violence from an intimate partner (Garcia-Moreno et al. 2006: 104). In Africa, studies have found that 26 % of females in Zimbabwe reported forced sexual intercourse and 23 % reported physical violence (Watts et al. 1998). Studies in Ethiopia have

N. De Wet (✉)
Demography and Population Studies, University of the Witwatersrand,
Johannesburg, South Africa
e-mail: nicole.dewet@wits.ac.za

© Springer International Publishing Switzerland 2015   33
Y.K. Djamba, S.R. Kimuna (eds.), *Gender-Based Violence*,
DOI 10.1007/978-3-319-16670-4_3

shown that about half to two-thirds of females experience a form of spousal abuse at least once in a lifetime (Yigzaw et al. 2010). According to a study carried out in three provinces in South Africa, preventing females from working is a form of abuse because it reduces female's ability to resist other abusive acts by undermining their self-esteem (Jewkes et al. 2001). Jewkes et al. (2001) also found that the prevalence of ever having been physically abused by a current or ex-partner were 26.8 %, 28.4 %, and 19.1 % in Eastern Cape, Mpumalanga, and Northern Cape province, respectively (Jewkes et al. 2001). The prevalence of rape were 4.5 % in Eastern Cape, 7.2 % in Mpumalanga, and 4.8 % in the Northern Cape province, while that of physical abuse during a pregnancy were 9.1 % in Eastern Cape, 6.7 % in Mpumalanga, and 4.7 % in Northern province (Jewkes et al. 2001).

The study of the different forms of violence against females (gender-based violence (GBV) and domestic violence) is marred by the challenge of underreporting, which results in a lack of quantitative and qualitative survey data addressing the issue specifically (Dunkle et al. 2004; Shannon et al. 2009). In addition, definition, attitude, and perceptions about the permissiveness of violence against females in Africa contribute to the ongoing challenge of researching its incidences and severities on the continent. Attempts to define violence against females have been made. Spousal violence is a pattern of behavior employed by a person in a relationship to control the other which could include battery, burning, emotional blackmail, mockery or ridicule, threats of abandonment, confinement to the home, and withholding of money and other family support (Yigzaw et al. 2010). It encompasses physical, sexual, psychological, and economic dimensions of different controlling behaviors (Yigzaw et al. 2010). Acts of violence are perceived by the potential harm it may inflict; use of weapons is seen as more violent or severe when compared to slaps and kicks, while verbal aggressions are also taken lightly unless they are perceived as unwarranted (Yigzaw et al. 2010). Moreover, the United Nations has defined violence against women to include but not be limited to the following:

1. Physical, sexual, and psychological violence occurring in the family, including battering, sexual abuse of female children in the household, dowry-related violence, marital rape, female genital mutilation, and other traditional practices harmful to women, such as non-spousal violence and violence related to exploitation.
2. Physical, sexual, and psychological violence occurring within the general community, including rape, sexual abuse, sexual harassment, and intimidation at work, in educational institutions and elsewhere, trafficking in women, and forced prostitution.
3. Physical, sexual, and psychological violence perpetrated or condoned by the state, wherever it occurs.
4. In addition, acts of violence against women also include forced sterilization and forced abortion, coercive/forced use of contraceptives, female infanticide, and prenatal sex selection (United Nations General Assembly 1993: 105).

The problem of definition is also complicated by the meaning some females attach to wife beating. Several studies suggest that many females believe wife beating signifies love and is justified. A South African study reported that 34 % of respondents personally agreed to the statement that beating signifies love (Jewkes et al. 2002a). An Ethiopian Demographic and Health Survey carried out in 2000 also indicated that the majority of females believed that a husband is justified to beat his wife for at least one reason (Central Statistical Authority [Ethiopia] and ORC Macro 2001). Another study conducted in Uganda reported that 70 % of men and 90 % of females believed that beating was justified in some situations (Koenig et al. 2003).

These challenges also contribute to the ineffectiveness of policies and programs on the continent aimed at reducing GBV. A recent evaluation of the new Domestic Violence Act in South Africa found that, although the number of requests for protection orders increased, there was no increase among applicants that are females (Outwater et al. 2005). This is despite the fact that violence against females has been acknowledged as both a social and public health concern in South Africa.

A study done in Soweto, south of Johannesburg, found that females with violent partners are more likely to contract HIV (Dunkle et al. 2004). A similar study also found intimate partner violence to be associated with HIV infection and the infection would most likely be the result of partner violence (Jewkes et al. 2010). Other than its relationship to HIV infection, research in South Africa has found violence against females to result in unwanted pregnancy, and incidents of violence against females are associated with alcohol consumption and low levels of education among victims and perpetrators (Jewkes et al. 2002a, b). Generally, it has been found that the consequences of violence extend beyond reproductive and sexual health of females to encompass their overall well-being, which extends to the households, communities, and the society as a whole (Izugbara et al. 2008). This applies to females of all ages, including youth who are entering intimate partner relationships for the first time.

In South Africa, youth constitute 42 % of the total population (UNFPA 2013). The liberal definition of youth contributes to this. The South African National Youth Policy 2009–2014 defines "youth" as young people whose age falls between 15 and 34 years old (Presidency of the Republic of South Africa 2009). This definition of "youth" is broader than the international definition by the World Health Organization which views youth as between the ages of 15 and 24 years old (United Nations 2002). The reason for South Africa adopting a broader age group is to allow previously disadvantaged persons to benefit from youth development programs that were previously unattainable during the Apartheid years (National Youth Development Agency 2012). These programs are aimed at improving young females' education, employment, development, health, and reproductive health statuses.

Other than the threat of violence from a partner, young females face the challenge of negative reproductive health outcomes such as the contraction of STIs (including HIV/AIDS) and maternal mortality in South Africa. Gender roles and expectations have been found to be associated with reproductive health outcomes such as poor sexual intercourse negotiation and early pregnancy (Varga 2003). Other challenges are social and economic, including unemployment, single parenthood, and poverty (Hallman 2004; Hunter 2007; Monasch and Boerma 2004).

Global and national reduction of violence against females has been acknowledged by the United Nations in the construction of the Millennium Development Goals (MDGs). Among other MDGs that address female's rights indirectly, goal number 8 recognizes the promotion of gender inequality and female empowerment globally (World Health Organization 2005).

In South Africa, the target for the promotion of gender inequality is to achieve a gender parity ratio 1:1 of girl-to-boy children enrolled in school (Chopra et al. 2009). However, with violence against females being as prevalent as it is, in the Gauteng province alone it is estimated that 51.2 % of females had experienced some form of violence in their lifetime, which makes it difficult to reach the educational gender parity goal. Therefore, there is a need for research to address the dynamics related to violence against young females in South Africa, in particular, to quantify the severe forms of violence against females which include physical and sexual assault, as well as mortality due to assault. In 2009 the rate of female homicides in the country was 12.9 per 100,000 population (Abrahams et al. 2012:106). With the population of young females being as high as it is currently (51.3 % according to the 2011 Census), women are potential social and economic assets to the country (Statistics South Africa 2012: 107). This study aims to estimate the current prevalence of violence against young females, 15–34 years old, and to examine the levels, trends, and determinants of young female mortality due to assault for the period of 1997–2009.

Theoretical Framework

Research has in many instances drafted and redrafted theoretical and conceptual frameworks for the study of GBV. Frameworks to map the understanding of health-seeking behavior of victims of violence have been created (Kishor and Johnson 2004). These frameworks explain the pathways through which females operate to seek curative medical and social support (Sokoloff and Dupont 2005). Some frameworks even describe the role of service providers in assisting victims of GBV (Crowell and Burgess 1997). An ecological framework for the understanding of community, household, and individual-level factors contributing to violence against females has also been developed (Heise 1998).

For this study, however, a framework for the risk factors of violence at an individual level is adapted. The World Bank (2009) developed the "Risk Factors for Violence based on the Ecological model" (see Table 3.1). This model is an adaptation of the work by several researchers, over several years, and the result is a comprehensive framework for understanding the risk of violence to females. The model shows factors identified at societal, community, relationship, and individual levels that are considered to be associated with violence against females (World Bank 2009).

For this study, the risk factors identified at the "individual" level are operationalized. Due to restrictions in the data sources, not all individual-level variables are used in this study. The variables that have been used are sex (gender), age, education, and employment status. As a proxy for the "relationship" level of the World Bank model, this study does consider "marital status" as a variable for analysis. In addition to the model, this study uses "relationship to the household head" and "province of residence" as possible risk factors for violence against females.

Table 3.1 Risk factors for violence based on the ecological model

Societal	Community	Relationship	Individual
Broad factors that reduce inhibitions against violence	Neighborhood, schools, and workplaces	With family, intimate partners, and friends	Personal factors that influence individual behavior
• Poverty	• High unemployment	• Family dysfunction	• Gender, age, and education
• Economic, social, and gender inequalities	• High population density	• Intergenerational violence poor parenting	• A family history of violence
• Poor social security	• Social isolation of females and family	• Parental conflict involving violence	• Witnessing GBV
• Masculinity linked to aggression and dominance	• Lack of information	• Association with friends who engage in violence or delinquent behavior	• Victim of child abuse or neglect
• Weak legal and criminal justice system	• Inadequate victim care	• Low socioeconomic status, socioeconomic stress	• Lack of sufficient livelihood and personal income
• Perpetrators not prosecuted	• Schools and workplaces not addressing GBV	• Friction over women's empowerment	• Unemployment
• No legal rights for victims	• Weak community sanctions against GBV	• Family honor more important than female health and safety	• Mental health and behavioral problems
• Social and cultural norms support violence	• Poor safety in public spaces		• Alcohol and substance abuse
• Small fire arms	• Challenging traditional gender roles		• Prostitution
• Conflict or post-conflict	• Blaming the victim		• Refugee internally displaced
• Internal displacement and refugee camps	• Violating victim confidentiality		• Disabilities
			• Small fire arms ownership

Source: World Bank (2009). Reprinted with permission granted by the World Bank on September 22, 2014

Data and Methods

This study uses two sources that collect data related to violence against females. The first is a survey, called the Victims of Crime Survey, which identifies persons who were victims of violent crimes in South Africa and asks that they report on their experiences. The second is Death Notification Forms (DNFs) which is a national database of medical death certificates which indicates, among others, the sex and cause of death of persons who died in the country. Together, these data sources are used to create a profile of current prevalence of assault against females, as well as to quantify the level of mortality due to violence against females in the past.

The Victims of Crime Survey (VOCS) of 2010 is used. The survey is conducted by the national statistics organization, Statistics South Africa (Statistics SA). The sample design for the VOCS is based on a master sample (MS) originally designed for the Quarterly Labor Force Survey (QLFS) as a sampling frame. The MS is based on information collected during the 2001 Population Census conducted by Statistics SA. The MS has been developed as a general-purpose household survey frame that can be used by all household-based surveys, irrespective of the sample size requirement of the survey. The VOCS, like all other household-based surveys, uses an MS of primary sampling units (PSUs) which comprises census enumeration areas (EAs) that are drawn from across the country. The sample size of 3,080 PSUs was selected. In each selected PSU a systematic sample of dwelling units was drawn. From this the sample size for the VOCS is approximately 30,000 dwelling units (Statistics South Africa 2012).

Out of these dwelling units, 862,921 females were identified as having reported being victims of physical assault and 126,207 females as having reported experiencing a sexual assault. These are the study population for the prevalence of violence against female section of the study.

For the objective of this study that addresses violence against females that results in death, DNF data are used. According to the Statistics SA (2008), DNF data are from the National Population Register which is updated following a death and the issuing of a death certificate. The Register in South Africa does not contain information of noncitizens and members who are not in possession of a legal identity number. However, Statistics SA collects the Register data and the information of individuals not captured and processes, analyzes, and disseminates the completed information for analytical use.

The data used for this study is the DNFs as collated by Statistics SA from 1997 to 2009. The data received from the organization are based on Form BI-1663 (Notification/Register of Deaths/Stillbirth), which was introduced in South Africa in 1998. Data collected prior to 1998 was fit into the new categories of data as far as possible. The only notable difference between the pre- and post-1998 forms is the classification of occupation groups, which does not affect this study, since specific occupations are not of interest but rather the broad employment status of females. In the event that a death is not certified by a medical practitioner in the country, a chief or headman of the community is asked to give information on the circumstances that led to the death (Statistics SA 2008). This has been an effort on Statistics SA's part to counter the problem of undercount.

Assault is defined as injuries inflicted by another person with intent to injure or kill by any means and includes the use of weapons (guns and explosive material), sharp (knives) and blunt (bricks, stones) objects, bodily force (pushing, strangulation), and motor vehicles (AAPC 2011: 74). For the first period (1997–2001), 935 females died from assault. In the second period (2002–2005) 1,011 and in the final period (2006–2009) 1,467 females died from assault. This is the study population for the part of the analysis which assesses mortality from violent causes among females in the country.

The study population selected for this chapter are females aged 15–34 years old who have been victims of physical and sexual assault (from VOCS) as well as females aged 15–34 years old who died from violent (assault) causes of death (from DNF). The broad age group of South African youth is aligned with the country's adoption of 15–34 years old.

Predictor Variables

The independent/predictor variables selected for this study relate to the conceptual framework outlined above. For each data source, there are similar demographic and socioeconomic variables as well as variables particular to the violence experienced. But the two samples are independent.

For the VOCS, the demographic and socioeconomic variables selected are age, race or population group, relationship to the household head, marital status, highest level of educational attainment, and employment status. For data from the DNFs, age, year of death, marital status, highest level of education, province of residence, and employment status are used.

Other variables included in the study pertain to the experiences of violence or crime. In the VOCS experiences of other crimes (thefts and fraud) are included for the purpose of generating a proportional measure of violence against females. Also, in the generation of a measure of assault mortality in proportion to all other causes in the DNF data, other causes of unnatural deaths (accidents, events of undetermined intent, and self-harm) among female youths are used.

Outcome Variables

This study is concerned with the outcome of violence against females. There are two particular facets of this outcome which this study focuses on: (1) prevalence of physical violence (which includes acts of physical only and sexual violence) and (2) mortality due to violence. The VOCS is used to identify the prevalence of physical and sexual violence and the DNFs are used to establish morality.

In the VOCS, victims were asked if they had experienced physical or sexual violence in the last 5 years (with particular emphasis on the last 12 months). Respondents who answered "yes" to either physical or sexual assault are included in the study. Respondents who did not answer this question or responded with a "no" were excluded from the analysis. A total of 989,128 females reported having experienced these forms of violence.

To identify causes of death, the ICD-10 code for assault (X85-Y09) was used in the DNF data (AAPC 2011). Only females whose broad underlying cause of death was a reported assault were included in the analysis. In total, 6,821 deaths reported in females of all ages and 3,143 in adolescent (youth) females were due to assault during the period of 1997–2009.

Analytical Strategy

In line with the study objectives, the analysis is conducted in two ways. First, the prevalence of violence against females is calculated to show the distribution of females who experienced assault by demographic and socioeconomic characteristics. Second, the rates of physical and sexual assault are created using the following formula:

$$\frac{\text{Number of female assaults}}{\text{Total number of females}} \times 10,000$$

where *number of female assaults* is physical assaults and sexual assaults, respectively, and *total number of females* is obtained from the Statistics South Africa Mid-Year Population Report (Statistics SA 2010). Due to underreporting, the number of cases is low, so the rate is set at 10,000.

A proportional rate of assaults is also generated. The purpose of this rate is to quantify the contribution of assault to the overall crime experience of female victims in the country. Thus the result is presented as a percentage (%) of all crimes. The formula used is

$$\frac{\text{Number of assaults}}{\text{Total number of other crimes}} \times 100$$

The numerator, number of assaults, is the sum of both physical and sexual assaults. Other crimes refer to thefts (muggings, house robbery, hijacking, and other forms of theft of property) and consumer fraud, which are the other forms of crimes reported in the VOCS.

The second objective of this study is to assess the mortality experience of females who died due to violence during the period of 1997–2009. For this, the distribution of females who died from assault is also shown. Then, a proportion of female mortality due to assault is generated using the following formula:

$$\frac{\text{Number of female deaths due to assaults}}{\text{Total number of female deaths from all causes}} \times 10,000$$

Both the *number of female deaths due to assault* and *total number of female deaths from all causes* are from the DNFs. Again, this measure is per 10,000, due to low numbers of events being reported.

The bivariate and multivariate logistic regression analyses are conducted to determine the relationship between selected demographic and socioeconomic characteristics and mortality due to assault.

The bivariate analysis of the variables was done to examine the association between each of the socioeconomic and demographic variables and the dependent variable (mortality due to assault). In order to examine such an association, adjusted odds ratios were calculated to explain the likelihood of mortality occurring per characteristic of the individual. For this, logistic regression analysis was used and the two different censored groups were selected. First, females who died from causes other than assault were chosen as the censored group and coded as 0. For the second, males of the same age who died from assault were selected and coded as 0. These censored groups and coding were also used in subsequent analysis which employed multivariate logistic regression models.

The basic logistic regression equation is

$$Li = \alpha + \beta 1 X 1i + \beta 2 X 2i + \ldots + \beta k X ki$$

where Li = dependent variables, α = constant, βk = regression coefficients, and X = independent variables.

Results

The results of the level of violence against females from the VOCS 2010 are shown in Table 3.2. All results are only for the female population. Overall, more females reported physical assault (862,921) than sexual assault (126,207). The age group that experienced the highest prevalence of physical (12.08 %) and sexual (11.97 %) assault are aged 20–24 years old. Alarmingly, 10.22 % and 9.51 % of female children aged 0–4 had been physically and sexually assaulted, respectively. Many young adolescents (10–14 years old) also experienced physical (10.18 %) and sexual (9.67 %) assault. For physical assault, there is constant fluctuation from one age group to the next. However what can be seen is a peak at age 50–54 years (4.85 %) followed by a decline to age 74 years (0.72 %) before assault mortality increases again among the elderly (75+ years old). A similar fluctuating trend is seen for sexual assault with highest percentages being among adolescents and young adults followed by a decline to 2.88 % among 50–54-year-olds.

Data on race or population group show that the majority of victims who reported violence are African/Black, with 76.78 % reporting physical and 87.62 % reporting sexual assault (in South Africa all Blacks are reported as African/Black or Black/African). Among the Indian population, only 2.6 % reported physical assault and none reported sexual assault. Equally low is the reporting of physical and sexual assault among the White population at 4.82 % and 1.1 %, respectively.

Table 3.2 Distribution of physical and sexual assault among females in South Africa, 2010

Characteristic	Physical assault		Sexual assault	
	N	%	N	%
All	862,921	100.00	126,207	100.00
Age group				
0–4 years	88,165	10.22	12,007	9.51
5–9	81451	9.44	11,483	9.10
10–14	87,822	10.18	12,202	9.67
15–19	72,631	8.42	14,101	11.17
20–24	104,207	12.08	15,105	11.97
25–29	86,022	9.97	11,594	9.19
30–34	66,062	7.66	11,854	9.39
35–39	50,880	5.90	6,615	5.24
40–44	39,407	4.57	4,054	3.21
45–49	40,634	4.71	2,717	2.15
50–54	41,875	4.85	3,639	2.88
55–59	31,210	3.62	3,953	3.13
60–64	15,355	1.78	2,657	2.11
65–69	12,856	1.49	271	0.21
70–74	6,249	0.72	1,005	0.80
75+	16,000	1.85	3,381	2.68
Unknown	22,095	2.56	9,569	7.58
Race				
African	662,556	76.78	110,578	87.62
Colored	136,328	15.80	14,240	11.28
Indian	22,417	2.60		
White	41,620	4.82	1,389	1.10
Relationship to household head				
Head	182,255	21.12	33,196	26.30
Spouse of head	153,060	17.74	10,166	8.06
Child of head	296,458	34.36	40,963	32.46
Sibling of head	22,565	2.61	6,660	5.28
Parent of head	3,822	0.44		
Grandparent of head	2,239	0.26	568	0.45
Grandchild of head	120,934	14.01	20,361	16.13
Head is other relative	59,117	6.85	13,958	11.06
Head is nonrelative	6,723	0.78		
Unknown	15,748	1.82	335	0.27
Marital status				
Married	198,197	22.97	15,772	12.50
Divorced/separated/widowed	88,005	10.20	12,594	9.98
Cohabiting	15,973	1.85	2,024	1.60
Never married	535,994	62.11	92,954	73.65
Unknown	24,752	2.87	2,863	2.27

(continued)

Table 3.2 (continued)

Characteristic	Physical assault		Sexual assault	
	N	%	N	%
Highest level of education				
None	140,864	16.32	27,555	21.83
Primary	250,929	29.08	37,580	29.78
Secondary with no diploma	416,262	48.24	49,401	39.14
Secondary with diploma	34,263	3.97	5,712	4.53
Tertiary	11,444	1.33	3,506	2.78
Other	2,750	0.32	887	0.70
Unknown	6,409	0.74	1,566	1.24
Employment status				
Working	166,437	19.29	21,196	16.79
Not working	433,372	50.22	63,379	50.22
Unknown	263,112	30.49	41,632	32.99
Province of residence				
Western Cape	141,505	16.40	12,003	9.51
Eastern Cape	93,340	10.82	32,081	25.42
Northern Cape	20,010	2.32	2,184	1.73
Free State	49,403	5.73	5,242	4.15
KwaZulu Natal	169,678	19.66	34,923	27.67
North West	63,021	7.30	6,438	5.10
Gauteng	162,523	18.83	8,284	6.56
Mpumalanga	69,377	8.04	8,148	6.46
Limpopo	94,064	10.90	16,904	13.39

Notes: Due to missing values some totals for some variables may be lower than the number reported in the first row. Also, percent for some variables may not add to 100 due to rounding

Relationship to the household head shows that most victims of violence against females are the children of the household head at 34.63 % and 32.46 % for physical and sexual assault, respectively. The second highest distribution of assaults is among the female heads of households themselves with 21.21 % reporting physical assault and 26.3 % reporting sexual assault. Grandchildren of the household head also reported prevalence of physical (14.01 %) and sexual (16.13 %) assault.

Married females reported more violence, both physical and sexual, than divorced, separated, or widowed females. More married females reported physical assault at almost 23 % than sexual assault at 12.5 %. Never-married females, however, reported the highest numbers of physical (62.11 %) and sexual (73.65 %) assaults. In addition, there is more sexual assault among never-married females than physical assault.

Data on education indicate that physical and sexual assault is more prevalent among females with a secondary education at 48.24 % and 39.14 %, respectively. Those with no education and primary education have lower rates of assault. However, females with tertiary education have the lowest reported physical (1.33 %) and sexual (2.78 %) assaults. The percentage distribution of sexual assaults, with

Table 3.3 Type of crimes on females in South Africa, 2010

Type of crime	Number of cases	Rate per 10,000 females[a]	Proportional ratio (%)
Sexual assault	126,207	49.18	4.82
Physical assault	862,921	336.26	32.93
Physical and sexual assaults	19,720	7.68	0.75
Other crimes	1,631,158	635.62	62.25
Total[b]	2,620,286	1,021.06	100.00

Note: Percent may not add to 100 due to rounding
[a]Total female population in 2010 was 25,662,300 (Statistics SA midyear population estimates)
[b]Excludes the third category (physical and sexual assaults) to avoid double counting these crimes

the exception of incomplete secondary education (secondary no diploma), is higher than the distribution of physical assaults by all education classifications.

There are some disparities by province of residence. For both physical (19.66 %) and sexual (27.67 %) assault, the highest distribution is found in the KwaZulu Natal province. For physical assault, the second highest distribution is found in Gauteng at almost 19 %, but for sexual assault, the second highest distribution is found in the Eastern Cape at 25.42 %. The lowest distribution for both physical and sexual assault is from the Northern Cape province.

Employment status shows that females with no employment are victims of physical and sexual assault, at 50.22 %, more than females who are employed. However, employed females are not exempt from experiencing physical assault (19.3 %) and sexual assault (almost 17 %).

The rate of sexual assaults as reported in the VOCS (2010) is 49.18 sexual assaults per 10,000 females in South Africa (Table 3.3). The overall rate for physical assault is higher at 336.26 per 10,000 female population. In addition to analyzing these forms of violence independently, the number of females who reported both physical and sexual assault was obtained. In 2010, 19,720 females reported experiencing both physical and sexual assault. The rate of "both" forms of assault is 7.86 per 10,000 female population in South Africa. All other crimes reported in the survey (thefts, burglaries, hijackings, consumer fraud, etc.) were then quantified to obtain a rate of "other crimes." The rate for other crimes is 635.62 per 10,000 female population. Finally, all crimes perpetrated against females, violent and other, were added together and a rate of 1,021 per 10,000 females was obtained.

Table 3.3 also shows the proportional ratio of assault for the other category and total crimes against females. Sexual assault contributed 4.82 % of all crimes. While physical assault is more prevalent at almost 33 % (32.93 %), the proportional ratio for all other crimes is 62.52 %. The proportion of both physical and sexual assault is 0.75 %.

Using the DNFs made it possible to examine the distribution of female deaths due to assault for the period 1997–2009. Table 3.4 shows that the number of female deaths due to assault increased from 935 in the 1997–2001 period to 1,011 in 2001–2005 and 1,467 in the 2006–2009 period. There are however fluctuations by characteristics over the years. For age, the number of deaths was higher in the age group 30–35-year-olds

Table 3.4 Distribution of assault mortality among young females in South Africa, 1997–2009

Characteristic	1997–2001		2002–2005		2006–2009	
	N	%	N	%	N	%
All	935	100.00	1,011	100.00	1,467	100.00
Age group						
15–19	144	15.40	146	14.44	232	15.81
20–24	213	22.78	295	29.18	408	27.81
25–29	279	29.84	252	24.93	417	28.43
30–35	299	31.98	318	31.45	410	27.95
Marital status						
Single	718	76.79	835	82.59	1,197	81.60
Married	150	16.04	105	10.39	141	9.61
Divorced	15	1.60	10	0.99	11	0.75
Unknown	52	5.56	61	6.03	118	8.04
Education						
None	37	3.96	36	3.56	34	2.32
Primary	185	19.79	224	22.16	254	17.31
Secondary	200	21.39	294	29.08	584	39.81
Tertiary	7	0.75	10	0.99	25	1.70
Unknown	506	54.12	447	44.21	570	38.85
Employment status						
Employed	9	81.82	12	75.00	831	56.65
Unemployed	2	18.18	4	25.00	636	43.35
Province of birth						
Western Cape	76	8.14	91	9.00	106	7.24
Eastern Cape	174	18.63	247	24.43	312	21.31
Northern Cape	54	5.78	71	7.02	82	5.60
Free State	49	5.25	70	6.92	133	9.08
KwaZulu Natal	129	13.81	179	17.71	234	15.98
North West	34	3.64	41	4.06	65	4.44
Gauteng	64	6.85	53	5.24	86	5.87
Mpumalanga	21	2.25	27	2.67	46	3.14
Limpopo	42	4.50	48	4.75	72	4.92
Unknown	5	0.54	3	0.30	282	19.26
Outside South Africa	17	1.82	11	1.09	33	2.25
Unspecified	269	28.8	170	16.82	13	0.89

Notes: Due to missing values some totals for some variables may be lower than the number reported in the first row. Also, percent for some variables may not add to 100 due to rounding

for the first two of the three periods considered here. There were some changes over time in the lower age groups.

Mortality by marital status shows that throughout the years, single females have had higher mortality than any other marital status category. In 2002–2005, mortality among single females due to assault was higher (82.59 %) than the other two periods. However, female mortality due to assault among married females appears to have

Table 3.5 Number and proportional mortality ratios of assault (broad-underlying cause of death) among young females in South Africa, 1997–2009

Cause of death	1997–2001		2002–2005		2006–2009	
	N	%	N	%	N	%
Assault	935	0.47	1,011	0.32	1,467	0.49
All other unnatural causes	24,049	12.13	19,325	6.18	18,042	6.07
All natural causes	173,225	87.40	292,545	93.50	277,805	93.44
Total	198,209	100.00	312,881	100.00	297,314	100.00

declined over the years with 16.04 % of deaths in 1997–2001, followed by 10.39 % in 2002–2005, and finally 9.61 % in 2006–2009.

Table 3.4 also shows that throughout the three study periods, deaths from assault among females are consistently higher in the Eastern Cape province of South Africa than any other province. In 1997–2001, 18.63 % deaths from assault occurred to females born in the province, in 2002–2005 almost 25 %, and in 2006–2009, 21.31 %. Equally high is the distribution of mortality in the KwaZulu Natal province which ranged from almost 14 % in 1997–2001 to 17.71 % in 2002–2005 and then about 16 % in 2006–2009. The area for "unspecified" province of birth accounted for 28.8 % of female deaths in 1997–2001 but declined to 0.89 % in 2006–2009.

Further, Table 3.4 shows that mortality is particularly high among females with secondary education across all periods. There is almost 20 % increase in the number of female deaths due to assault over the study period, 1997–2009, with 21.39 % at the start of the period and almost 40 % in the last period. Data for the employment status category show a decline in trend over the study period. In the initial period (1997–2001), 81.82 % of deaths were among employed females and this declined to about 57 % in 2006–2009.

The proportions of mortality due to assault in relation to all other unnatural (or non-disease) and natural (disease) causes of death are given in Table 3.5. Data show that disease-related mortality (all natural causes) was a major contributor to youth mortality in South Africa from 1997 to 2009. All other unnatural causes, which exclude assault, show a downward trend. In 1997–2001 there were 12.13 % deaths due to unnatural causes, 6.18 % deaths in 2002–2005, and 6.07 % deaths in 2006–2009. While deaths due to assault have remained relatively low throughout the period, there are fluctuations. In the initial period, the proportion of young female mortality due to assault was 0.47 %, which then declined to 0.32 % in 2005–2009 before increasing to 0.49 % in the last period of analysis.

To determine an association between each predictor variable and mortality due to assault, odds ratios from bivariate logistic regression models are analyzed (see Table 3.6). Independently, the odds of mortality due to assault among females aged 20 and over are consistently lower than the reference category of adolescent females (15–19 years old). These decreased odds are lower in the years post-2001 than in the initial period (1997–2001).

No significant difference was found between never- and ever-married females. Only those whose marital statuses were unknown appeared significantly less likely to die from assault. This was consistent over all the three periods analyzed in this study.

Table 3.6 Adjusted (bivariate) odds ratios showing the likelihood of young females dying from assault by demographic and socioeconomic characteristics in South Africa, 1997–2009

Characteristic	1997–2001		2002–2005		2006–2009	
	Odds ratio	[95 % C.I.]	Odds ratio	[95 % C.I.]	Odds ratio	[95 % C.I.]
Age group						
15–19 (ref.)	1.00		1.00		1.00	
20–24	0.55*	[0.439–0.683]	0.63*	[0.513–0.769]	0.60*	[0.500–0.719]
25–29	0.45*	[0.363–0.553]	0.28*	[0.223–0.344]	0.33*	[0.271–0.390]
30–35	0.43*	[0.347–0.525]	0.28*	[0.231–0.344]	0.23*	[0.188–0.272]
Marital status						
Single (ref.)	1.00		1.00		1.00	
Married	1.11	[0.923–1.338]	0.80	[0.647–0.981]	0.91	[0.747–1.097]
Divorced	0.86	[0.463–1.617]	0.56	[0.264–1.173]	0.72	[0.371–1.383]
Unknown	0.50*	[0.370–0.666]	0.38*	[0.290–0.494]	0.40*	[0.323–0.497]
Education						
None (ref.)	1.00		1.00		1.00	
Primary	1.44	[0.993–2.096]	1.38	[0.963–1.971]	1.59*	[1.053–2.391]
Secondary	0.96	[0.661–1.391]	0.93	[0.651–1.315]	1.41	[0.946–2.089]
Tertiary	0.56	[0.235–1.341]	0.72	[0.359–1.465]	1.15	[0.629–2.096]
Unknown	0.68*	[0.474–0.964]	0.73	[0.517–1.033]	0.95	[0.637–1.405]
Province of birth						
Western Cape (ref.)	1.00		1.00		1.00	
Eastern Cape	0.44*	[0.334–0.586]	0.35*	[0.270–0.450]	0.30*	[0.233–0.379]
Northern Cape	0.84	[0.580–1.208]	0.82	[0.591–1.146]	0.66	[0.476–0.907]
Free State	0.19*	[0.128–0.270]	0.19*	[0.136–0.261]	0.26*	[0.193–0.338]
KwaZulu Natal	0.19*	[0.142–0.257]	0.18*	[0.138–0.234]	0.16*	[0.124–0.207]
North West	0.17*	[0.109–0.258]	0.14*	[0.094–0.204]	0.15*	[0.107–0.216]
Gauteng	0.22*	[0.153–0.308]	0.12*	[0.086–0.177]	0.14*	[0.102–0.194]
Mpumalanga	0.11*	[0.067–0.190]	0.09*	[0.059–0.144]	0.08*	[0.050–0.114]
Limpopo	0.25*	[0.166–0.369]	0.17*	[0.120–0.249]	0.13*	[0.095–0.187]
Unknown	0.76	[0.304–1.891]	0.30*	[0.096–0.968]	0.19*	[0.147–0.242]
Outside South Africa	0.37*	[0.206–0.650]	0.16*	[0.083–0.311]	0.23*	[0.149–0.354]
Unspecified	0.16*	[0.126–0.215]	0.19*	[0.146–0.249]	0.15*	[0.081–0.286]

Notes: *ref.* reference category
*P-value < 0.05

The association between education attainment and female mortality due to assault was not statistically significant except for females with primary education in 2006–2009. During that period, females with a primary education were 1.59 times more likely to die from assault than females with no education ($p < 0.05$). Also, data in Table 3.6 show decreased odds of dying from assault in all provinces except the Western Cape (reference category).

Table 3.7 shows the unadjusted (multivariate) odds ratios indicating the likelihood of dying from assault (for females only and for males and females) by

Table 3.7 Unadjusted (multivariate) odds ratios showing the likelihood of dying from assault (for females only and for males and females) by demographic and socioeconomic characteristics in South Africa, 1997–2009

	1997–2001		2002–2005		2006–2009	
Characteristic	Females only	Males and females	Females only	Males and females	Females only	Males and females
Sex						
Male (ref.)		1.00		1.00		1.00
Female		0.61*		0.95		1.20
Age group						
15–19 (ref.)	1.00	1.00	1.00	1.00	1.00	1.00
20–24	0.56*	1.06*	0.67*	1.26	0.63*	0.94
25–29	0.45*	1.12*	0.30*	1.13	0.34*	0.78
30–35	0.42*	1.10*	0.31*	1.06	0.24*	0.71*
Marital status						
Single (ref.)	1.00	1.00	1.00	1.00	1.00	1.00
Married	0.90	0.78	0.65	1.00	0.89	1.00
Divorced	0.61*	0.49	0.44*	0.22*	0.47*	0.45
Unknown	0.97	0.73	0.74	0.69*	0.54	1.07
Education						
None (ref.)	1.00	1.00	1.00	1.00	1.00	1.00
Primary	1.41	1.06	1.30	0.54	1.50	1.16
Secondary	0.94	1.18	0.89	0.57	1.38	1.05
Tertiary	0.56	0.67	0.71	1.23	1.00	4.79
Unknown	0.72	0.89	0.73	0.52	0.99	1.34
Province of birth						
Western Cape (ref.)	1.00	1.00	1.00	1.00	1.00	1.00
Eastern Cape	0.46*	0.71	0.36*	1.77*	0.30*	1.25
Northern Cape	0.79	0.44	0.79	0.37*	0.62*	1.24
Free State	0.18*	0.81	0.18*	1.49	0.24*	1.55
KwaZulu Natal	0.19*	0.59*	0.18*	1.68	0.15*	1.83
North West	0.17*	0.57*	0.14*	0.79	0.16*	1.31
Gauteng	0.22*	0.41*	0.13*	1.17	0.15*	1.33
Mpumalanga	0.11*	0.47*	0.09*	2.26*	0.07*	1.12
Limpopo	0.24*	0.55*	0.18*	1.04	0.14*	0.93
Unknown	0.84	1.00	0.33	1.00	0.21*	1.16
Outside South Africa	0.37*	0.99	0.18*	1.00	0.26*	1.84
Unspecified	0.19*	0.64*	0.22*	2.53*	0.20*	1.31

Notes: ref. reference category
*P-value < 0.05

demographic and socioeconomic characteristics in South Africa, 1997–2009. In the years 1997–2001, compared to young females aged 15–19, young females in all other age groups are statistically significantly less likely to die from assault. This outcome is consistent in the other two study periods, 2002–2005 and 2006–2009.

Further, for all the study periods, compared to single females, divorced females are statistically significantly less likely to die from assault during all the three periods considered here. In 2002–2005, females whose marital statuses were unknown were significantly more likely to die of assault than single women. The significant impact of place of birth changed slightly over time. In 1997–2001 and 2002–2005, compared to young females whose province of birth is Western Cape, those born in the following provinces were significantly less likely to die from assault: Eastern Cape, Free State, KwaZulu Natal, North West, Gauteng, Mpumalanga, and Limpopo, including those born outside South Africa or with unspecified place of birth. No significant differences were found between Western Cape natives and their counterparts born in Northern Cape or those with unknown birthplace in the first two periods. In contrast, females born in all provinces, including those with unspecified and unknown birthplaces, were significantly less likely to die from assault in 2006–2009.

Table 3.7 also contains the results for both males and females for all the three periods. In the initial period, compared to young males, young females were 0.61 times less likely to die from assault in South Africa. No significant gender differences were observed in 2002–2005 and 2006–2009. For 2006–2009, compared to youth of both sexes aged 15–19 years, youth of both sexes aged 30–35 years were 0.71 times less likely to die from assault in South Africa. In 2002–2005, compared to youth of both sexes who were single, youth of both sexes who were married were 0.22 times less likely, while those who were divorced were 0.69 times less likely to die from assault in South Africa.

Discussion

The aim of this study is to identify the prevalence of physical and sexual assault against females in South Africa, and to quantify the trends and determinants of assault mortality among females over time. The results show that more physical assaults are reported by females than sexual assaults (862,921 vs. 126,207). Nonetheless, the rate of sexual assault is high at about 49 females per 10,000 population (Table 3.3). This high rate of sexual assault is consistent with a United Nations study using data from the year 2000, which found that 53,008 rape cases were reported to the police, representing a rate of 123 female rapes per 100,000 population in the country for the same year (United Nations 2003). This is far higher than rapes in other parts of the world such as Australia (81/100,000), the UK (16/100,000), and Zimbabwe (44/100,000) (United Nations 2003).

Despite this high rate of sexual assaults that are reported by females, rapes and intimate partner violence are said to be underreported. Research has found that the sexual assault of children, females with mental illness, and females assaulted while under the influence of alcohol are among the main types of sexual assault that are underreported in the world (Abbey et al. 2001; Goodman et al. 1997; Widom and Morris 1997). In South Africa, reasons for underreporting include fear of not being believed by the police, lack of physical access to the police, and fear of retaliation by the perpetrator (Artz 1999; CIET Africa 1998; Stanton 1993).

This study showed that a high number of female heads of households reported physical (21.12 %) and sexual (26.3 %) assaults (Table 3.2). The number of female-headed households in South Africa is estimated to be half the number of households in the country (Department of Health, Medical Research Council and OrcMacro 2007). Researchers have argued that this is historically due to non-marriage and labor migration of men in the country (Posel 2001). In more recent times, premature male mortality from AIDS is noted as the reason for decreasing marriage rates (Walker and Gilbert 2002). It is also acknowledged that female-headed households are among the poorest households in the country, with these households having a 48 % chance of being poor compared to male-headed households which have a 28 % chance of being poor (Woolard 2002). If this is the case, females heading households may engage in transactional sexual relationships which make them more vulnerable to assault from their partners (Ferguson and Morris 2007; Maganja et al. 2007).

This study has found that fewer married females report assault than never-married or single females. This again could be a reporting issue. There have, in the past, been debates over the acceptability of husband violence and if rape can occur within a marriage (Bergen 1998; Khan et al. 1996; Stark and Flitcraft 1988). In the event that it is believed that physical assault from a spouse is permitted and accept-able and that a "husband cannot rape his wife," then it is clear why the statistic for married females is lower than for single females. This also gives insight into the greater challenge of females recognizing domestic violence and intimate partner violence as a problem (Heise 1992; Heise et al. 1994; Straus and Gelles 1986).

Related to the problem of recognition is the issue of female education. In South Africa, 18.8 % of females have at least a secondary education (Statistics South Africa 2012). This study has found that most females who report assault have a secondary education. This is because the level of education of females in the country is high compared to Malawi, where it has been suggested that only 7 % of children with a primary education will complete secondary school (UNESCO 2008). Given then that the majority of assault victims have at least some education, we speculate that there are more influential determinants of female assaults in South Africa, such as the effect of culture and patriarchy.

To a great extent, the roots of violence against females lie in the patriarchal nature of African societies, where females are often seen as inferior compared to men (Jewkes et al. 2001). The effect of patriarchy on violence against females in South Africa has been researched and the relationship between patriarchy and vio-lence against females has been established (Hester et al. 1996; Hunnicutt 2009; Schuler et al. 1996). In the KwaZulu Natal province of South Africa, the patriarchal practice of polygyny (having more than one wife) is common (Hunter 2005). It is more than just coincidence that violence against females is also high in this patriar-chal setting. Research has also found that there is a high number of sexual assaults in that province with almost 46 % of young females reporting that their first sexual encounter was coerced (Maharaj and Munthree 2007). Similarly, this study found high prevalence of sexual and physical assault in the KwaZulu Natal province.

Females from other parts of the country, such as the Eastern Cape and Gauteng, have also reported high rates of sexual and physical assault. In addition to cultural practices that are male dominant, there are other factors that could explain the violence against females in these places. One such reason is frustration due to unemployment and poor service delivery in those parts of the country. An example of this is the Eastern Cape where unemployment is as high as 28.3 % (Statistics SA 2012). Furthermore, service delivery is poor in this province as indicated by the infant mortality rate (61.2 per 1,000 live births) which is the highest in the country (Woolard 2002). Some research has suggested that when men feel frustrated or overwhelmed by circumstances which they cannot control, such as being unable to find suitable employment, a resulting behavior is violence against females (Browne 1993; Heise 1998).

The employment status of females in this study shows two different results. The study shows higher prevalence of assault (physical and sexual) among unemployed females in the country; however, mortality is higher for employed females than among their unemployed counterparts. Employment status of females in South Africa is moderate with 5,902,000 females employed and 2,265,000 unemployed (Statistics SA 2012). With more females being employed than unemployed in the country, the result found in this study requires more in-depth analysis. Unemployed females have been reported to be at a higher risk of intimate partner violence and endure it more due to financial dependence on their abusers (Brownridge 2006). However, in order to better understand the assault mortality of employed females, there is need for research to address the employment discordant couples, whereby abusers (partners) are unemployed and females are employed. This would aid in the understanding of this finding because research has found that unemployed partners can be more aggressive (Brownridge 2006).

Overall, mortality in South Africa is low in comparison to other sub-Saharan African countries, with 572,673 deaths reported in 2009 (Statistics SA 2012). Despite overall mortality being moderate, this study has shown that female mortality due to assault has increased over time. Overall, females have higher odds of mortality due to assault than males. Research shows that mortality trends of the youth in South Africa show higher rates of death among older youth males, than younger ones, while female mortality increases with age (Kahn et al. 2007). The causes of these deaths are mostly diseases, or "natural" causes of death. Mortality due to "unnatural" causes or non-disease deaths is generally higher among males (De Wet et al. 2014). These causes include transport accidents, violence, and injuries which are caused by high-risk behaviors which men are more likely to engage in than females (Turner and McClure 2003). This study has shown however that an important "unnatural" cause of death—assault mortality—is higher among females, which suggests a high prevalence of severe violence against females in the country.

Conclusion

Violence against females in South Africa is a social and public health concern. The magnitude of violence presented in this chapter shows high rates of physical and sexual assault as well as increasing female mortality due to assault. Females (and children) in any society are the most vulnerable populations. Females in particular carry the burden of being caretakers to children and the elderly, a role that they may be prevented from fulfilling in instances of severe violence. Needless to say then, females need to be protected from violence perpetrated by the opposite sex, whether these men are partners and spouses or complete strangers.

This study did not examine any particular type of violence against females, but rather looked more generally at female victims of assault. This broad overview is useful in two ways. First, it gives a general indication of the level and determinants of violence against females. Second, it identifies subpopulations of females that can be targeted for in-depth research and specialized program intervention. For example, contrary to other studies, this study found a high number of victims to have a secondary education. This shows that programs, such as the United Nations Girls' Education Initiative which aims to improve education of girls and females in an effort to reduce violence, would not work in South Africa, since much of the female population is educated. Therefore, there is a need for qualitative research to address other aspects of educated females' lives which place them at a higher risk of violence from partners, relatives, and strangers. This chapter suggests that cultural norms and practices play a fundamental role in violence against females and data pertaining to particularly harmful practices need to be examined.

From this chapter, violence against females has health consequences and impacts various aspects of social life, including increasing female mortality which should be acknowledged as working against gender equality in the country. For example, the National Development Plan, which among others aims to create a safe and secure country for all citizens, should take note that with an overall crime rate of 1,021 per 10,000 female population, the country is not a safe place for females. Further, the National Development Plan should also take note of the physical assault rate of 336 per 10,000 female population and cautiously proceed with interventions to reduce this rate. Finally, interventions at a "ground level" should be mindful of the determinants of mortality produced in this work. The finding that females are more likely to die from assault than males could be useful to the "Africa Fatherhood Initiative" which works with men to address issues such as violence against females and gender-based violence.

References

AAPC. (2011). ICPD-10 overview. http://www.aapc.com/ICD-10/icd-10.aspx. Accessed 24 Sept 2014.

Abbey, A., Zawacki, T., Buck, P. O., Clinton, A. M., & McAuslan, P. (2001). Alcohol and sexual assault. *Alcohol Research and Health, 25*(1), 43–51.

Abrahams, N., Mathews, S., Jewkes, R., Martin, L., & Lombard, C. (2012). *Every eight hours: Intimate femicide in South Africa 10 years later!* Cape Town: Medical Research Centre.

Artz, L. (1999). *Access to justice for rural females: Special focus on violence against females.* Cape Town: University of Cape Town.

Bergen, R. K. (1998). The reality of wife rape: Females experiences of sexual violence in marriage.

Browne, A. (1993). Violence against females by male partners: Prevalence, outcomes, and policy implications. *American Psychologist, 48*(10), 1077.

Brownridge, D. A. (2006). Partner violence against females with disabilities: Prevalence, risk, and explanations. *Violence Against Females, 12*(9), 805–822.

Central Statistical Authority [Ethiopia] and ORC Macro. (2001). *Ethiopia Demographic and Health Survey 2000.* Addis Ababa, Ethiopia and Calverton, Maryland, USA: Central Statistical Authority and ORC Macro.

Chopra, M., Lawn, J. E., Sanders, D., Barron, P., Karim, S. S. A., Bradshaw, D., et al. (2009). Achieving the health Millennium Development Goals for South Africa: Challenges and priorities. *The Lancet, 374*(9694), 1023–1031.

CIET Africa. (1998). *Prevention of sexual violence. A social audit of the role of the police in the jurisdiction of Johannesburg's Southern Metropolitan Local Council.* Johannesburg: CIET Africa.

Crowell, N. A., & Burgess, A. W. (1997). *Understanding violence against females.* Washington, DC: National Academies Press.

De Wet, N., Oluwaseyi, S., & Odimegwu, C. (2014). Youth mortality due to HIV/AIDS in South Africa, 2001 to 2009: An analysis of the levels of mortality using life table techniques. *African Journal of AIDS Research, 13*(1), 13–20. Forthcoming.

Department of Health, Medical Research Council & OrcMacro. (2007). *South Africa Demographic and Health Survey 2003.* Pretoria: Department of Health, Medical Research Council & OrcMacro.

Dunkle, K. L., Jewkes, R. K., Brown, H. C., Gray, G. E., McIntryre, J. A., & Harlow, S. D. (2004). Gender-based violence, relationship power, and risk of HIV infection in females attending antenatal clinics in South Africa. *The Lancet, 363*(9419), 1415–1421.

Ferguson, A. G., & Morris, C. N. (2007). Mapping transactional sex on the Northern Corridor highway in Kenya. *Health and Place, 13*(2), 504–519.

Garcia-Moreno, C., Jansen, H. A., Ellsberg, M., Heise, L., & Watts, C. H. (2006). Prevalence of intimate partner violence: Findings from the WHO multi-country study on women's health and domestic violence. *The Lancet, 368*(9543), 1260–1269.

Goodman, L. A., Rosenberg, S. D., Mueser, K. T., & Drake, R. E. (1997). Physical and sexual assault history in females with serious mental illness. *Schizophrenia Bulletin, 23*(4), 685–696.

Hallman, K. (2004). Socioeconomic disadvantage and unsafe sexual behaviors among young females and men in South Africa. Population Council Working Paper No. 190. http://www.popcouncil.org/uploads/pdfs/wp/190.pdf. Accessed 24 Sept 2014.

Heise, L. (1992). Violence against females: The hidden health burden. *World Health Statistics Quarterly, 46*(1), 78–85.

Heise, L. L. (1998). Violence against females an integrated, ecological framework. *Violence Against Females, 4*(3), 262–290.

Heise, L. L., Raikes, A., Watts, C. H., & Zwi, A. B. (1994). Violence against females: A neglected public health issue in less developed countries. *Social Science and Medicine, 39*(9), 1165–1179.

Hester, M., Kelly, L., & Radford, J. (1996). *Females, violence, and male power: Feminist activism, research, and practice.* Buckingham: Open University Press.

Hunnicutt, G. (2009). Varieties of patriarchy and violence against females resurrecting "patriarchy" as a theoretical tool. *Violence Against Females, 15*(5), 553–573.

Hunter, M. (2005). Cultural politics and masculinities: Multiple-partners in historical perspective in KwaZulu-Natal. *Culture Health and Sexuality, 7*(4), 389–403.

Hunter, M. (2007). The changing political economy of sex in South Africa: The significance of unemployment and inequalities to the scale of the AIDS pandemic. *Social Science and Medicine, 64*(3), 689–700.

Izugbara, C. O., Duru, E., & Dania, P. O. (2008). Females and male-partner dating violence in Nigeria. *Indian Journal of Gender Studies, 15*, 461–484.

Jewkes, R., Levin, J., & Penn-Kekana, L. (2002a). Risk factors for domestic violence: Findings from a South African cross-sectional study. *Social Science and Medicine, 55*(9), 1603–1617.

Jewkes, R., Levin, J., Mbananga, N., & Bradshaw, D. (2002b). Rape of girls in South Africa. *The Lancet, 359*(9303), 319–320.

Jewkes, R., Penn-Kekana, L., Levin, J., Ratsaka, M., & Schrieber, M. (2001). Prevalence of emotional, physical and sexual abuse of females in three South African Provinces. *South African Medical Journal, 91*(5), 421–428.

Jewkes, R. K., Dunkle, K., Nduna, M., & Shai, N. (2010). Intimate partner violence, relationship power inequity, and incidence of HIV infection in young females in South Africa: A cohort study. *The Lancet, 376*(9734), 41–48.

Khan, M., Townsend, J. W., Sinha, R., & Lakhanpal, S. (1996). *Sexual violence within marriage.* Paper presented at the Seminar-New Delhi.

Kahn, K., Garenne, M. L., Collinson, M. A., & Tollman, S. M. (2007). Mortality trends in a new South Africa: Hard to make a fresh start. *Scandinavian Journal of Public Health, 35*(Suppl 69), 26–34.

Kishor, S., & Johnson, K. (2004). Profiling domestic violence: A multi-country study.

Koenig, M., Lutalo, T., Zhao, F., Nalugoda, F., Wabwire-Mangen, F., et al. (2003). Domestic violence in rural Uganda: Evidence from a community-based study. *Bulletin of World Health Organization, 81*(1), 53–60.

Maganja, R. K., Maman, S., Groves, A., & Mbwambo, J. K. (2007). Skinning the goat and pulling the load: Transactional sex among youth in Dar es Salaam, Tanzania. *AIDS Care, 19*(8), 974–981.

Maharaj, P., & Munthree, C. (2007). Coerced first sexual intercourse and selected reproductive health outcomes among young females in KwaZulu-Natal, South Africa. *Journal of Biosocial Science, 39*(2), 231.

Monasch, R., & Boerma, J. T. (2004). Orphanhood and childcare patterns in sub-Saharan Africa: An analysis of national surveys from 40 countries. *Aids, 18*, S55–S65.

National Youth Development Agency. (2012). *The Integrated Youth Development Strategy (IYDS) of South Africa 2012–2016.* Johannesburg: National Youth Development Agency Policy and Research Cluster.

Outwater, A., Abrahams, N., & Campbell, J. C. (2005). Women in South Africa intentional violence and HIV/AIDS: Intersections and prevention. *Journal of Black Studies, 35*(4), 135–154.

Posel, D. R. (2001). Who are the heads of household, what do they do, and is the concept of headship useful? An analysis of headship in South Africa. *Development Southern Africa, 18*(5), 651–670.

Presidency of the Republic of South Africa. (2009). *National Youth Policy.* Pretoria.

Schuler, S. R., Hashemi, S. M., Riley, A. P., & Akhter, S. (1996). Credit programs, patriarchy and men's violence against females in rural Bangladesh. *Social Science and Medicine, 43*(12), 1729–1742.

Shannon, K., Kerr, T., Strathdee, S. A., Shoveller, J., Montaner, J. S., & Tyndall, M. W. (2009). Prevalence and structural correlates of gender based violence among a prospective cohort of female sex workers. *British Medical Journal, 339*, b2939.

Sokoloff, N. J., & Dupont, I. (2005). Domestic violence at the intersections of race, class, and gender challenges and contributions to understanding violence against marginalized females in diverse communities. *Violence Against Females, 11*(1), 38–64.

Stanton, S. (1993). *A qualitative and quantitative analysis of empirical data on violence against females in greater Cape Town from 1989 to 1991.* Cape Town, South Africa: University of Cape Town.

Stark, E., & Flitcraft, A. (1988). Violence among intimates. In V. B. van Hasselt et al. (Eds.), *Handbook of family violence* (pp. 293–317). New York: Springer.

Statistics South Africa. (2010). *Mid- year population estimates 2010.* Pretoria: Statistics South Africa.

Statistics South Africa. (2012). *South African Statistics, 2012.* Pretoria: Statistics South Africa.

Stats, S. A. (2008). *Community survey 2007: Unit records, metadata.* Report No. 03-01-21 (2007). Pretoria: Statssa.

Straus, M. A., & Gelles, R. J. (1986). Societal change and change in family violence from 1975 to 1985 as revealed by two national surveys. *Journal of Marriage and the Family, 48*, 465–479.

Turner, C., & McClure, R. (2003). Age and gender differences in risk-taking behaviour as an explanation for high incidence of motor vehicle crashes as a driver in young males. *Injury Control and Safety Promotion, 10*(3), 123–130.

UNESCO. (2008). The development of education: National Report of Malawi. http://www.ibe.unesco.org/National_Reports/ICE_2008/malawi_NR08.pdf. Accessed 24 Sept 2014.

UNFPA. (2013). *Fact sheet: Young people, South Africa.* Pamphlet. South Africa. http://countryoffice.unfpa.org/southafrica/2013/04/22/6609/youth/. Accessed 29 Sept 2014..

United Nations. (2002). The United Nations Programme on Youth.

United Nations. (2003). *The Seventh United Nations survey on crime trends and the operations of criminal justice systems (1998/2000).* http://www.unodc.org/pdf/crime/seventh_survey/7sc.pdf. Accessed 29 Sept 2014.

United Nations General Assembly. (1993). *Declaration on the elimination of violence against women.* Geneva, Switzerland: United Nations General Assembly.

Varga, C. A. (2003). How gender roles influence sexual and reproductive health among South African adolescents. *Studies in Family Planning, 34*(3), 160–172.

Walker, L., & Gilbert, L. (2002). HIV/AIDS: South African females at risk. *African Journal of AIDS Research, 1*(1), 75–85.

Watts, C., Keogh, E., Ndlovu, M., & Kwaramba, R. (1998). Withholding of sex and forced sex: Dimensions of violence against Zimbabwean females. *Reproductive Health Matters, 6*(12), 57–65.

Widom, C. S., & Morris, S. (1997). Accuracy of adult recollections of childhood victimization, part 2: Childhood sexual abuse. *Psychological Assessment, 9*(1), 34.

Woolard, I. (2002). An overview of poverty and inequality in South Africa. Unpublished briefing paper. Pretoria: HSRC.

World Bank. (2009). *Gender-based violence, health and the role of the health sector at a glance.* Sweden: The World Bank.

World Health Organization. (2005). *Addressing violence against females and achieving the millennium development goals.* Geneva, Switzerland: World Health Organization.

Yigzaw, T., Berhane, Y., Deyessa, N., & Kaba, M. (2010). Perceptions and attitude towards violence against females by their spouses: A quantitative study in Northwest Ethiopia. *Ethiopia Journal of Health Development, 1*, 39–45.

Chapter 4
Exploring the Linkages Between Spousal Violence and HIV in Five Sub-Saharan African Countries

Kerry L.D. MacQuarrie, Rebecca Winter, and Sunita Kishor

Abstract There has been increasing recognition that spousal violence and HIV are overlapping vulnerabilities for many women. Yet a direct effect of most forms of spousal violence on women's HIV status is unlikely, as there is no apparent causal pathway leading from one to the other. This study examines the relationship between spousal violence and women's HIV status using Demographic and Health Surveys from five African countries: Kenya, Malawi, Rwanda, Zambia, and Zimbabwe. It uses couples data and nuanced measures of five separate forms of spousal violence. We adopt a gender-based framework in which a woman's experience of spousal violence and her HIV status are mediated by her husband's and her own behavioral and situational HIV risk factors, factors which are also shown to be associated with spousal violence. A series of regression models test for the direct effect of spousal violence, controlling for risk factors. An initial significant relationship with women's HIV status is found for suspicion and isolation controlling behaviors in Zambia and Zimbabwe; for emotional violence in Kenya, Rwanda, and Zimbabwe; and for physical violence, in Kenya, Rwanda, and Zimbabwe. Sexual violence is not associated with women's HIV status. Multiple associations between spousal violence and risk factors, and between these risk factors and women's HIV status, suggest several possible mediators. When they are added to our base model, spousal violence no longer significantly predicts women's HIV status with one exception: physical violence retains its association with women's HIV status in Kenya and Zimbabwe.

Keywords Spousal violence • HIV • Sub-Saharan Africa

K.L.D. MacQuarrie (✉)
The DHS Program, Avenir Health, Glastonbury, CT, USA
e-mail: Kerry.Macquarrie@icfi.com

R. Winter • S. Kishor
The DHS Program, ICF International, Rockville, MD, USA
e-mail: Rebecca.Winter@icfi.com; Sunita.Kishor@icfi.com

© Springer International Publishing Switzerland 2015   57
Y.K. Djamba, S.R. Kimuna (eds.), *Gender-Based Violence*,
DOI 10.1007/978-3-319-16670-4_4

Introduction

Over the past decade there has been increasing international interest in how women's experience of spousal violence affects the risk of acquiring HIV, and consensus is growing that women's experience of intimate partner violence—alongside gender inequality more broadly—contributes to vulnerability to HIV infection. In 2011 the World Health Organization (WHO) included the reduction of gender-based vulnerability to HIV infection as part of its Global Health Sector Strategy on HIV/AIDS 2011–2015 (World Health Organization 2011).

It is not intuitively obvious, however, that there should be a relationship between women's experience of intimate partner violence and their risk of HIV. With the exception of sexual violence, there is no direct causal pathway leading from most forms of spousal violence to HIV infection. This study examines the direct or indirect linkage between spousal violence—a key component of intimate partner violence—and women's HIV status. It also explores the association between spousal violence and wives' and husbands' risk factors, which may more directly influence women's HIV status. The study is based on data from recent Demographic and Health Surveys (DHS) in five sub-Saharan African countries—Kenya, Malawi, Rwanda, Zambia, and Zimbabwe.

A diverse body of literature, mostly in the developing world, has explored the association between intimate partner violence, with various degrees of emphasis on causal pathways. With a few notable exceptions, these studies have reported a significant association between some form of violence and women's HIV status. To date, the studies that have suggested a positive association between women's experience of intimate partner violence and risk of HIV fall into two categories: studies using clinic-based samples or other nonrepresentative samples, or cross-sectional studies using population-based samples.

Studies based on women who attend health clinics (ranging from antenatal care clinics to voluntary counseling and testing (VCT) clinics to enrollees in HIV-prevention interventions) often have reported a significantly higher prevalence of violence among HIV-positive women compared with HIV-negative women (Dunkle et al. 2004; Fonck et al. 2005; Maman et al. 2002, 2010; Prabhu et al. 2011). These clinic-based studies have found women's HIV status to be associated with their experience of physical violence (Maman et al. 2002), physical or sexual violence (Maman et al. 2002), any intimate partner violence (Dunkle et al. 2004), and spousal control (Dunkle et al. 2004). In a recent study that sought to isolate the direction of causality in the association between intimate partner violence and HIV status, Maman and colleagues (2010) followed a cohort of South African women (age 15–26) enrolled in an HIV-prevention intervention. They found that a woman's report at baseline of one or more incidents of intimate partner violence was a significant predictor of HIV incidence during the follow-up period.

Several rigorous, non-household-based studies have also examined the association between forms of spousal violence and women's HIV status. One cohort study among young women in South Africa (Jewkes et al. 2010) reported a significant association between incidence of HIV infection and both intimate partner violence and relationship power inequity. A second cohort study in seven African countries, however, reported no evidence of an association between seroconversion and the experience of intimate partner violence prior to acquiring HIV, based on an analysis of discordant couples enrolled in a clinical trial of a herpes simplex virus type 2 suppressive therapy (Were et al. 2011). Finally, a cluster randomized control trial of an HIV behavioral intervention among women aged 15–26 in South Africa reported that the significant bivariate association between women's experience of intimate partner violence and HIV status did not retain its significance after adjusting for HIV risk behaviors (including risk factors for both the female and male partners) (Jewkes et al. 2006a).

Most studies using population-based cross-sectional data have found a significant association between women's experience of intimate partner violence and HIV status. For example, within Indian couples where the man is HIV positive the odds that the female partner contracts HIV are higher where the male partner has perpetrated intimate partner violence (Decker et al. 2009a). Overall, of the seven studies identified that use nationally representative samples, six reported a significant association between some form of violence and HIV status (Andersson and Cockcroft 2012; Decker et al. 2009a; Ghosh et al. 2011; Kayibanda et al. 2012; Sareen et al. 2009; Silverman et al. 2008). Three of these six studies used data from India's third National Family Health Survey (NFHS-3) (Decker et al. 2009a; Ghosh et al. 2011; Silverman et al. 2008). One study used data from the Rwanda DHS (Kayibanda et al. 2012), another examined a non-DHS nationally representative sample from Botswana, Namibia, and Swaziland (Andersson and Cockcroft 2012), and the sixth study reporting a positive association used data from the USA (Sareen et al. 2009). The only nationally representative study identified that did not report a significant association between some form of spousal violence and HIV status used DHS data on ever-married women from ten developing countries (Harling et al. 2010).

While six of the seven studies reported significant findings, their samples, methodologies, and findings are noteworthy for their differences. As mentioned above, three of the six studies with significant findings relied on the same data from India, and the experience of couples in India may not be representative of couples' experience in other countries or cultures. Also, while all studies were population based, the analytic samples varied considerably, ranging from all men and women regardless of marital status (Andersson and Cockcroft 2012) to currently married women (Silverman et al. 2008), ever-married women (Harling et al. 2010), women who were in any romantic relationship in the last year (Sareen et al. 2009), and currently cohabitating couples (Decker et al. 2009a; Ghosh et al. 2011; Kayibanda et al. 2012).

Definitions of violence varied as well, from bivariate measures of any violence versus none (Decker et al. 2009b) to summary scales counting the number of violent items experienced (Kayibanda et al. 2012), and to categorical variables identifying women who experienced no violence, just physical violence, or physical and sexual violence (Silverman et al. 2008), just to name a few variations. Some studies looked only at sexual violence (Ghosh et al. 2011), others physical and sexual violence (Sareen et al. 2009; Silverman et al. 2008), while some included emotional violence

(Kayibanda et al. 2012), and a few included spousal controlling behaviors as well (Kayibanda et al. 2012). The manner in which these studies assessed intimate partner violence and the forms of violence they examined may have influenced both the reporting of violence and the detection of associations with other factors, including HIV prevalence (Lary et al. 2004; O'Leary and Kar 2010). Finally, the inconsistent inclusion of HIV risk behaviors across studies makes it difficult to compare their findings.

Given that the studies' methodologies and definitions vary substantially, it is not surprising that their findings also vary. Silverman et al. (2008) found that women who have experienced both physical and sexual spousal violence were 3.92 times more likely ($p=0.01$) to be HIV positive, but found no significant association between the experience of other combinations of spousal violence and HIV status. In contrast, Kayibanda et al. (2012) found that emotional violence—but not physical violence, sexual violence, or controlling behaviors—was significantly associated with women's HIV status, among currently married/cohabitating women in Rwanda, after adjusting for socio-demographic characteristics. Harling et al. (2010) examined combinations of physical and sexual violence among ever-married women and found no association. The range in findings may well depend on variations across studies in the conceptualization of violence (for example, the study by Harling and colleagues did not consider domains of emotional violence and controlling behaviors), differences in analytic methodologies, and range of covariates included in multivariate models (such as the problematic inclusion of risk factors that could be part of the pathways between spousal violence and HIV).

Our study adds to the literature on the association between spousal violence and HIV status by focusing on cross-sectional data from married couples in five countries. A focus on couples permits a more comprehensive examination of the link between HIV and spousal violence, since information is available on not only women at risk of spousal violence but also the spouses who perpetrate the violence, as well as risk factors for each member of the couple. Specifically, this research considers information on both spouses' characteristics, HIV status, and risk behaviors in assessing the mechanisms through which women who experience spousal violence may have increased risk of being HIV positive.

Conceptual Framework: Gendered Clustering of HIV Risk Factors and Spousal Violence

Many of the population-based studies exploring the link between forms of intimate partner violence and HIV status have not explicitly articulated, let alone modeled, the pathways through which intimate partner violence influences HIV status. The conclusions from these studies may differ due to the inclusion or exclusion of intervening factors through which violence affects HIV status. This framework seeks to clarify the ways in which the experience of spousal violence may lead to increased odds of having HIV among married women, either directly or indirectly.

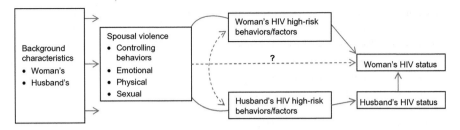

Fig. 4.1 Conceptual pathways from spousal violence to HIV

As illustrated in Fig. 4.1, we consider multiple forms of spousal violence: emotional, physical, and sexual violence. We also consider controlling behaviors by husbands toward their wives—such as acting jealous or suspicious, or trying to limit their actions—which the literature alternately conceptualizes as a separate form or a predictor of spousal violence or as a component of (usually emotional) spousal violence (Tjaden 2004; Watts and Mayhew 2004).

The usual interpretation given to an association, if detected, is that spousal violence increases the risk of HIV for women.[1] We question the plausibility of a direct effect of spousal violence on women's HIV status and instead posit two indirect mechanisms for such an association: husbands' HIV high-risk behaviors/factors and wives' high-risk behaviors/factors.

In the gender-based conceptual framework we present here, the association between a woman's experience of spousal violence and her HIV status is mediated by two primary pathways. First, among men, the well-documented association between men's perpetration of violence and HIV behavioral risk factors points to an underlying traditional masculinity, associated with violent behavior toward female partners, male-dominant attitudes, multiple sexual partners, potential infidelity, risk-taking tendencies, and alcohol consumption, among other "male" behaviors (Townsend et al. 2011). In this view, men who are violent toward their spouses are also more likely to exhibit other behaviors associated with traditional masculine identity, and thereby are more likely to have acquired HIV.

Indeed, the literature demonstrates that husbands who perpetrate violence against their wives are more likely to exhibit riskier sexual behaviors, abuse alcohol or drugs, or be HIV positive (Campbell et al. 2008; Decker et al. 2009a; Dunkle and Decker 2013; Fals-Stewart and Kennedy 2005; Lary et al. 2004; Makayoto et al. 2013; Maman et al. 2010; Silverman et al. 2008; Teti et al. 2006). This association may be the result of adherence to these traditional masculine norms or gender-inequitable attitudes that devalue women and perpetuate sexual double standards (Dunkle and Decker 2013). These are co-occurring behaviors, manifestations of a common gendered system, rather than causally linked—being violent is not likely

---

[1] The reverse causal direction, that having HIV leads to spousal violence, cannot be ruled out with cross-sectional data, and a spurious correlation also is a possibility. However, the panel study conducted by Maman et al. (2010) lends credibility to the standard interpretation.

to *cause* sexual risk-taking, nor is engaging in risky sexual behaviors likely to *cause* spousal violence [except insofar as certain risk behaviors, such as infidelity, may be a source of marital conflict that may trigger incidents of spousal violence (Lary et al. 2004; Schensul et al. 2006)]. Therefore, no causal direction is implied in the Conceptual Framework, as indicated by the curved line in Fig. 4.1.

Second, women who experience violence may engage in riskier behaviors of their own. As Jewkes et al. (2006a, p. 1462) note: "the experience of violence ... reinforces gendered power inequalities that impact on women's HIV risk." Women who experience spousal violence are likely to experience lower levels of personal empowerment and agency, and thus be compromised in their ability to demand fidelity from their partner. They also may be less able to negotiate the terms of sexual activity, such as insisting upon condom use or refusing sex when the husband has a sexually transmitted infection (STI) or its symptoms. That is, women who experience spousal violence face diminished self-efficacy or power in the relationship, a context defined by "choice disability" (Andersson et al. 2008; Jewkes et al. 2006b; Mittal et al. 2011; Raj et al. 2004; Stockman et al. 2013). For example, one study that examined the association between women's experience of violence and condom negotiation efficacy in a sample of incarcerated women in three states in the USA (Delaware, Kentucky, and Virginia) found that women who had experienced violence had significantly lower confidence to negotiate condom use with a partner (Swan and O'Connell 2011).

Furthermore, the experience of spousal violence is associated with poor mental health outcomes, low self-esteem and self-worth, and alcohol and drug use, which are in turn associated with riskier sexual behaviors (González-Guarda et al. 2011; Meyer et al. 2001; Teti et al. 2006). In a sample of women in the USA, the experience of intimate partner violence in the last three months was found to be associated with having had more episodes of unprotected sex with a steady partner, with drug use before sex, and with depressive symptoms (Mittal et al. 2011). Pitpitan et al. (2013) found that the experience of physical violence was strongly associated with women's alcohol consumption and with women's sexual risk behaviors, including the number of male sex partners, the likelihood of unprotected sex, the occurrence of sex under the influence of alcohol, and the occurrence of a recent STI. Several studies have noted that sexual abuse, in particular, earlier in life is associated with riskier sexual behaviors in adulthood (Andersson et al. 2008; Stockman et al. 2013), behaviors that lead to an increased likelihood of a woman herself being HIV positive. Therefore, the second indirect pathway portrayed in Fig. 4.1 is through the association of spousal violence with women's risk factors for HIV.

Some authors highlight the potential for direct transmission of HIV via forced sex (Andersson and Cockcroft 2012; Stockman et al. 2013). Sexual violence is the only form of spousal violence which implicates a clear biological mechanism; the other forms do not. While incidents of sexual violence could lead directly to HIV infection, the low rate of transmission in any given sexual encounter makes unlikely a large, statistically significant direct association between sexual violence and a woman's HIV status unless that violence is perpetual and frequent. It is more likely that sexual violence affects a woman's HIV status indirectly via similar mechanisms as emotional or physical violence or controlling behaviors: through some intervening mechanism, by association with her own risk behaviors or those of her spouse.

This study addresses the following questions about the potential pathways through which the experience of spousal violence may affect women's HIV status:

- Are all forms of spousal violence equally and similarly associated with women's HIV status? For which forms of spousal violence does this association exist?
- How strong is the relationship between spousal violence and individual/partner risk factors?
- Does the relationship between spousal violence and women's HIV status disappear when risk factors and their husbands' HIV status are accounted for?

Data, Measures, and Analytical Approach

Data

The data for this study come from six recent DHS in sub-Saharan Africa: Kenya 2008–2009, Malawi 2010, Rwanda 2005, Rwanda 2010, Zambia 2007, and Zimbabwe 2010–2011. DHS surveys are nationally representative, population-based household surveys that employ standardized questionnaires and biomarker protocols, enabling comparative analysis across countries and over time. Surveys were considered for inclusion in the study if (1) they were conducted in 2005 or later and the data were publicly available by June 2013; (2) they included the domestic violence module; (3) they included HIV testing for both women and men; and (4) there was an overlap between the HIV-tested subsample and the subsample selected for the domestic violence module. Of the nine countries that met these criteria, four were excluded due to the small sample size available for analysis, which greatly limited the power to detect key associations (Burkina Faso, Liberia, Mali, and São Tomé and Príncipe). We include both the Rwanda 2005 and Rwanda 2010 DHS surveys since the 2010 survey did not collect information on several violence measures contained in the 2005 survey.

The DHS uses multistage cluster sampling techniques to obtain nationally representative samples. In the first sampling stage each country is stratified into regions from which census-based enumeration areas are selected, with a probability proportional to size. Enumeration areas are then mapped and all households listed. In the second sampling stage, households are randomly selected from the household list within each selected enumeration area. Urban and less populous areas are typically oversampled. All analyses are weighted using the domestic violence weight calculated in the DHS datasets. This weight accounts for sampling probability and survey nonresponse. Additionally, we use the survey (svy) commands available within Stata to account for the complex sampling design and estimate robust standard errors.

From the total number of eligible women aged 15–49 with completed interviews, the sample is first restricted to women who were administered the domestic violence module. In Kenya, Zambia, and Zimbabwe, the domestic violence module was administered in all households. In Malawi, however, it was administered in every third household, and in both Rwanda surveys, in every second household. Further, only one randomly selected eligible woman per household was administered the domestic violence module, in order to maintain confidentiality and maximize the safety of the respondents in accordance with WHO guidelines on the ethical conduct of domestic violence research (World Health Organization 2001).

The sample for analysis is further restricted to women who provided blood for HIV testing and has a valid test result. HIV testing was conducted for all eligible women who provided consent in all households in the Zambia and Zimbabwe surveys, in every second household in the Kenya and both Rwanda surveys, and in every third household in the Malawi survey. Finally, the sample is restricted to matched married couples for whom the husband also has a valid HIV test result, and both spouses have complete information on variables in the analysis.

The final analytical sample includes 873 Kenyan couples, 2,627 Malawian couples, 1,452 Rwandan couples (2005 DHS), 2,013 Rwandan couples (2010 DHS), 1,611 Zambian couples, and 1,711 Zimbabwean couples. Couples include both those who are married and those who are cohabiting as if married.

Measures

The outcome measure in this study is *women's current HIV status*. A standard DHS protocol provides for anonymous, informed, and voluntary testing of women and men. Response rates for HIV testing in study countries range from 79.4 % among men in Zambia to 99.6 % among women in Rwanda (2010). Blood spots for HIV testing are collected on filter paper from a finger prick and are then transported to a laboratory. The laboratory protocol is typically based on an initial ELISA test and a retest of all positive samples with a second ELISA. Between 5 and 10 % of samples that are negative on the first ELISA test are retested. For samples with discordant results on the two ELISA tests, a third ELISA or a Western blot is performed. The protocol for HIV testing undergoes ethical reviews in survey countries and in the USA.

Spousal violence, the key predictor variables, is measured using five domains of violence and controlling behaviors that consistently emerge in factor analyses across all study countries. The five domains are women's report of spousal emotional violence, spousal physical violence, and spousal sexual violence ever perpetrated by their current husbands, and women's report of two domains of controlling behaviors ever exhibited by their current husbands, which we label "suspicion" and "isolation." For all regression models, the five domains of violence and controlling behavior are measured as continuous factor scores. For several descriptive tables, dichotomous summary variables are used to identify couples in which the wife reported any experience of each type of spousal violence by her husband. Throughout this study, the term "husband" refers to partners who are legally married to the respondent or partners cohabiting as if married.

The study also examines wives' and husbands' HIV risk factors, insofar as these could be important intermediary variables that might partially explain the observed association between spousal violence and HIV status. The HIV risk behaviors listed below all have been associated with HIV-positive status for women and men in the extant literature:

- *Lifetime number of sexual partners.* This indicator has three categories for women who report that they had sex with (1) one partner, (2) two partners, and (3) three or more partners in their lifetime. For their husbands, the indicator has five categories: men who report having had sex with (1) one partner, (2) two partners, (3) three partners, and (4) four or more partners, and (5) men who reported that they do not know how many partners they had. A substantial number of husbands in several countries report "don't know," which could indicate having many lifetime partners. Because our analysis is restricted to couples, and all respondents report at least one sexual partner, there is no category for zero partners for either women or men. Women and men with missing responses are excluded from the analysis.
- *Had an STI or STI symptoms in last 12 months.* During the interview, male and female respondents are asked three questions about STI: whether in the 12 months preceding the survey they had (a) an STI; (b) a bad smelling abnormal genital discharge; and (c) a genital sore or ulcer. This summary variable identifies women/men who report that they experienced one of these in the past 12 months. Respondents with missing information for all three questions are excluded.
- *Sex with nonspousal, noncohabiting partner.* This variable identifies women/ men who report sexual partners in the past 12 months other than their spouse or cohabitating partner. This measure is included for men only because reports of this behavior among women were exceedingly rare in most study countries. Men with missing information or who responded that they did not know are excluded from the analysis.

For an additional two high-risk behaviors included in the analysis, information is available only for men:

- *Ever paid for sex.* Men who report that they have ever paid for sex are compared with men who report that they have never paid for sex. In the Kenya and Zambia surveys, information is only collected about whether men paid for sex *in the last 12 months.* In these two cases, paying for sex in the last 12 months is used as a proxy for having ever paid for sex.
- *Husband's alcohol use.* This indicator, based on the wife's report, has three categories: (1) husband does not drink or drinks but never gets drunk, (2) husband drinks and sometimes gets drunk, and (3) husband drinks and often gets drunk. Alcohol consumption has been associated with both perpetrating spousal violence and being infected with HIV. Couples in which the wife did not provide information on her husband's drinking habits are excluded.

Our analysis adjusts for demographic variables that, per the literature, would be likely to confound the association between spousal violence and women's HIV status.

In selecting control variables, we avoid variables that could be part of indirect pathways between spousal violence and HIV, such as men's and women's HIV risk factors. From a full list of potential confounders, variables are selected for inclusion only if they had a significant bivariate association with women's HIV status and at least one violence factor in at least one country. Four variables did not meet these criteria and are not included in the analysis: marital status (married versus cohabiting), whether the wife's father beat her mother, spousal age difference, and wife's employment status. Included controls are household wealth quintiles, household place of residence (urban/rural), geographic region of the country, wife's educational attainment (none, primary, secondary, or higher), husband's educational attainment (none, primary, secondary, or higher), wife's total number of children ever born (measured continuously), and wife's age at first marriage (measured continuously).

Analytical Approach

The DHS domestic violence module uses a modified version of the conflict tactics scales (CTS) (Straus 1979, 1990). One benefit of a CTS-style instrument for comparative research is that these items refer to specific acts, regardless of whether they are understood to constitute violence in a given cultural setting (Kishor and Bradley 2012). The many different types of acts and behaviors asked about in the DHS are organized into categories of physical, emotional, and sexual violence and controlling behaviors. Assigning different acts/behaviors into these four categories is based on the face validity of the items according to experts in the field. However, we are unaware of any analysis that determines conclusively whether these groupings are validated by the data in the range of cultural settings in which the DHS module has been applied—for example, whether acts that other researchers consider to be physical violence share more in common with each other than with acts that we consider to be emotional or sexual violence.

Additionally, these different items have to be summarized into one or more indicators of violence. One common approach has been to assume that women in DHS surveys can be counted as having experienced violence if they respond yes to having experienced even one act (or some other predefined number of acts), thereby converting a large number of questions into a single dichotomous indicator. This indicator is based on the assumption that the experience of any act/behavior versus no act/behavior is more meaningful than the specific act/behavior or how many acts/behaviors are experienced. Another approach with similar assumptions uses a simple additive index (sometimes referred to as a naïve index), which gives equal weight to each act/behavior (DiStefano et al. 2009).

We use factor analysis to understand the underlying structure of items related to spousal violence and determine if these structures are similar or dissimilar across study countries. We then define violence measures derived from the factor scores resulting from this analysis. A factor score is essentially a weighted index in which the respondent's value on each item is weighted by the importance or influence of that item in the overall factor, as measured by its factor loading score (Pett et al. 2003). These factor scores hold several advantages for measuring violence compared with other commonly used summary indicators. By assessing the shared variance and uniqueness of items, factor scores eliminate the need for arbitrary assumptions about how to combine the different items and how to weight them (DiStefano et al. 2009).

The factor analysis is conducted on the full sample of women to whom the domestic violence module is administered, rather than the restricted sample of women in couples in which both members have valid HIV test results so as to uncover the relationship among observed spousal violence variables in the broadest population possible.

We conduct exploratory factor analysis (EFA) using principal component factor extraction technique with oblique (Promax) rotation of factor loadings, as no strong assumptions about the independence of factors could be asserted (Pett et al. 2003). Separate EFA solutions are sought for each survey sample, rather than pooling countries together. Factors are retained based on a combination of scree plots and a minimum eigenvalue of approximately 1.0 (Pett et al. 2003). A strict restriction of an eigenvalue ≥ 1.0 is relaxed so as to detect any common structure across countries that might lie just below this threshold. Sixteen spousal violence items, including six describing controlling behaviors, are included in the factor analysis, as follows:

Husband

- Is jealous or angry if wife talks with other men.
- Frequently accuses wife of being unfaithful.
- Insists on knowing where wife is at all times.
- Does not permit wife to meet her female friends.
- Tries to limit wife's contact with family.
- Does not trust wife with any money.
- Ever says or does something to humiliate wife in front of others.
- Ever threatens to hurt or harm wife or someone close to her.
- Ever insults wife or makes her feel bad about herself.
- Ever pushes, shakes, or throws something at wife.
- Ever slaps wife.
- Ever punches wife with his fist or hits with something that could hurt her.
- Ever kicks, drags, or beats up wife.
- Ever tries to choke or burn wife on purpose.
- Ever physically forces wife to have sexual intercourse with him even when she does not want to.
- Ever forces wife to perform any sexual acts she does not want to.

A seventeenth item describing violence with a weapon[2] is excluded from the analysis because the wording of the question is inconsistent across countries; the

---

[2] Some DHS questionnaires had an item about "*threats or attacks* with a knife or gun or any other weapon," while others asked about "*threats* with a knife or gun" only. In one survey, respondents were asked about threats and attacks in separate items.

loading score for this item is both poor and sensitive to the variation in wording. The Rwanda 2010 survey includes neither items describing controlling behaviors nor the three items describing humiliation, threats, and insults.

Items with factor loadings >0.40 are retained (Kootstra 2004; Pett et al. 2003). Cronbach's alpha is calculated for each factor as a measure of inter-item reliability. Finally, factors were tested for correlation and, since they are slightly correlated, the oblique rotation is retained (Kootstra 2004). The final factor scores are estimated for each case and saved as new variables in the dataset. These factor scores, generated from the sample of women completing the domestic violence module, are subsequently used as latent variables in the regression analyses of spousal violence and HIV, which uses the more restricted sample of matched couples with spousal violence data from the wife and HIV status data for both members of the couple.

Using the factor regression scores as the key independent spousal violence variables, we analyze the relationship, if any, between spousal violence and women's HIV status. We run a sequence of multivariate regression models separately for each of the six surveys. For each, we first run unadjusted models by regressing women's HIV status on each of the spousal violence variables, and then we run adjusted models with controls for urban/rural residence, region, wealth quintile, wife's education, husband's education, wife's occupation, husband's occupation, wife's age, husband's age, total number of children ever born, and wife's age at first birth (Table 4.3). The adjusted model serves as the base model for each country and indicates whether there is a relationship between the dependent variable—women's HIV-positive status—and the independent variables of interest.

We then run partial logistic regressions that model, in sections, each pathway of our conceptual model. Each of these models includes the same socio-demographic control variables as the corresponding base model. In sequence, we regress women's HIV status on (a) their husbands' HIV status and HIV risk factors and (b) women's HIV risk factors (Table 4.4). We then regress women's risk factors on the spousal violence variables (Table 4.5), and the spousal violence variables on their husbands' risk factors (Table 4.6), with the spousal violence variables expressed as factor scores in both sets of regressions. This sequence of models helps to establish relationships between variables in each segment of the pathway(s) through which we expect spousal violence to affect women's HIV status.

A preferable analytical strategy to adopt for this purpose might be to simultaneously estimate a system of regression equations, but the cross-sectional nature of the survey data does not allow us to temporally sequence each of the variables to facilitate such an analysis. Therefore, we are restricted to making conclusions about associations rather than causation between HIV status, spousal violence, and factors along the conceptual pathway.

Next, we run a series of additive models. To our base model of women's experience of spousal violence (again expressed as factor scores) and socio-demographic controls (Model 1), we first add husbands' HIV status and risk factors (Model 2). In Model 3 we replace husbands' risk factors with women's risk factors and in Model 4 we include both sets of risk factors. This modeling approach allows us to distinguish any direct effect of spousal violence variables on women's HIV status from their indirect effects through HIV risk factors with which they are associated. A weakening of the significance of and/or reduction in the magnitude of the odds ratio for spousal violence variables in the presence of risk factors is taken as evidence of an indirect effect. Any residual significant odds ratio after controlling for risk factors is taken as evidence of a direct association between spousal violence and women's HIV status.

Results

Forms of Spousal Violence

We conducted factor analysis to determine how many violence-related factors emerge and if the same factors emerge in different settings. The results of the factor analysis using 16 violence-related items reveal a strikingly common structure of what constitutes different types of violence across the five countries included in this study.

Five factors emerge, which we label as (1) suspicion, (2) isolation, (3) emotional violence, (4) physical violence, and (5) sexual violence. These five factors account for 57–66 % of the variance among the items in each country. All items load onto these factors in an identical pattern across the countries. In the Rwanda 2010 survey, which did not include all 16 items, just two factors emerge—physical violence and sexual violence—but with the same items loading onto these factors as in the other countries.

Table 4.1 shows the Cronbach's alpha internal reliability measure for each of the factors and the eigenvalue for the five-factor solution, all of which approach 1.0, among the six surveys. Physical violence is composed of five items, with a sixth item, "husband/partner ever spit in respondent's face," included only in the Rwanda 2005 survey, also loading on the physical violence factor in that sample. The Cronbach's alpha for this factor ranges from 0.73 in Zimbabwe to 0.84 in Malawi.

Table 4.1 Internal reliability and eigenvalues for five spousal violence factors

		Kenya	Malawi	Rwanda 2005	Rwanda 2010	Zambia	Zimbabwe
Cronbach's alpha	Suspicion	0.6759	0.6546	0.6088	na	0.6815	0.6277
Cronbach's alpha	Isolation	0.5815	0.6609	0.6750	na	0.5765	0.6375
Cronbach's alpha	Emotional violence	0.7619	0.7963	0.6844	na	0.7423	0.6466
Cronbach's alpha	Physical violence	0.7795	0.8384	0.8312	0.7801	0.7437	0.7273
Cronbach's alpha	Sexual violence	0.5821	0.6474	0.6700	0.6653	0.7530	0.7079
Eigenvalue for the five-factor solution		*0.8618*	*1.0077*	*1.0364*	*0.9811*	*0.9344*	*0.8997*

na not available

Emotional violence is composed of three items capturing whether a woman's husband ever humiliated her in front of others, threatened to hurt her, or insulted her. The Cronbach's alpha for this factor ranges from 0.65 in Zimbabwe to 0.80 in Malawi. Sexual violence, with its two items, consistently remains as a separate factor, and its alpha ranges from 0.58 in Kenya to 0.75 in Zambia. This apparent structure regarding these three factors largely validates the three forms of violence commonly conceptualized by experts in this field.

Two factors, rather than one, consistently emerge to capture controlling behaviors. The first, termed "suspicion," includes three items for husband is jealous if respondent talks with other men, accuses her of infidelity, and insists on knowing where she is. For this factor, the Cronbach's alpha ranges from 0.61 in Rwanda (2005) to 0.68 in Zambia. The second controlling behavior factor, "isolation," includes three items for husband prevents respondent from meeting with female friends, limits her contact with family, and does not trust her with money; and its alpha ranges from 0.58 in Zambia and Kenya to 0.68 in Rwanda (2005).

This finding of two factors for the controlling behaviors offers new insight into the nature of spousal violence, in two ways. First, it indicates that controlling behaviors are separate factors from emotional violence or any other violence factor, rather than being a component of any of these forms of violence. Second, it suggests that suspicion and isolation are distinct forms of controlling behaviors.

Most factors are only modestly correlated with one another, with a correlation coefficient ranging from 0.2 to 0.6 (not shown). Correlations are weakest between the sexual violence factor and either of the two controlling behavior factors, suspicion and isolation. They are highest between physical violence and emotional violence, ranging from 0.54 in Rwanda (2005) to 0.61 in Kenya. This pattern persists in all five countries. Because factors are somewhat correlated, an oblique rotation is retained for the solution that produced the factor scores for these five factors.

Profile of Spousal Violence and HIV

Table 4.2 presents the prevalence of each domain of spousal violence, as established by the factor analyses, as well as HIV prevalence among women in the study population (married couples with complete information on spousal violence and HIV status). Prevalence of violence is here defined as experiencing at least one item in that domain of spousal violence.

Of the five domains of violence, suspicion-related controlling behaviors is the most prevalent form among couples in the five countries studied, ranging from 46 % of wives in Rwanda (2005) to 75 % in Zambia who report that their husbands exhibit at least one of the three controlling behaviors in this domain (the husband is jealous or angry if she talks with other men, the husband accuses her of unfaithfulness, or insists on knowing where she is at all times). The second domain of controlling behaviors, which identifies women whose husbands do not permit them to meet their female friends, try to limit their contact with their family, or do not trust them with money,

Table 4.2 Prevalence of spousal violence, controlling behaviors, and women's HIV status in the analytic sample

	Kenya	Malawi	Rwanda 2005	Rwanda 2010	Zambia	Zimbabwe
	N=873	N=2,627	N=1,452	N=2,013	N=1,611	N=1,711
	%	%	%	%	%	%
Prevalence of spousal violence						
Controlling behaviors						
Suspicion[a]	55.9	58.1	46.1	na	74.9	62.2
Isolation[b]	33.0	18.3	24.5	na	36.2	21.3
Emotional violence[c]	27.6	23.2	9.3	na	22.2	26.5
Physical violence[d]	33.7	19.6	32.9	53.9	44.8	30.0
Sexual violence[e]	14.5	15.3	11.7	14.8	16.7	16.6
Women's HIV prevalence	6.1	9.5	1.9	3.0	12.6	15.1

na not available

[a]Identifies couples for whom the wife reports that her current husband exhibits at least one of the following behaviors: he is jealous if she talks with other men, accuses her of unfaithfulness, or insists on knowing where she is

[b]Identifies couples for whom the wife reports that her current husband exhibits at least one of the following behaviors: he does not permit her to meet her female friends, tries to limit her contact with her family, or does not trust her with money

[c]Identifies couples for whom the wife reports any lifetime experience of the following items of violence with her current husband: the partner ever said or did something to humiliate the respondent in front of others, threatened to hurt or harm respondent or someone close to her, or ever insulted respondent or made her feel bad

[d]Identifies couples for whom the wife reports any lifetime experience of the following items of violence by her current husband: he ever pushed, shook her, or threw something at her; ever slapped her; ever punched respondent with his fist or hit with something that could hurt her; ever kicked, dragged, or beat up respondent; ever twisted respondent's arm or pulled hair; ever spit on her, or tried to choke or burn respondent on purpose

[e]Identifies couples for whom the wife reports any lifetime experience of the following items of violence by her current husband: ever physically forced her to have sexual intercourse with him even when she did not want to, or ever forced her to perform any sexual acts she did not want to

is far less prevalent, ranging from 18 % of wives in Malawi to 36 % in Zambia who report that their husbands exhibit at least one of these controlling behaviors.

Of the three traditional forms of spousal violence, physical violence is consistently the most prevalent among study couples, followed by emotional violence and then sexual violence. Women's reported lifetime experience of any spousal physical violence ranges from 20 % in Malawi to 54 % in Rwanda (2010). About one-third of women in Kenya, Rwanda (2005), and Zimbabwe report experiencing any physical violence, and nearly half of women in Zambia do. In all countries except Rwanda, between 20 and 30 % of women report any lifetime experience of spousal emotional violence; in Rwanda less than 10 % of women report any spousal emotional violence. In the five study countries, the percentage of women who report any lifetime experience of spousal sexual violence ranges from 12 % in Rwanda (2005) to 17 % in Zambia and Zimbabwe.

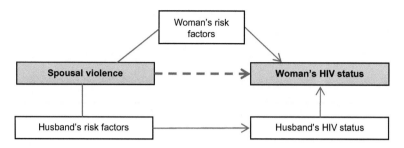

Fig. 4.2 Direct association between spousal violence and women's HIV status

Table 4.2 also presents HIV prevalence among women in the study couples. HIV prevalence varies across the six surveys—at 2 % in Rwanda 2005 and 3 % in Rwanda 2010, 6 % in Kenya, 10 % in Malawi, 13 % in Zambia, and 15 % in Zimbabwe. Recall that these estimates are not representative of all women in the study countries, but rather a subsample of couples of reproductive age with both spouses successfully interviewed and tested for HIV with a valid result.

Associations Between Spousal Violence and HIV (Fig. 4.2)

Table 4.3 presents unadjusted and adjusted odds ratios for women's HIV status regressed on different forms of spousal violence. In the adjusted models the associations between each form of violence and women's HIV status are modeled separately, controlling for the couple's place of residence, geographic region, and wealth quintile; both spouses' level of education, occupation, and age; the total number of children born to the wife; and the woman's age at first marriage/cohabitation.

In four of the six surveys, a significant bivariate association is observed between at least one form of violence and women's HIV status. In the adjusted model, spousal physical violence is significantly associated with women's HIV status in three of the six surveys (Kenya, Rwanda 2010, and Zimbabwe). In Zimbabwe, notably, four of the five violence domains are significant. In Rwanda 2005 and Zambia, the association is not significant but the direction and magnitude of association are consistent, such that in all six surveys the odds of being HIV positive are greater among women with higher scores on the physical violence scale. In Kenya, for example, each unit increase on the physical violence scale is associated with a 36 % increase in the adjusted odds of being HIV positive.

Emotional violence is significantly associated with women's HIV status in the adjusted model in Zimbabwe, and is borderline significant ($p < 0.10$) in Kenya and Rwanda 2005, such that scoring higher on the spousal emotional violence scale is associated with increased adjusted odds of being HIV positive. In Zimbabwe each one unit increase on the emotional violence scale is associated with a 21 % increase in the odds of being HIV positive.

Table 4.3 Unadjusted and adjusted associations between forms of spousal violence and women's HIV status in the analytic sample: Odds ratios from separate logistic regressions

| | Kenya | | Malawi | | Rwanda 2005 | | Rwanda 2010 | | Zambia | | Zimbabwe | |
| | N=873 | | N=2,627 | | N=1,452 | | N=2,013 | | N=1,611 | | N=1,711 | |
	uOR	aOR	uOR	aOR	uOR	aOR	uOR	aOR	uOR	aOR	uOR	aOR
Controlling behaviors												
Suspicion	1.02	1.05	1.00	0.95	1.11	0.94	na	na	1.22*	1.18†	1.20**	1.31***
Isolation	1.03	1.10	1.00	1.02	1.23	1.00	na	na	1.23*	1.19†	1.13†	1.20*
Emotional	1.23	1.31†	1.02	0.97	1.41*	1.32†	na	na	1.28**	1.19	1.13†	1.21**
Physical	1.27*	1.36*	1.11	1.08	1.15	1.28	1.18	1.38*	1.18†	1.16	1.28***	1.39***
Sexual	1.05	1.00	0.95	0.97	1.13	1.01	1.03	1.12	1.10	1.04	1.05	1.13

Note: The adjusted model controls for place of residence (urban/rural), region, wealth (quintiles), women's education (none/primary/secondary+), men's education (none/primary/secondary+), women's occupation (unemployed/employed in agriculture/employed in non-agriculture), men's occupation (unemployed/employed in agriculture/employed in non-agriculture), women's age (four categories), men's age (four categories), total children ever born (continuous), women's age at first cohabitation (continuous)

uOR unadjusted odds ratio; *aOR* adjusted odds ratio; *na* not available

***p ≤ 0.001; **p ≤ 0.01; *p ≤ 0.05; †*p* ≤ 0.10

The association between spousal sexual violence—the least prevalent form of violence among study couples—and women's HIV status is not statistically significant in any of the six surveys.

The two domains of controlling behaviors are strongly and significantly associated with women's HIV status in Zimbabwe only. With each one-unit increase on the suspicion and isolation scales, the odds that a Zimbabwean woman is HIV positive increase by 31 % (suspicion) and 20 % (isolation), respectively. In Zambia, too, suspicion and isolation are associated with women's HIV status, but the significance is marginal.

In summary, after adjusting for likely confounders, at least one domain of spousal violence remains significantly associated with women's HIV status in Kenya, Rwanda (2010), and Zimbabwe. The most consistent associations appear to be between spousal physical and emotional violence and women's HIV status. Given that there is no direct causal pathway between any of the forms of spousal violence and women's HIV status, the remainder of the study will attempt to better understand indirect pathways that could explain these observed significant associations.

Indirect Relationship Between Spousal Violence and HIV Status Through Risk Factors

In order for spousal violence to potentially influence women's HIV status indirectly through wives' and husbands' risk factors, these risk factors must simultaneously hold an association with women's HIV status on the one hand and with spousal violence on the other (Fig. 4.3).

Table 4.4 presents adjusted odds ratios obtained by regressing the wife's HIV status on known HIV risk behaviors and factors reported by women and by their husbands, controlling for background characteristics. Table 4.5 shows the adjusted associations between spousal violence and women's HIV risk factors. For each risk factor, the effect of each form of spousal violence is estimated in separate models, controlling for background characteristics. Table 4.6 shows the adjusted coefficients in ordinary least square models in which women's spousal violence factor scores (one adjusted model for each factor) are regressed on husbands' risk factors, with background characteristics as covariates.

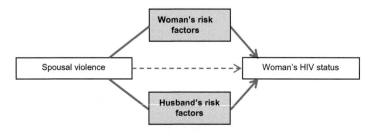

Fig. 4.3 Indirect pathway between spousal violence and women's HIV status

Table 4.4 Adjusted associations between women's HIV status (dependent variable) and wives' risk factors and husbands' risk factors in the analytic sample: Odds ratios from separate logistic regressions

	Kenya	Malawi	Rwanda 2005	Rwanda 2010	Zambia	Zimbabwe
	$N=873$	$N=2,627$	$N=1,452$	$N=2,013$	$N=1,611$	$N=1,711$
	aOR	aOR	aOR	aOR	aOR	aOR
Women's risk factors[a]						
Lifetime number of partners						
One (reference)	1.00	1.00	1.00	1.00	1.00	1.00
Two	1.71	3.47***	2.38*	3.88***	2.44***	4.02***
Three or more	4.14***	9.13***	2.31	6.32***	3.16***	6.78***
STI symptoms in last 12 months						
No STI (reference)	1.00	1.00	1.00	1.00	1.00	1.00
STI	3.42*	1.83**	4.55**	4.06***	1.87	2.87***
Men's risk factors						
Lifetime number of partners						
One (reference)	1.00	1.00	1.00	1.00	1.00	1.00
Two	0.83	2.60*	1.78	4.62**	5.04**	1.78†
Three	0.97	5.32***	2.40†	5.60**	4.67*	2.27*
Four or more	0.66	6.12***	2.62†	7.84***	8.20***	3.29***
Don't know	2.12	10.62***		63.10**	7.25**	5.67***
Sex with nonspousal, noncohabiting partner in last 12 months						
No (reference)	1.00	1.00	1.00	1.00	1.00	1.00
Yes	0.83	0.81	0.79	5.75***	2.09**	0.89
STI symptoms in last 12 months						
No STI (reference)	1.00	1.00	1.00	1.00	1.00	1.00
STI	1.06	2.33**	12.68***	4.16***	2.73**	2.60***
Ever paid for sex						
No (reference)	na	1.00	1.00	1.00	1.00	1.00
Yes	na	1.02	1.42	4.03***	1.80	1.57**
Alcohol use						
Husband doesn't drink or drinks but never drunk (reference)	1.00	1.00	1.00	na	1.00	1.00
Husband drinks and sometimes drunk	1.29	1.28	0.99	na	1.58*	1.18
Husband drinks and often drunk	2.54†	1.64†	0.63	na	2.14**	1.56†

***p ≤ 0.001; **p ≤ 0.01; *p ≤ 0.05; †*p* ≤ 0.10

[a]Women's risk factors are each run in separate models, adjusting for the following key control variables: place of residence (urban/rural), region, wealth (quintiles), women's education (none/primary/secondary+), men's education (none/primary/secondary+), women's occupation (unemployed/employed in agriculture/employed in non-agriculture), men's occupation (unemployed/employed in agriculture/employed in non-agriculture), women's age (four categories), men's age (four categories), total children ever born (continuous), women's age at first cohabitation (continuous)

Table 4.5 Adjusted associations[a] between women's HIV risk factors and spousal violence in the analytic sample: Odds ratios from separate logistic regressions

	Kenya	Malawi	Rwanda 2005	Rwanda 2010	Zambia	Zimbabwe
	$N=873$	$N=2,627$	$N=1,452$	$N=2,013$	$N=1,611$	$N=1,711$
Dependent variable 1: woman had STI or STI symptoms in last 12 months						
Controlling behaviors						
Suspicion	0.88	1.41***	1.37**	na	1.32*	1.32**
Isolation	0.98	1.32***	1.31*	na	1.12	1.24*
Emotional	1.46*	1.47***	1.33*	na	1.50***	1.33**
Physical	1.28†	1.24**	1.45***	1.51***	1.51***	1.41***
Sexual	1.37**	1.27***	1.29**	1.39***	1.33**	1.32***
Dependent variable 2: woman reported two or more lifetime sexual partners[b]						
Controlling behaviors						
Suspicion	1.49***	1.20***	1.24**	na	1.20**	1.38***
Isolation	1.16	1.07	1.20*	na	1.19**	1.16*
Emotional	1.38**	1.12*	1.15†	na	1.29***	1.21**
Physical	1.40**	1.13*	1.17*	1.33***	1.34***	1.25***
Sexual	1.00	1.17**	0.91	1.11†	1.15*	1.09

***$p \leq 0.001$; **$p \leq 0.01$; *$p \leq 0.05$; †$p \leq 0.10$

[a]Forms of violence are run in separate logistic models, adjusting for the following key control variables: place of residence (urban/rural), region, wealth (quintiles), women's education (none/primary/secondary+), men's education (none/primary/secondary+), women's occupation (unemployed/employed in agriculture/employed in non-agriculture), men's occupation (unemployed/employed in agriculture/employed in non-agriculture), women's age (four categories), men's age (four categories), total children ever born (continuous), women's age at first cohabitation (continuous)

[b]Women's lifetime number of sexual partners was collapsed to create a binary indicator comparing women with two or more lifetime sexual partners to women with one reported sexual partner, so that comparable logistic regression models could be run for both risk factors

Women's Risk Factors

In four of the six surveys, both of the HIV risk factors for women that we examine are significantly associated with women being HIV positive in Table 4.4 and at least one form of spousal violence in Table 4.5. In Zambia, wives' number of sexual partners maintains these dual associations, but having an STI or STI symptoms in the past 12 months does not. In Malawi, neither women's risk factor is associated with any form of spousal violence.

Women's HIV risk factors are associated with either or both *emotional* violence and *physical* violence as well as women's HIV status in Kenya, Rwanda 2005, Rwanda 2010, and Zimbabwe. In Zambia and Zimbabwe, the *suspicion* and *isolation* controlling behaviors are also simultaneously associated with women's HIV status and women's number of sexual partners and, in Zimbabwe only, with experience of an STI or STI symptoms.

Table 4.6 Adjusted linear associations[a] between spousal violence (dependent variable) and husbands' HIV risk factors in the analytic sample: Coefficients from linear regressions

	Kenya	Malawi	Rwanda 2005	Rwanda 2010	Zambia	Zimbabwe
	aβ	aβ	aβ	aβ	aβ	Aβ
Dependent variable 1: suspicion controlling behavior						
Husband's lifetime number of partners						
One (reference)	1.00	1.00	1.00	na	1.00	1.00
Two	−0.18	0.21**	0.04	na	0.03	0.26**
Three	−0.24	0.10	0.04	na	0.17†	0.22*
Four or more	0.01	0.16*	0.03	na	0.20*	0.15†
Don't know	0.02	0.35*	na	na	0.10	0.39**
Husband had sex with nonspousal, noncohabiting partner in last 12 months (Y/N)	−0.03	−0.07	0.15†	na	−0.06	−0.02
Husband had STI symptoms in last 12 months (Y/N)	0.30	0.15	0.05	na	0.12	0.13
Husband ever paid for sex (Y/N)	0.34	0.05	0.10	na	0.05	0.05
Husband's alcohol use						
Husband doesn't drink or drinks but never drunk (reference)	1.00	1.00	1.00	na	1.00	1.00
Husband drinks and sometimes drunk	0.28*	0.12*	0.12*	na	0.20**	0.19***
Husband drinks and often drunk	0.52***	0.49***	0.65***	na	0.42***	0.55***
Dependent variable 2: isolation controlling behavior						
Husband's lifetime number of partners						
One (reference)	1.00	1.00	1.00	na	1.00	1.00
Two	−0.22	0.14**	0.04	na	−0.07	0.19*
Three	−0.33	0.17*	0.06	na	−0.05	0.14†
Four or more	−0.31	0.17**	0.01	na	−0.02	0.14†
Don't know	−0.31	0.01	na	na	0.01	0.38*
Husband had sex with nonspousal, noncohabiting partner in last 12 months (Y/N)	−0.05	−0.06	0.24*	na	0.14*	−0.06
Husband had STI symptoms in last 12 months (Y/N)	−0.09	0.03	0.01	na	0.00	0.12
Husband ever paid for sex (Y/N)	−0.03	0.01	0.11	na	−0.19	0.01
Husband's alcohol use						
Husband doesn't drink or drinks but never drunk (reference)	1.00	1.00	1.00	na	1.00	1.00
Husband drinks and sometimes drunk	0.10	0.08	0.06	na	0.03	0.10†
Husband drinks and often drunk	0.56***	0.39***	0.53***	na	0.22**	0.41***

(continued)

Table 4.6 (continued)

	Kenya	Malawi	Rwanda 2005	Rwanda 2010	Zambia	Zimbabwe
	aβ	aβ	aβ	aβ	aβ	Aβ
Dependent variable 3: emotional spousal violence						
Husband's lifetime number of partners						
One (reference)	1.00	1.00	1.00	na	1.00	1.00
Two	−0.11	0.10†	0.07	na	−0.02	0.07
Three	−0.09	0.00	0.09	na	0.01	0.08
Four or more	0.11	0.08	0.16*	na	0.10	0.09
Don't know	0.19	0.05	na	na	0.10	0.30
Husband had sex with nonspousal, noncohabiting partner in last 12 months (Y/N)	−0.10	0.07	0.13	na	0.01	0.04
Husband had STI symptoms in last 12 months (Y/N)	0.38	0.27**	0.09	na	−0.04	0.02
Husband ever paid for sex (Y/N)	0.00	−0.05	−0.13	na	0.24	−0.06
Husband's alcohol use						
Husband doesn't drink or drinks but never drunk (reference)	1.00	1.00	1.00	na	1.00	1.00
Husband drinks and sometimes drunk	0.01	0.16**	0.08*	na	0.08	0.17**
Husband drinks and often drunk	0.96***	0.84***	0.47***	na	0.69***	0.76***
Dependent variable 4: physical spousal violence						
Husband's lifetime number of partners						
One (reference)	1.00	1.00	1.00	1.00	1.00	1.00
Two	0.00	0.10†	0.11*	0.15**	0.03	0.16*
Three	−0.01	0.04	0.19**	0.05	0.05	0.16†
Four or more	0.14	0.09†	0.26***	0.14*	0.10	0.17*
Don't know	0.00	0.03	na	0.60*	0.19	0.45**
Husband had sex with nonspousal, noncohabiting partner in last 12 months (Y/N)	0.14	0.23*	0.05	0.41***	0.04	0.12
Husband had STI symptoms in last 12 months (Y/N)	0.11	0.19†	−0.02	0.01	0.19	0.05
Husband ever paid for sex (Y/N)	−0.25	−0.02	−0.16†	−0.15†	0.34	−0.15*
Husband's alcohol use						
Husband doesn't drink or drinks but never drunk (reference)	1.00	1.00	1.00	Na	1.00	1.00
Husband drinks and sometimes drunk	0.05	0.10*	0.17***	Na	0.10*	0.09†
Husband drinks and often drunk	1.10***	0.85***	1.01***	Na	0.72***	0.65***

(continued)

Table 4.6 (continued)

	Kenya	Malawi	Rwanda 2005	Rwanda 2010	Zambia	Zimbabwe
	aβ	aβ	aβ	aβ	aβ	Aβ
Dependent variable 5: sexual spousal violence						
Husband's lifetime number of partners						
One (reference)	1.00	1.00	1.00	1.00	1.00	1.00
Two	−0.04	0.12*	0.03	0.08	−0.07	−0.05
Three	0.06	0.15*	0.16*	−0.04	0.09	0.24*
Four or more	−0.15	0.18**	−0.03	0.00	0.11	0.01
Don't know	−0.12	0.16		−0.23	0.30	0.32*
Husband had sex with nonspousal, noncohabiting partner in last 12 months (Y/N)	−0.06	−0.11	0.14	0.11	0.02	−0.13†
Husband had STI symptoms in last 12 months (Y/N)	0.02	0.08	0.30†	0.09	0.23	0.02
Husband ever paid for sex (Y/N)	0.07	0.13†	0.14	0.16	0.06	−0.07
Husband's alcohol use						
Husband doesn't drink or drinks but never drunk (reference)	1.00	1.00	1.00	Na	1.00	1.00
Husband drinks and sometimes drunk	0.13	0.05	0.10*	Na	0.01	−0.01
Husband drinks and often drunk	0.87***	0.51***	0.39***	Na	0.39***	0.41***

***$p <= 0.001$; **$p <= 0.01$; * $p <= 0.05$; †$p <= 0.10$
na not available
[a]Husband's risk factors are run together in one model, adjusting for the following key control variables: place of residence (urban/rural), region, wealth (quintiles), women's education (none/primary/secondary+), men's education (none/primary/secondary+), women's occupation (unemployed/employed in agriculture/employed in non-agriculture), men's occupation (unemployed/employed in agriculture/employed in non-agriculture), women's age (four categories), men's age (four categories), total children ever born (continuous), women's age at first cohabitation (continuous)

Men's Risk Factors

Husbands' HIV risk factors are far less consistent across surveys in their adjusted associations with their wives' HIV status than are women's risk factors (Table 4.4). In general, the association between women's experience of spousal violence and husbands' HIV risk factors is also weaker and less consistent than with women's HIV risk factors (Table 4.6). These findings combine such that men's risk factors are associated with either spousal violence or women's HIV status, but not always both. In Malawi and Rwanda (2005), no risk factor for husbands is simultaneously associated with a form of spousal violence and women's HIV status. In Kenya, only husbands' alcohol use is significantly associated with their wives being HIV positive (but marginally so with $p < 0.10$) and with one form of spousal violence: *physical* violence. There are more significant linkages among forms of spousal violence, men's risk factors, and women's HIV status in Rwanda (2010), Zambia, and Zimbabwe. For example, husbands' reported number of partners, having a non-marital sexual partner, and having ever paid for sex are each associated with both their wives' HIV status and perpetuation of *physical* violence in Kenya. In Zambia, husbands' alcohol use and reports of a nonmarital sexual partner are associated with one or both controlling behaviors and wives' HIV status. In Zimbabwe, having paid for sex is simultaneously associated with wives' HIV status and *physical* violence while lifetime number of sexual partners and alcohol use are associated with wives' HIV status and *suspicion* and *isolation* controlling behaviors, *physical* violence, and, for alcohol use only, *emotional* violence.

Nuanced Relationship Between Spousal Violence and HIV (Fig. 4.4)

In order to determine whether the experience of spousal violence exerts an indirect effect on women's HIV status through their own or their husbands' risk factors, or has a net direct effect even controlling for these factors, a sequence of logistic regression models was run. In the first model women's HIV status is regressed on the experience of spousal violence and a range of background characteristics (also shown in Table 4.3). In Model 2 we add to this base model husbands' HIV status and HIV risk factors. We substitute women's own risk factors for their husbands' risk factors in Model 3; and in Model 4 we combine both sets of risk factors in a complete model of the projected pathways through which the experience of spousal violence may influence women's HIV status. Rather than presenting an exhaustive series of regressions for all five forms of violence and controlling behaviors for all five countries, we estimate this series of four models only for those forms of violence that initially have a significant association with women's HIV status in the base model (Model 1).

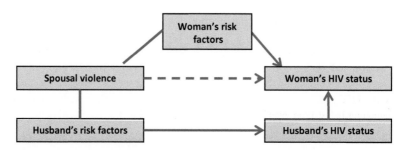

Fig. 4.4 Complete pathway between spousal violence and women's HIV status

Suspicion and Women's HIV Status

As Table 4.7 shows, the odds of a woman being HIV positive are 18 % higher in Zambia and 31 % higher in Zimbabwe with each unit increase in her suspicion factor score. However, in Zambia, this observed association disappears with the inclusion

Table 4.7 Multivariate associations[a] between women's HIV status (dependent variable) and suspicion in the analytic sample: Odds ratios from a sequence of logistic regressions[b]

	Model 1	Model 2	Model 3	Model 4
	aOR	aOR	aOR	aOR
Zambia (WN = 1,611)				
Controlling behavior–suspicion factor score	1.18[†]	1.11	1.13	1.08
Male partner's HIV status				
Negative (reference)		1.00	1.00	1.00
Positive		15.85***	16.25***	15.72***
Men's risk factors				
Lifetime number of partners				
One (reference)		1.00		1.00
Two		3.13		2.68
Three		2.26		1.87
Four or more		3.49[†]		2.85
Don't know		2.83		2.43
Sex with nonspousal, noncohabiting partner in last 12 months				
No (reference)		1.00		1.00
Yes		1.47		1.41
STI symptoms in last 12 months				
No STI (reference)		1.00		1.00
STI		1.31		1.18
Ever paid for sex				
No (reference)		1.00		1.00
Yes		1.32		1.47
Alcohol use				
Husband doesn't drink or drinks but never drunk (reference)		1.00		1.00
Husband drinks and sometimes drunk		1.48		1.44
Husband drinks and often drunk		1.86**		1.71*
Women's risk factors				
Lifetime number of partners				
One (reference)			1.00	1.00
Two			2.28***	2.09**
Three or more			2.80***	2.47**
STI symptoms in last 12 months				
No STI (reference)			1.00	1.00
STI			1.32	1.12

(continued)

Table 4.7 (continued)

	Model 1 aOR	Model 2 aOR	Model 3 aOR	Model 4 aOR
Zimbabwe (WN = 1,711)				
Controlling behavior–suspicion factor score	1.31***	1.23*	1.14	1.11
Male partner's HIV status				
Negative (reference)		1.00	1.00	1.00
Positive		31.89***	33.30***	34.01***
Men's risk factors				
Lifetime number of partners				
One (reference)		1.00		1.00
Two		1.23		1.12
Three		2.32*		2.40†
Four or more		2.44*		1.83
Don't know		4.34**		4.19**
Sex with nonspousal, noncohabiting partner in last 12 months				
No (reference)		1.00		1.00
Yes		0.54*		0.52*
STI symptoms in last 12 months				
No STI (reference)		1.00		1.00
STI		2.10**		2.18**
Ever paid for sex				
No (reference)		1.00		1.00
Yes		0.88		1.00
Alcohol use				
Husband doesn't drink or drinks but never drunk (reference)		1.00		1.00
Husband drinks and sometimes drunk		1.08		1.07
Husband drinks and often drunk		1.52		1.42
Women's risk factors				
Lifetime number of partners				
One (reference)			1.00	1.00
Two			4.37***	4.43***
Three or more			6.23***	5.99***
STI symptoms in last 12 months				
No STI (reference)			1.00	1.00
STI			2.62***	2.70***

***$p \leq 0.001$; **$p \leq 0.01$; *$p \leq 0.05$; †$p \leq 0.10$

[a]Models control for the following key control variables: place of residence (urban/rural), region, wealth (quintiles), women's education (none/primary/secondary+), men's education (none/primary/secondary+), women's occupation (unemployed/employed in agriculture/employed in non-agriculture), men's occupation (unemployed/employed in agriculture/employed in non-agriculture), women's age (four categories), men's age (four categories), total children ever born (continuous), women's age at first cohabitation (continuous). Model 1: Adjusts only for the control variables. Model 2: Adjusts for control variables, husband's HIV risk factors, and husband's HIV status. Model 3: Adjusts for control variables, the wife's HIV risk factors, and husband's HIV stats. Model 4: Adjusts for control variables, the husband's and wife's HIV risk factors, and husband's HIV status

[b]The model sequence is presented for all surveys in which the suspicion factor score was significantly associated with women's HIV status ($p < 0.10$) after adjusting for key control variables (see Table 4.3)

of either or both her own risk factors and her husband's risk factors and HIV status. This is in spite of the fact that few risk factors are independently associated with women's HIV status in either the spouse-specific models (Models 2 and 3) or the combined model (Model 4). While wives' number of partners and husbands' alcohol use are significantly associated with both women's HIV status and suspicion in separate models that do not control for other risk behaviors, women's number of partners is not significant net of the other risk factors presented in Table 4.7. Only women whose husbands are often drunk and who themselves have had more than two sexual partners in their lifetime have increased odds of being HIV positive.

The findings appear to be slightly different in Zimbabwe. The highly significant direct effect of the experience of suspicious controlling behaviors is explained away not by the husbands' HIV risk factors but by women's own risk factors. Additionally, Models 2 and 3 indicate that more risk factors for both members of the couple are associated with women's HIV status. Both of the women's risk factors, and three of their husbands' risk factors—lifetime number of partners, having had an STI or STI symptoms, and having had a nonmarital sexual partner—but not husbands' alcohol use—are associated with higher odds of women being HIV positive. In both Zambia and Zimbabwe, their husbands' HIV status is, unsurprisingly, a significant predictor of women's own HIV status, and the odds ratios indicate this effect to be sizable.

Isolation and Women's HIV Status

As Table 4.8 shows for Zambia and Zimbabwe, women's experience of isolating controlling behaviors by their husbands is associated with higher odds of having HIV. The pattern of this association across the series of models is much the same as it is the case for suspicion. While women in both countries face approximately 20 % greater odds of being HIV positive with a unit increase in isolation scores when controlling only for background characteristics, this effect is no longer significant in models that control for women's own HIV risk factors and their husbands' risk factors.

In these models a similar set of women's and husbands' HIV risk factors are associated with women's HIV status, as is the case for the models for the suspicion factor.

Emotional Violence and Women's HIV Status

The emotional violence factor is significantly associated with having HIV for women in Kenya, Rwanda (2005), and Zimbabwe (Table 4.9). The odds of being HIV positive are roughly 30 % higher in Kenya and Rwanda (2005) and 20 % higher in Zimbabwe with each unit increase in the emotional violence factor score.

In both Kenya and Rwanda (2005), any independent effect of the experience of emotional violence is absent in models controlling for either husbands' HIV risk

Table 4.8 Multivariate associations[a] between women's HIV status (dependent variable) and isolation in the analytic sample: Odds ratios from a sequence of logistic regressions[b]

	Model 1 aOR	Model 2 aOR	Model 3 aOR	Model 4 aOR
Zambia (WN=1,611)				
Controlling behavior–isolation factor score	1.19[†]	1.11	1.11	1.08
Male partner's HIV status				
Negative (reference)	1.00	1.00	1.00	
Positive	15.69***	16.13***	15.61***	
Men's risk factors				
Lifetime number of partners				
One (reference)	1.00	1.00		
Two	3.17	2.69		
Three	2.33	1.91		
Four or more	3.58[†]	2.89		
Don't know	2.83	2.41		
Sex with nonspousal, noncohabiting partner in last 12 months				
No (reference)	1.00	1.00		
Yes	1.45	1.39		
STI symptoms in last 12 months				
No STI (reference)	1.00	1.00		
STI	1.31	1.18		
Ever paid for sex				
No (reference)	1.00	1.00		
Yes	1.35	1.49		
Alcohol use				
Husband doesn't drink or drinks but never drunk (reference)	1.00	1.00		
Husband drinks and sometimes drunk	1.51[†]	1.46		
Husband drinks and often drunk	1.89**	1.73*		
Women's risk factors				
Lifetime number of partners				
One (reference)	1.00	1.00		
Two	2.28***	2.08**		
Three or more	2.83***	2.48**		
STI symptoms in last 12 months				
No STI (reference)	1.00	1.00		
STI	1.32	1.12		
Zimbabwe (WN=1,711)				
Controlling behavior–isolation factor score	1.2*	1.14	1.11	1.08
Male partner's HIV status				
Negative (reference)	1.00	1.00	1.00	
Positive	32.04***	33.37***	33.98***	

(continued)

Table 4.8 (continued)

	Model 1	Model 2	Model 3	Model 4
	aOR	aOR	aOR	aOR
Men's risk factors				
Lifetime number of partners				
One (reference)	1.00	1.00		
Two	1.29	1.15		
Three	2.43*	2.46*		
Four or more	2.48*	1.84		
Don't know	4.43**	4.21**		
Sex with nonspousal, noncohabiting partner in last 12 months				
No (reference)	1.00	1.00		
Yes	0.56*	0.53*		
STI symptoms in last 12 months				
No STI (reference)	1.00	1.00		
STI	2.14**	2.2**		
Ever paid for sex				
No (reference)	1.00	1.00		
Yes	0.9	1.01		
Alcohol use				
Husband doesn't drink or drinks but never drunk (reference)	1.00	1.00		
Husband drinks and sometimes drunk	1.12	1.09		
Husband drinks and often drunk	1.56	1.43		
Women's risk factors				
Lifetime number of partners				
One (reference)	1.00	1.00		
Two	4.44***	4.49***		
Three or more	6.43***	6.14***		
STI symptoms in last 12 months				
No STI (reference)	1.00	1.00		
STI	2.63***	2.71***		

***$p \leq 0.001$; **$p \leq 0.01$; *$p \leq 0.05$; †$p \leq 0.10$

[a]Models control for the following key control variables: place of residence (urban/rural), region, wealth (quintiles), women's education (none/primary/secondary+), men's education (none/primary/secondary+), women's occupation (unemployed/employed in agriculture/employed in non-agriculture), men's occupation (unemployed/employed in agriculture/employed in non-agriculture), women's age (four categories), men's age (four categories), total children ever born (continuous), women's age at first cohabitation (continuous). Model 1: Adjusts only for the control variables. Model 2: Adjusts for control variables, husband's HIV risk factors, and husband's HIV status. Model 3: Adjusts for control variables, the wife's HIV risk factors, and husband's HIV stats. Model 4: Adjusts for control variables, the husband's and wife's HIV risk factors, and husband's HIV status

[b]The model sequence is presented for all surveys in which the suspicion factor score was significantly associated with women's HIV status ($p < 0.10$) after adjusting for key control variables (see Table 4.3)

Table 4.9 Multivariate associations[a] between women's HIV status (dependent variable) and emotional violence in the analytic sample: Odds ratios from a sequence of logistic regressions[b]

	Model 1	Model 2	Model 3	Model 4
	aOR	aOR	aOR	aOR
Kenya (WN = 873)				
Emotional violence factor score	1.31[†]	1.34	1.39	1.28
Male partner's HIV status				
Negative (reference)	1.00	1.00	1.00	
Positive	126.72***	82.3***	144.66***	
Men's risk factors				
Lifetime number of partners				
One (reference)	1.00	1.00		
Two	0.59	0.69		
Three	0.79	1.05		
Four or more	0.28	0.28		
Don't know	1.08	1.03		
Sex with nonspousal, noncohabiting partner in last 12 months				
No (reference)	1.00	1.00		
Yes	0.30	0.21		
STI symptoms in last 12 months				
No STI (reference)	1.00	1.00		
STI	1.63	1.18		
Alcohol use				
Husband doesn't drink or drinks but never drunk (reference)	1.00	1.00		
Husband drinks and sometimes drunk	1.08	1.02		
Husband drinks and often drunk	4.52*	4.26[†]		
Women's risk factors				
Lifetime number of partners				
One (reference)	1.00	1.00		
Two	1.59	2.06		
Three or more	4.09**	5.64***		
STI symptoms in last 12 months				
No STI (reference)	1.00	1.00		
STI	2.91	2.44		
Rwanda 2005 (WN = 2,013)				
Emotional violence factor score	1.32[†]	1.18	0.98	1.1
Male partner's HIV status				
Negative (reference)	1.00	1.00	1.00	
Positive	259.07***	349.97***	401.37***	
Men's risk factors				
Lifetime number of partners				
One (reference)	1.00	1.00		
Two	1.90	1.68		
Three	2.38	2.41		

(continued)

Table 4.9 (continued)

	Model 1	Model 2	Model 3	Model 4
	aOR	aOR	aOR	aOR
Four or more	2.13	1.53		
Don't know				
Sex with nonspousal, noncohabiting partner in last 12 months				
No (reference)	1.00	1.00		
Yes	0.49	0.56		
STI symptoms in last 12 months				
No STI (reference)	1.00	1.00		
STI	12.53***	11.31***		
Ever paid for sex				
No (reference)	1.00	1.00		
Yes	1.11	1.48		
Alcohol use				
Husband doesn't drink or drinks but never drunk (reference)	1.00	1.00		
Husband drinks and sometimes drunk	0.65	0.57		
Husband drinks and often drunk	0.19*	0.18†		
Women's risk factors				
Lifetime number of partners				
One (reference)	1.00	1.00		
Two	5.27**	5.23**		
Three or more	1.61	1.61		
STI symptoms in last 12 months				
No STI (reference)				
STI	3.01	2.79		
Zimbabwe (WN = 1,711)				
Emotional violence factor score	1.21**	1.19*	1.16†	1.12
Male partner's HIV status				
Negative (reference)	1.00	1.00	1.00	
Positive	32.36***	33.71***	34.18***	
Men's risk factors				
Lifetime number of partners				
One (reference)	1.00	1.00		
Two	1.30	1.14		
Three	2.38*	2.40†		
Four or more	2.46*	1.82		
Don't know	4.43**	4.18**		
Sex with nonspousal, noncohabiting partner in last 12 months				
No (reference)	1.00	1.00		
Yes	0.55*	0.53*		
STI symptoms in last 12 months				
No STI (reference)	1.00	1.00		
STI	2.13**	2.21**		

(continued)

Table 4.9 (continued)

	Model 1	Model 2	Model 3	Model 4
	aOR	aOR	aOR	aOR
Ever paid for sex				
No (reference)	1.00	1.00		
Yes	0.90	1.01		
Alcohol use				
Husband doesn't drink or drinks but never drunk (reference)	1.00	1.00		
Husband drinks and sometimes drunk	1.08	1.07		
Husband drinks and often drunk	1.45	1.35		
Women's risk factors				
Lifetime number of partners				
One (reference)	1.00	1.00		
Two	4.39***	4.45***		
Three or more	6.34***	6.10***		
STI symptoms in last 12 months				
No STI (reference)	1.00	1.00		
STI	2.60***	2.70***		

***$p \leq 0.001$; **$p \leq 0.01$; *$p \leq 0.05$; †$p \leq 0.10$

[a]Models control for the following key control variables: place of residence (urban/rural), region, wealth (quintiles), women's education (none/primary/secondary+), men's education (none/primary/secondary+), women's occupation (unemployed/employed in agriculture/employed in non-agriculture), men's occupation (unemployed/employed in agriculture/employed in non-agriculture), women's age (four categories), men's age (four categories), total children ever born (continuous), women's age at first cohabitation (continuous). Model 1: Adjusts only for the control variables. Model 2: Adjusts for control variables, husband's HIV risk factors, and husband's HIV status. Model 3: Adjusts for control variables, the wife's HIV risk factors, and husband's HIV stats. Model 4: Adjusts for control variables, the husband's and wife's HIV risk factors, and husband's HIV status

[b]The model sequence is presented for all surveys in which the suspicion factor score was significantly associated with women's HIV status ($p < 0.10$) after adjusting for key control variables (see Table 4.3)

factors or women's risk factors, or both. This is the case although only a few risk factors predict women's HIV status. These are women's lifetime number of partners, husbands' alcohol use, and, in Rwanda only, husbands' reports of STI or STI symptoms.

Zimbabwe shows slightly different results: the odds ratio for emotional violence remains little changed with the addition of either husbands' or women's HIV risk factors, and it maintains its significant association with women's HIV status. Only when both sets of risk factors are controlled for is the experience of emotional violence no longer significantly associated with women's HIV status. Zimbabwe is also set apart by the fact that both of the women's risk factors and a greater number of and different husbands' risk factors are associated with women's HIV status.

Physical Violence and Women's HIV Status

In Kenya, Rwanda (2010), and Zimbabwe, the odds of women being HIV positive are 36–39 % higher with each unit increase in their physical violence score (Table 4.10).

In Kenya and Zimbabwe the experience of spousal physical violence maintains its significant association with women's HIV status as their husbands' HIV status and husbands' or women's HIV risk factors are added to the model, either separately

Table 4.10 Multivariate associations[a] between women's HIV status (dependent variable) and physical violence in the analytic sample: Odds ratios from a sequence of logistic regressions[b]

	Model 1	Model 2	Model 3	Model 4
	aOR	aOR	aOR	aOR
Kenya (WN=873)				
Physical violence factor score	1.36*	1.51*	1.59**	1.44[†]
Male partner's HIV status				
Negative (reference)	1.00	1.00	1.00	
Positive	126.67***	87.31***	138.98***	
Men's risk factors				
Lifetime number of partners				
One (reference)	1.00	1.00		
Two	0.63	0.75		
Three	0.82	1.10		
Four or more	0.31	0.32		
Don't know	1.29	1.26		
Sex with nonspousal, noncohabiting partner in last 12 months				
No (reference)	1.00	1.00		
Yes	0.29	0.22		
STI symptoms in last 12 months				
No STI (reference)	1.00	1.00		
STI	1.77	1.24		
Alcohol use				
Husband doesn't drink or drinks but never drunk (reference)	1.00	1.00		
Husband drinks and sometimes drunk	1.05	1.00		
Husband drinks and often drunk	3.52	3.33		
Women's risk factors				
Lifetime number of partners				
One (reference)	1.00	1.00		
Two	1.68	2.06		
Three or more	4.07**	5.43***		
STI symptoms in last 12 months				
No STI (reference)	1.00	1.00		
STI	2.87	2.48		

(continued)

Table 4.10 (continued)

	Model 1	Model 2	Model 3	Model 4
	aOR	aOR	aOR	aOR
Rwanda 2010 (WN=2,013)				
Physical violence factor score	1.38*	0.92	0.90	0.85
Male partner's HIV status				
Negative (reference)	1.00	1.00	1.00	
Positive	448.69***	340.68***	363.11***	
Men's risk factors				
Lifetime number of partners				
One (reference)	1.00	1.00		
Two	2.07	1.81		
Three	1.97	1.62		
Four or more	1.06	0.77		
Don't know	0.49	0.40		
Sex with nonspousal, noncohabiting partner in last 12 months				
No (reference)	1.00	1.00		
Yes	6.67**	6.59**		
STI symptoms in last 12 months				
No STI (reference)	1.00	1.00		
STI	1.20	1.36		
Ever paid for sex				
No (reference)	1.00	1.00		
Yes	1.46	1.60		
Women's risk factors				
Lifetime number of partners				
One (reference)	1.00	1.00		
Two	3.19*	3.36**		
Three or more	2.20	2.53		
STI symptoms in last 12 months				
No STI (reference)	1.00	1.00		
STI	2.29†	2.10		
Zimbabwe (WN=1,711)				
Physical violence factor score	1.39***	1.54***	1.47***	1.45***
Male partner's HIV status				
Negative (reference)	1.00	1.00	1.00	
Positive	34.68***	36.73***	36.48***	
Men's risk factors				
Lifetime number of partners				
One (reference)	1.00	1.00		
Two	1.21	1.06		
Three	2.19†	2.18†		
Four or more	2.35*	1.73		
Don't know	3.65**	3.40*		

(continued)

Table 4.10 (continued)

	Model 1	Model 2	Model 3	Model 4
	aOR	aOR	aOR	aOR
Sex with nonspousal, noncohabiting partner in last 12 months				
No (reference)	1.00	1.00		
Yes	0.54*	0.52*		
STI symptoms in last 12 months				
No STI (reference)	1.00	1.00		
STI	2.18**	2.29**		
Ever paid for sex				
No (reference)	1.00	1.00		
Yes	0.97	1.10		
Alcohol use				
Husband doesn't drink or drinks but never drunk (reference)	1.00	1.00		
Husband drinks and sometimes drunk	1.05	1.03		
Husband drinks and often drunk	1.11	1.06		
Women's risk factors				
Lifetime number of partners				
One (reference)	1.00	1.00		
Two	4.34***	4.37***		
Three or more	6.15***	5.97***		
STI symptoms in last 12 months				
No STI (reference)	1.00	1.00		
STI	2.43***	2.56***		

***$p \leq 0.001$; **$p \leq 0.01$; *$p \leq 0.05$; †$p \leq 0.10$

[a]Models control for the following key control variables: place of residence (urban/rural), region, wealth (quintiles), women's education (none/primary/secondary+), men's education (none/primary/secondary+), women's occupation (unemployed/employed in agriculture/employed in non-agriculture), men's occupation (unemployed/employed in agriculture/employed in non-agriculture), women's age (four categories), men's age (four categories), total children ever born (continuous), women's age at first cohabitation (continuous). Model 1: Adjusts only for the control variables. Model 2: Adjusts for control variables, husband's HIV risk factors, and husband's HIV status. Model 3: Adjusts for control variables, the wife's HIV risk factors, and husband's HIV stats. Model 4: Adjusts for control variables, the husband's and wife's HIV risk factors, and husband's HIV status

[b]The model sequence is presented for all surveys in which the suspicion factor score was significantly associated with women's HIV status ($p < 0.10$) after adjusting for key control variables (see Table 4.3)

or combined (although the level of significance diminishes somewhat in Kenya). Furthermore, a comparison of the odds ratios across the models shows that the effect of the physical violence factor increases when incorporating HIV risk factors. In the comprehensive model (Model 4) in Kenya and Zimbabwe, the odds of women being HIV positive are 44 % and 45 % higher, respectively, with each unit increase in their physical violence score.

The results from these two countries differ from one another in minor ways. In Kenya none of the HIV risk factors of husbands are significant predictors of women's HIV status in the presence of women's experience of physical violence and husbands' HIV status (Models 2 and 4). However, several of the husbands' risk factors remain significant in Model 4 in Zimbabwe. These are lifetime number of sexual partners, nonmarital sex, and STI or STI symptoms. Additionally, women's HIV risk factors are more strongly predictive of their HIV status in Zimbabwe than in Kenya.

Compared with Kenya and Zimbabwe, results of the 2010 Rwanda survey indicate a different pattern altogether. Initially significant, the association between women's HIV status and experience of physical violence loses its association when either husbands' or women's HIV risk factors and husbands' HIV status are entered into the model. The only HIV risk factor for husbands that predicts women's HIV status is sex with a nonmarital partner in the last 12 months (Models 2 and 4). Women's lifetime number of partners and their experience of an STI or STI symptoms in the last 12 months are both associated with women's HIV status, although only women's lifetime number of partners (specifically, having two partners) retains significance in the comprehensive model (Model 4).

Sexual Violence and Women's HIV Status

In none of the five countries is there an initially significant relationship between sexual violence and women's HIV status, controlling for basic background characteristics. Therefore, no further analysis is performed to examine its association while controlling for women's and their husbands' HIV risk factors.

Conclusions and Discussion

In spite of variation in the prevalence of the various forms of spousal violence reported by married women among sampled couples in the five countries studied, there is remarkable consistency in the *structure* of spousal violence across countries. Notably, our factor analysis, under a relaxed eigenvalue criterion, upholds the face validity of the categories of emotional, physical, or sexual violence that experts have assigned to the different acts of violence asked about in the DHS domestic violence module. Correlations suggest that emotional and physical violence are more similar to each other than other forms. The factor analysis provides another important insight: that the six items typically categorized as controlling behaviors may represent not one but two separate concepts, which we label "suspicion" and "isolation" in this study. These terms describe husbands' behaviors that represent suspicion of their wives and behaviors that aim to isolate them. Both are distinct from any of the three categories of emotional, physical, and sexual spousal violence.

The items in these two controlling behavior factors are similar to those in the dominance/isolation subscale of the Psychological Maltreatment of Women Inventory (PMWI) (Tolman 1999). While they may be similar in underlying construct to the "jealousy" and "dominance" factors identified in other research using PMWI-type measures (Kar and O'Leary 2013; Kasian and Painter 1992), we apply different labels because the sets of items comprising "suspicion" and "isolation" differ both in number and in wording from those comprising "jealousy" and "dominance." Additional psychometric testing would be needed to determine whether these differences are meaningful and represent distinct constructs, or whether they are immaterial to assessing the same latent construct.

Despite the consistency in the structure of spousal violence across countries, there is substantial variation in the relationships between the various forms of violence and women's HIV status, and in their associations with the two pathways through which violence exerts influence. No single form of spousal violence is consistently associated with a woman's risk of HIV in all five countries studied. In Malawi no form of violence is associated with a wife's risk of having HIV. A significant relationship is found with women's HIV status for the factors of suspicion and isolation in Zambia and Zimbabwe; for emotional violence in Kenya, Rwanda, and Zimbabwe; and for physical violence in Kenya, Rwanda, and Zimbabwe; and in no country is a significant relationship found between sexual violence and women's HIV status.

It is somewhat surprising that there is no apparent association in any of the countries in this study between spousal sexual violence and women's HIV status, even in the base model, as this form of violence is the only one for which there is a conceptual basis for a direct effect on women's HIV status. Of all the forms of violence and controlling behaviors, sexual violence is the least prevalent in all countries. One possibility is that, given the low prevalence, the sample sizes are insufficient to detect any significant effect. Another possibility is that there is truly no relationship between sexual violence and women's HIV status, either directly or indirectly. Sexual violence is associated with women's experience of an STI or STI symptom in the last 12 months, women's lifetime number of sexual partners, husbands' alcohol use, and husbands' lifetime number of partners in multiple countries. However, compared with other forms of spousal violence, sexual violence is associated with fewer HIV risk factors for women and their husbands, and in fewer countries. Where an association is found, the magnitude of the odds ratio is smaller than for other forms of violence. These findings suggest that, if sexual violence is to influence women's HIV status through the same pathways as other forms of violence, these linkages are relatively weak.

The investigation into the pathways through which the different forms of violence may be associated with a woman's risk of HIV is also revealing. For almost all forms of spousal violence, with the exception of physical violence, and in all countries, any observed significant relationship between spousal violence and a woman's risk of HIV is explained away by women's or their husbands' HIV risk factors, or both. In other words, a woman's experience of different forms of spousal violence is positively associated with her risk of HIV because either (a) her own high-risk behaviors or STI status are affected by her experience of violence and in turn affect her risk of HIV, or (b) her husband's HIV and STI status along with his high-risk behaviors is also positively associated with her risk of violence and her risk of HIV, or because of both (a) and (b). Thus, this study provides evidence that there is no direct effect of most forms of spousal violence on women's HIV status, only an indirect effect through selected behavioral and other factors commonly considered to put an individual at high risk of HIV.

The only form of violence that appears to have a direct net association with HIV is physical violence. Physical violence remains significant in all models in Kenya and Zimbabwe. In Zimbabwe, even with controls for all high-risk factors, a unit increase in the physical violence factor score increases the odds of the wife being HIV positive by 45 %, and this relationship remains highly significant for the entire analysis. In Kenya, by contrast, although a similar relationship is observed, the significance is greatly reduced if all risk factors are controlled for.

Several potential explanations can be proposed for this finding. It could be that the net positive direct association of the experience of physical violence with the risk of having HIV remains because some key variables that represent additional indirect pathways through which physical violence influences women's HIV status are absent from this analysis. Alternately, perhaps, the direct relationship is capturing a simultaneous association between spousal violence and women's HIV status in the reverse causal direction. That is, at the same time that the experience of physical violence increases the risk of a woman having HIV (through multiple risk factors), being HIV positive may be a trigger for episodes of physical violence. Or, finally, it may be that physical violence does in fact have a direct effect, perhaps by triggering increased levels of stress that compromise a woman's immune system, leaving her more susceptible to HIV infection (Campbell et al. 2008).

This study has some limitations, primarily the limitations imposed by the cross-sectional nature of DHS data. We use retrospective measures of the experience of spousal violence and data on the prevalence—but not incidence—of HIV. As such, and like the vast majority of empirical research on this question, we do not know whether experience of spousal violence precedes infection with HIV or if infection with HIV precedes spousal violence. This constraint prevents us from interpreting any causal direction to the associations we find between spousal violence and women's HIV status, or between spousal violence and wives' and husbands' HIV risk factors.

The use of data on both members of a couple is a strength of this study. However, the use of couple data presents some trade-offs. These data rely on couples in which both members could be successfully interviewed and for whom there are valid HIV test results and in which the wife was administered the domestic violence module of the DHS questionnaire. Thus, we exclude couples in which either the wife or the husband was not present in the household, was unavailable for interview, or declined HIV testing. Additionally, both HIV and spousal violence may contribute to dissolution of marriages, through death of one spouse, divorce, or separation. As a result, our sample of couples may or may not be fully representative of all marriages in which spousal violence occurs. Finally, spousal violence and several of the personal risk factors included in our analyses may be subject to underreporting, due to recall error, embarrassmeht, or social desirability bias. It is not fully known how any underreporting of these variables may impact the results we observe.

Despite these limitations, the study contributes to an understanding of the relationship between spousal violence and HIV. It takes advantage of data from both members of a couple and uses discrete, nuanced measures of violence to better specify the associated pathways through which the various forms of spousal violence influence women's HIV status.

References

Andersson, N., & Cockcroft, A. (2012). Choice-disability and HIV infection: a cross sectional study of HIV status in Botswana, Namibia and Swaziland. *AIDS and Behavior, 16*(1), 189–198. doi:10.1007/s10461-011-9912-3.

Andersson, N., Cockcroft, A., & Shea, B. (2008). Gender-based violence and HIV: Relevance for HIV prevention in hyperendemic countries of southern Africa. *AIDS, 22*(Suppl 4), S73–S86. doi:10.1097/01.aids.0000341778.73038.86.

Campbell, J. C., Baty, M. L., Ghandour, R. M., Stockman, J. K., Francisco, L., & Wagman, J. (2008). The intersection of intimate partner violence against women and HIV/AIDS: A review. *International Journal of Injury Control and Safety Promotion, 15*(4), 221–231. doi:10.1080/17457300802423224.

Decker, M. R., Seage, G. R., Hemenway, D., Gupta, J., Raj, A., & Silverman, J. G. (2009a). Intimate partner violence perpetration, standard and gendered STI/HIV risk behaviour, and STI/HIV diagnosis among a clinic-based sample of men. *Sexually Transmitted Infections, 85*(7), 555–560. doi:10.1136/sti.2009.036368.

Decker, M. R., Seage, G. R. I., Hemenway, D., Raj, A., Saggurti, N., Balaiah, D., et al. (2009b). Intimate partner violence functions as both a risk marker and risk factor for women's HIV infection: findings from Indian husband-wife dyads. *Journal of Acquired Immune Deficiency Syndromes, 51*(5), 593–600. doi:10.1097/QAI.0b013e3181a255d6.

DiStefano, C., Zhu, M., & Mindrila, D. (2009). Understanding and using factor scores: considerations for the applied researcher. *Practical Assessment, Research & Evaluation, 14*(20), 1–11.

Dunkle, K. L., & Decker, M. R. (2013). Gender-based violence and HIV: reviewing the evidence for links and causal pathways in the general population and high-risk groups. *American Journal of Reproductive Immunology, 69*, 20–26. doi:10.1111/aji.12039.

Dunkle, K. L., Jewkes, R. K., Brown, H. C., Gray, G. E., McIntryre, J. A., & Harlow, S. D. (2004). Gender-based violence, relationship power, and risk of HIV infection in women attending antenatal clinics in South Africa. *Lancet, 363*(9419), 1415–1421.

Fals-Stewart, W., & Kennedy, C. (2005). Addressing intimate partner violence in substance-abuse treatment. *Journal of Substance Abuse Treatment, 29*(1), 5–17. doi: http://dx.doi.org/10.1016/j.jsat.2005.03.001.

Fonck, K., Leye, E., Kidula, N., Ndinya-Achola, J., & Temmerman, M. (2005). Increased risk of HIV in women experiencing physical partner violence in Nairobi, Kenya. *AIDS and Behavior, 9*(3), 335–339.

Ghosh, P., Arah, O. A., Talukdar, A., Sur, D., Babu, G. R., Sengupta, P., et al. (2011). Factors associated with HIV infection among Indian women. *International Journal of STD and AIDS, 22*(3), 140–145. doi:10.1258/ijsa.2010.010127.

González-Guarda, R. M., Florom-Smith, A. L., & Thomas, T. (2011). A syndemic model of substance abuse, intimate partner violence, HIV infection, and mental health among Hispanics. *Public Health Nursing, 28*(4), 366–378. doi:10.1111/j.1525-1446.2010.00928.x.

Harling, G., Msisha, W., & Subramanian, S. V. (2010). No association between HIV and intimate partner violence among women in 10 developing countries. *PLoS One, 5*(12), e14257. doi:10.1371/journal.pone.0014257.

Jewkes, R., Dunkle, K., Nduna, M., Levin, J., Jama, N., Khuzwayo, N., et al. (2006a). Factors associated with HIV sero-status in young rural South African women: Connections between intimate partner violence and HIV. *International Journal of Epidemiology, 35*(6), 1461–1468.

Jewkes, R. K., Dunkle, K., Nduna, M., & Shai, N. (2010). Intimate partner violence, relationship power inequity, and incidence of HIV infection in young women in South Africa: A cohort study. *The Lancet, 376*(9734), 41–48.

Jewkes, R., Nduna, M., Levin, J., Jama, N., Dunkle, K., Khuzwayo, N., et al. (2006b). A cluster randomized-controlled trial to determine the effectiveness of Stepping Stones in preventing HIV infections and promoting safer sexual behaviour amongst youth in the rural Eastern Cape, South Africa: trial design, methods and baseline findings. *Tropical Medicine & International Health, 11*(1), 3–16. doi:10.1111/j.1365-3156.2005.01530.x.

Kar, H., & O'Leary, K. D. (2013). Patterns of psychological aggression, dominance, and jealousy within marriage. *Journal of Family Violence, 28*(2), 109–119. doi:10.1007/s10896-012-9492-7.

Kasian, M., & Painter, S. L. (1992). Frequency and severity of psychological abuse in a dating population. *Journal of Interpersonal Violence, 7*(3), 350–364. doi:10.1177/088626092007003005.

Kayibanda, J. F., Bitera, R., & Alary, M. (2012). Violence toward women, men's sexual risk factors, and HIV infection among women: Findings from a national household survey in Rwanda. *AIDS, 59*(3), 300–307. doi:10.1097/QAI.0b013e31823dc634.

Kishor, S., & Bradley, S. E. K. (2012). *Women's and men's experience of spousal violence in two African countries: does gender matter?* DHS Analytical Studies No. 27. Calverton, MD: ICF International.

Kootstra, G. J. (2004). Exploratory factor analysis: Theory and applications. Retrieved November 12, 2012 from: http://www.let.rug.nl/~nerbonne/teach/rema-stats-meth-seminar/Factor-Analysis-Kootstra-04.PDF.

Lary, H., Maman, S., Katebalila, M., McCauley, A., & Mbwambo, J. (2004). Exploring the association between HIV and violence: Young people's experiences with infidelity, violence and forced sex in Dar es Salaam, Tanzania. *International Family Planning Perspectives, 30*(4), 200–206.

Makayoto, L. A., Omolo, J., Kamweya, A. M., Harder, V. S., & Mutai, J. (2013). Prevalence and associated factors of intimate partner violence among pregnant women attending Kisumu District Hospital, Kenya. *Maternal Child Health Journal, 17*(3), 441–447. doi:10.1007/s10995-012-1015-x.

Maman, S., Mbwambo, J. K., Hogan, N. M., Kilonzo, G. P., Campbell, J. C., Weiss, E., et al. (2002). HIV-positive women report more lifetime partner violence: Findings from a voluntary counseling and testing clinic in Dar es Salaam, Tanzania. *American Journal of Public Health, 92*(8), 1331–1337.

Maman, S., Yamanis, T., Kouyoumdjian, F., Watt, M., & Mbwambo, J. (2010). Intimate partner violence and the association with HIV risk behaviors among young men in Dar es Salaam, Tanzania. *Journal of Interpersonal Violence, 25*(10), 1855–1872. doi:10.1177/0886260509354498.

Meyer, J. P., Springer, S. A., & Altice, F. L. (2001). Substance abuse, violence, and HIV in women: A literature review of the syndemic. *Journal of Women's Health, 20*(7), 991–1006. doi:10.1089/jwh.2010.2328.

Mittal, M., Senn, T. E., & Carey, M. P. (2011). Mediators of the relation between partner violence and sexual risk behavior among women attending a sexually transmitted disease clinic. *Sexually Transmitted Disease, 38*(6), 510–515. doi:10.1097/OLQ.0b013e318207f59b.

O'Leary, K. D., & Kar, H. L. (2010). Partner abuse. In J. C. Thomas & M. Hersen (Eds.), *Handbook of clinical psychology competencies* (pp. 1039–1062). New York: Springer.

Pett, M. A., Lackey, N. R., & Sullivan, J. J. (2003). *Making sense of factor analysis: The use of factor analysis for instrument development in health care research.* Thousand Oaks, CA: Sage Publications.

Pitpitan, E. V., Kalichman, S. C., Eaton, L. A., Cain, D., Sikkema, K. J., Skinner, D., et al. (2013). Gender-based violence, alcohol use, and sexual risk among female patrons of drinking venues in Cape Town, South Africa. *Journal of Behavioral Medicine, 36*(3), 295–304. doi:10.1007/s10865-012-9423-3.

Prabhu, M., McHome, B., Ostermann, J., Itemba, D., Njau, B., Thielman, N., et al. (2011). Prevalence and correlates of intimate partner violence among women attending HIV voluntary counseling and testing in northern Tanzania, 2005–2008. *International Journal of Gynaecology & Obstetrics, 113*(1), 63–67. doi:10.1016/j.ijgo.2010.10.019.

Raj, A., Silverman, J. G., & Amaro, H. (2004). Abused women report greater male partner risk and gender-based risk for HIV: Findings from a community-based study with Hispanic women. *AIDS Care, 16*(4), 519–529.

Sareen, J., Pagura, J., & Grant, B. (2009). Is intimate partner violence associated with HIV infection among women in the United States? *General Hospital Psychiatry, 31*(3), 274–278. doi:10.1016/j.genhosppsych.2009.02.004.

Schensul, S. L., Mekki-Berrada, A., Nastasi, B. K., Singh, R., Burleson, J. A., & Bojko, M. (2006). Men's extramarital sex, marital relationships and sexual risk in urban poor communities in India. *Journal of Urban Health, 83*(4), 614–624. doi:10.1007/s11524-006-9076-z.

Silverman, J. G., Decker, M. R., Saggurti, N., Balaiah, D., & Raj, A. (2008). Intimate partner violence and HIV infection among married Indian women. *JAMA, 300*(6), 703–710. doi:10.1001/jama.300.6.703.

Stockman, J. K., Lucea, M. B., Draughon, J. E., Sabri, B., Anderson, J. C., Bertrand, D., et al. (2013). Intimate partner violence and HIV risk factors among African-American and African-Caribbean women in clinic-based settings. *AIDS Care, 25*(4), 472–480. doi:10.1080/09540121.2012.722602.

Straus, M. A. (1979). Measuring intrafamily conflict and violence: The conflict tactics (CT) scales. *Journal of Marriage and Family, 41*(1), 75–88. doi:10.2307/351733.

Straus, M. A. (1990). Measuring intrafamily conflict and violence; the conflict tactic (CT) scales. In M. A. Straus & R. Gelles (Eds.), *Physical violence in American families: Risk factors and adaptations to violence in 8,145 families* (pp. 29–47). New Brunswick, NJ: Transaction Publishers.

Swan, H., & O'Connell, D. J. (2011). The impact of intimate partner violence on women's condom negotiation efficacy. *Journal of Interpersonal Violence, 27*(4), 775–792. doi:10.1177/0886260511423240.

Teti, M., Chilton, M., Lloyd, L., & Rubinstein, S. (2006). Identifying the links between violence against women and HIV/AIDS: Ecosocial and human rights frameworks offer insight into US prevention policies. *Health and Human Rights, 9*(2), 40–61.

Tjaden, P. (2004). What is violence against women: Defining and measuring the problem. *Journal of Interpersonal Violence, 19*(11), 1244–1251.

Tolman, R. M. (1999). The validation of the psychological maltreatment of women inventory. *Violence and Victims, 14*(1), 25–37.

Townsend, L., Jewkes, R., Mathews, C., Johnston, L. G., Flisher, A. J., Zembe, Y., et al. (2011). HIV risk behaviours and their relationship to intimate partner violence (IPV) among men who have multiple female sexual partners in Cape Town, South Africa. *AIDS and Behavior, 15*(1), 132–141. doi:10.1007/s10461-010-9680-5.

Watts, C., & Mayhew, S. (2004). Reproductive health services and intimate partner violence: Shaping a pragmatic response in Sub-Saharan Africa. *International Family Planning Perspectives, 30*(4), 207–213.

Were, E., Curran, K., Delany-Moretlwe, S., Nakku-Joloba, E., Mugo, N. R., Kiarie, J., et al. (2011). A prospective study of frequency and correlates of intimate partner violence among African heterosexual HIV serodiscordant couples. *AIDS, 25*(16), 2009–2018. doi:10.1097/QAD.0b013e32834b005d.

World Health Organization. (2001). *Putting women first: Ethical and safety recommendations for research on domestic violence against women*. Geneva, Switzerland: Department of Gender and Women's Health.

World Health Organization. (2011). *Global Health Sector Strategy on HIV/AIDS 2011–2015*. Geneva, Switzerland: WHO Press.

Part II
Gender-Based Violence:
Perspectives from the Middle East

Chapter 5
Consanguineous Marriage: Protective or Risk Factor for Intimate Partner Violence?

Jinan Usta, Marwan Khawaja, Dima Dandachi, and Mylene Tewtel

Abstract Consanguinity is still common in the Middle East. This chapter uses the Demographic and Health Surveys (DHS) from Egypt (2005; $N=5,240$) and Jordan (2007; $N=3,444$) to examine the relationship between consanguinity and intimate partner violence (IPV). Binary logistic regression models used to assess the association revealed that IPV, namely physical, emotional, and sexual violence during the past year to the survey, was fairly similar in both countries. Physical violence was 18 % in Egypt and 12 % in Jordan; emotional violence was 10 % in both countries, while sexual violence was lower: 6 % in Jordan and 4 % in Egypt. Jordan has a higher rate of consanguinity (39 %) compared to Egypt (33 %). Findings show significant association between consanguinity and experience of emotional, but not physical, or sexual IPV in the past year in both countries. Duration of marriage, education, and wealth were also found to be important determinants.

Keywords Intimate partner violence • Arab world • Consanguinity • Physical violence • Emotional violence • Sexual violence

J. Usta (✉) • D. Dandachi
American University of Beirut, Family Medicine Department, Beirut, Lebanon
e-mail: ju00@aub.edu.lb; dr.dimadandachi@gmail.com

M. Khawaja
UN-ESCWA, Beirut, Lebanon
e-mail: khawaja@un.org

M. Tewtel
Qatar Biomedical Research Institute, Qatar Foundation, Doha, Qatar
e-mail: mtewtel@qf.org.qa

© Springer International Publishing Switzerland 2015   101
Y.K. Djamba, S.R. Kimuna (eds.), *Gender-Based Violence*,
DOI 10.1007/978-3-319-16670-4_5

Introduction

It is estimated that over six million people in the world have consanguineous parents. Although first-cousin marriage is illegal in certain areas (Bittles and Black 2010), many countries, especially the Arab world, continue to have high rates of consanguineous marriages when compared to Western countries (Bras et al. 2009; Freire-Maia 1968; Stoltenberg et al. 1998). However, it is difficult to compare rates of consanguinity among different countries given the various methodologies used and the differences in years and in populations studied; yet, it might be possible to obtain from available literature a general idea about estimates of consanguinity across the Arab world and the changing pattern over time.

Several studies have found differences in consanguinity prevalence across the Arab world. For instance, in Egypt, Hafez and colleagues' 1983 study showed a general prevalence of consanguinity of 28.9 % (Hafez et al. 1983). A study conducted in Beirut, Lebanon, showed a 25 % general incidence (Khlat 1988). A more representative and recent study across different regions of Lebanon in 2009 showed an overall consanguinity rate of 35.5 % (Barbour and Salameh 2009), comparable to the 35.4 % rate reported from Syria (Othman and Saadat 2009), but lower than the rates reported elsewhere: 40 % in Yemen (Jurdi and Saxena 2003), 40.6 % among Israeli Arabs (Vardi-Saliternik et al. 2002), 50.5 % in the United Arab Emirates (UAE) (Al-Gazali et al. 1997), 51.2 % in Jordan (Khoury and Massad 1992), and 54 % in Qatar (Bener and Alali 2006). A study published from the Kingdom of Saudi Arabia (KSA) revealed an overall rate of consanguinity of 57.7 % (El-Hazmi et al. 1995). Another national study from KSA conducted over 2 years (2004–2005) from each of the 13 regions of the Kingdom showed a national prevalence of 56 % (El-Mouzan et al. 2007). The percentage is even higher in north Jordan at 63.7 % (Al-Salem and Rawashdeh 1993).

Most of the studies agreed that first-cousin marriage is the most common type of inbreeding (Hafez et al. 1983; Barbour and Salameh 2009; Othman and Saadat 2009; Jurdi and Saxena 2003; Al-Gazali et al. 1997; Khoury and Massad 1992; Bener and Alali 2006; El-Hazmi et al. 1995; El-Mouzan et al. 2007; Al-Salem and Rawashdeh 1993). However, uncle-niece and aunt–nephew mating is prohibited by Islamic law and is not encountered in Arab countries.

Several factors including sociocultural, religious, economic, degree of isolation of the population, and current laws are assumed to play a role in the rate differences observed among countries of the Arab world. The influence of modernization on the practice of consanguineous marriage seems not to be identical in different areas. Whereas the practice of consanguineous marriage has steadily declined in some countries like Jordan (Hamamy et al. 2005), Palestinian territories (Assaf and Khawaja 2009) and Israeli Arabs (Jaber et al. 2000; Sharkia et al. 2008), and non-Bedouin communities in Kuwait (Radovanovic et al. 1999), the rate of consanguineous marriages has increased in Yemen (Jurdi and Saxena 2003), the UAE (Al-Gazali et al. 1997), and Qatar (Bener and Alali 2006).

Consanguineous marriage is more common in those who get married at younger ages (Jurdi and Saxena 2003; Assaf and Khawaja 2009; Sharkia et al. 2008), among those residing in rural areas (Hafez et al. 1983; Vardi-Saliternik et al. 2002; Bener and Alali 2006; Bener et al. 2009; Assaf and Khawaja 2009), and within Bedouin communities (Vardi-Saliternik et al. 2002; Radovanovic et al. 1999). Further, other factors that determine consanguineous unions include Muslim affiliation (Khlat 1988; Barbour and Salameh 2009; Vardi-Saliternik et al. 2002; Khoury and Massad 1992), husbands with low occupational status (Khlat 1988), women out of labor force (Barbour and Salameh 2009; Assaf and Khawaja 2009), lower socioeconomic status, and individuals with lower wealth index (Assaf and Khawaja 2009; Sharkia et al. 2008). However, the role of education in consanguineous marriage is not clear. Although some studies have shown that women and men with low educational level are more likely to be in consanguineous marriage (Khlat 1988; Barbour and Salameh 2009; Jurdi and Saxena 2003; Khoury and Massad 1992), this was not evident in other studies (Al-Salem and Rawashdeh 1993; Hamamy et al. 2005; Assaf and Khawaja 2009; Gunaid et al. 2004). Actually, the opposite was true in Yemen regarding the husband's education (Jurdi and Saxena 2003).

The effect of consanguineous marriage on pregnancy outcomes, congenital malformations, genetic diseases, and cancer risks has been well documented (Denic et al. 2005; Bener et al. 2009, 2010; Pedersen 2002; Kanaan et al. 2008; Tadmouri et al. 2009; Hamamy et al. 2011). However, the effect of such marriage on the family dynamic and sociological factors has not been well studied. A recent study examined the association between consanguinity and susceptibility to drug abuse among offspring (Saadat and Vakili-Ghartavol 2010). Saadat's study revealed an association between drug abuse and parental consanguinity in non-alcohol drinkers, but the relationship between consanguinity and domestic violence has not been well studied.

The few studies from the region that document intimate partner violence prevalence and consanguinity as a covariate report mixed results. For example, Fikree and colleagues examined postnatal women in Pakistan about intimate partner violence and its determinants (Fikree et al. 2006). The study showed that 44 % of interviewed women reported marital abuse and consanguinity was found to be a significant risk for violence. In contrast, a research study of pregnant women attending a family planning clinic in Jordan showed that 15.4 % reported physical abuse during pregnancy. Being married to a first or second cousin was a protective factor against violence in the multivariate model compared to unrelated or distantly related marriage (Clark et al. 2009). These findings were in line with another study from Egypt (El-Zanaty and Way 2006). However, a study from the city of Aleppo, Syria, showed that the prevalence of physical abuse was not statistically different between women who were married to a relative vs. a nonrelative (Maziak and Asfar 2003). Similarly, consanguinity was associated, but not significantly, with lower rates of sexual coercion among pregnant Palestinian refugees in Lebanon (Khawaja and Hammoury 2008).

Thus, the aim of this study is to analyze the existing data on intimate partner violence and evaluate its relation to consanguinity taking into account the various types of domestic violence and the confounding factors (educational level, rural vs. urban settlement, wealth index, religious affiliation, occupational status, and working females).

The availability of national-level survey data on intimate partner violence and consanguinity with comparable instruments and survey methodology from two countries in the region provides a unique opportunity to assess this association in detail.

Methods

This study is based on two fairly comparable household survey data sets from the Demographic Health Survey (DHS) program: The first is the 2005 EDHS (Egypt Demographic and Health Survey) in Egypt (El-Zanaty and Way 2006) and the second is the 2007 PFHS (Population and Family Health Survey) from Jordan (Department of Statistics [Jordan] and Macro International Inc. 2008). Both of these surveys include a module on domestic violence and questions on consanguinity for ever-married women aged 15–49 years. The 2005 EDHS is the latest survey to include data on domestic violence in Egypt and, for comparative purposes, the 2007 PFHS survey from Jordan is the closest to the 2005 EDHS.

The 2007 PFHS is a stratified sample selected in two stages from the 2004 census frame. A total of 30 sampling strata were constructed for urban and rural areas of the 12 governorates in Jordan. In the first stage, 890 sampling clusters were selected randomly with probabilities proportional to population size and independently in each stratum. In the second stage, 16 households were selected from each sampling cluster. All ever-married women aged 15–49 years in the selected households were interviewed. The final sample included 11,113 women, with a response rate of 97.9 %. This study is based on one-third subsample of the total clusters. Only one woman in each cluster was selected randomly for the domestic violence module, resulting in a total sample of 3,444 ever-married women for analysis.

The 2007 EDHS data are stratified, three-stage probability samples based on the 1996 census frame. In the first stage, a total of 682 primary sampling units (PSUs) consisting mainly of towns and villages were selected from rural and urban areas. In the second stage, the PSUs were divided into sampling segments of approximately equal size: one was selected from smaller towns (PSUs) and two from larger ones. In the third stage, a systematic sample of 22,807 households was selected from the chosen segments. The final sample included 19,565 eligible women with a response rate of 99.5 %. As in the Jordan sample, a subsample consisting of one-third of the sampled households were selected for anemia testing and domestic violence module. One eligible woman was selected from each of this subsample, yielding a total of 5,240 women for the domestic violence module.

The outcome variable is exposure to violence by an intimate partner (IPV) during the past year before the survey. Measures of physical, emotional, and sexual violence against women were included. Physical violence is considered present if the woman answered yes to any of the seven physical attacks (by her husband) included in the instrument from the standard Conflict Tactics Scales (Straus et al. 1996). Emotional violence was considered present if the woman answered yes to any of the two questions, "Did your husband say or do something to humiliate you in front of others?" and "Did your husband threaten to hurt or harm you or someone close to you?" Sexual violence was considered present if the woman answered yes to the question, "Did your husband physically force you to have sexual intercourse with him even when you did not want to?"

The main independent variable is consanguinity. Although the two survey instruments are generally similar, as typical of DHS surveys, the question on consanguinity is not strictly comparable in the EDHS and JPFHS. In the EDHS, the answer categories consist of first and second cousins (from both father's and mother's side), other relative, or no relation. The answer categories for this question in the JPFHS in contrast are more detailed, consisting of six possible combinations for first-cousin marriage, depending on father's, mother's, and both sides, in addition to second cousin and marriage to other relatives. After checking frequencies of this variable in the two settings, we decided to measure consanguinity by a simple binary variable distinguishing if the woman was married to relative (consanguinity) or to nonrelative.

A range of demographic and socioeconomic risk factors were included as control variables, including age group (15–29, 30–39,40–49), age at marriage (<16, 16–19, 20–22, 22+), duration of marriage in years (<5, 5–19, 20+), educational level completed (less than secondary, secondary, more than secondary), residence (rural, urban), employment status (working, not working), and household wealth (quintiles). After bivariate analyses, multivariate analyses were conducted in the form of logistic regression models to assess the net effect of each of the independent variables on the IPV variables. These analyses were performed using the statistical package, Stata (version 12.0).

Results

Overall, the prevalence of physical violence reported during the past year was relatively higher in Egypt than in Jordan (Table 5.1). Nearly one woman out of five suffered from physical violence in Egypt and about one out of ten in Jordan. More than 10 % of women reported being emotionally abused within the past year in both countries. Sexual violence was lower at 6 % in Jordan and 4 % in Egypt. Over a third of women were married to relatives in both countries, with Jordan having a higher rate of consanguinity (39 %) than Egypt (33 %).

The age profile of women interviewed was fairly similar in both countries, with Egypt having a slightly younger sample. About 38 % of Egyptian women were aged less than 30 years old compared to 33 % in Jordan. On the other hand, Egyptian women were much less educated than their Jordanian counterparts. About one out of two Egyptian women had less than secondary education compared to one in ten in Jordan. Despite their higher educational level, Jordanian women were less likely to be employed (12 %) than Egyptian women (22 %). On average, most women were married before age 20 years in both countries. However, more women married at a younger age in Egypt than in Jordan. Marital duration was fairly similar in both countries, with about a fifth of women being married for less than 5 years. The vast

Table 5.1 Sample
characteristics and prevalence
of violence during past year,
Jordan (2007) and Egypt
(2005)

Variable	No. of women (%)	
	Jordan	Egypt
Physical violence		
Yes	412 (12.0)	1,022 (18.2)
No	3,032 (88.0)	4,591 (81.8)
Emotional violence		
Yes	354 (10.4)	575 (10.2)
No	3,054 (89.6)	5,038 (89.8)
Sexual violence		
Yes	193 (5.6)	217 (3.9)
No	3,229 (94.4)	5,396 (96.1)
Consanguinity		
Relative	1,332 (38.7)	1,861 (33.2)
Nonrelative	2,112 (61.3)	3,45 (66.7)
Age		
15–29	1,151 (33.4)	2,122 (37.8)
30–39	1,361 (39.5)	1,876 (33.4)
40–49	932 (27.1)	1,614 (28.8)
Education		
Less than secondary	346 (10.1)	2,812 (50.1)
Secondary	2,060 (59.8)	2,178 (38.8)
Higher than secondary	1,037 (30.1)	624 (11.1)
Employment		
Not working	3,024 (87.8)	4,365 (77.8)
Working	420 (12.2)	1,248 (22.2)
Age at first marriage		
<16	245 (7.1)	887 (15.8)
16–19	1,288 (37.4)	2,138 (38.1)
20–22	951 (27.6)	1,420 (25.3)
23+	959 (27.8)	1,168 (20.8)
Marital duration		
<5	728 (21.1)	1,175 (20.9)
5–19	1,907 (55.4)	2,822 (50.3)
20+	809 (23.5)	1,617 (28.8)
Place of residence		
Urban	2,938 (85.3)	2,339 (41.7)
Rural	506 (14.7)	3,274 (58.3)
Wealth index		
Poorest	646 (18.7)	1,048 (18.7)
Poorer	761 (22.1)	1,018 (18.1)
Middle	707 (20.5)	1,129 (20.1)
Richer	701 (20.4)	1,226 (21.8)
Total	3,444 (100.0)	5,613 (100.0)

majority of Jordanian women resided in urban areas (85 %) while more than 50 % of Egyptian women lived in rural areas. The wealth index distribution frequency looks similar in both countries.

Table 5.2 displays the bivariate (unadjusted) associations between physical violence and background variables. Consanguinity was significantly associated with physical violence in Jordan but not in Egypt, with women married to relatives

Table 5.2 Prevalence of physical violence during past year by selected background variables, Jordan (2007) and Egypt (2005)

Variable	Jordan		Egypt	
	N (%)	P-values*	N (%)	P-values*
Consanguinity				
Relative	136 (10.2)	0.012	350 (18.8)	0.388
Nonrelative	276 (13.1)		669 (17.9)	
Age				
15–29	156 (13.6)	0.052	440 (20.7)	0.000
30–39	162 (11.9)		358 (19.1)	
40–49	94 (10.9)		224 (13.1)	
Education				
Less than secondary	56 (16.1)	0.001	624 (22.2)	0,000
Secondary	260 (12.6)		358 (16.4)	
Higher than secondary	95 (9.2)		40 (6.4)	
Employment				
Not working	363 (12.0)	0.731	821 (10.1)	0.509
Working	48 (11.4)		201 (10.7)	
Age at first marriage				
<16	37 (15.1)	0.024	173 (19.5)	0.000
16–19	159 (12.3)		457 (21.4)	
20–22	90 (9.5)		221 (15.6)	
23+	126 (13.1)		171 (14.6)	
Marital duration				
<5	95 (13.0)	0.010	198 (16.9)	0.000
5–19	244 (12.8)		590 (20.9)	
20+	72 (8.9)		235 (14.5)	
Place of residence				
Urban	352 (12.0)	0.925	355 (15.2)	0.000
Rural	60 (11.8)		667 (20.4)	
Wealth index				
Poorest	97 (15.0)	0.002	240 (22.9)	0.000
Poorer	105 (13.8)		227 (22.3)	
Middle	66 (9.3)		229 (20.3)	
Richer	85 (12.1)		200 (16.3)	
Richest	59 (9.4)		127 (10.7)	
Total	412 (100.0)		1,022 (100.0)	

*P-values of chi-square statistics

in Jordan being less at risk for physical violence than women married to nonrelatives. Younger age, low education, low age at marriage, shorter marital duration, and low level of wealth were also associated with physical violence in both countries. It should be noted that marital duration was not consistently related to physical violence in Egypt, but longer marital duration (>20 years) was associated with lower rates of physical violence. Finally, Egyptian women residing in rural areas were more likely to suffer from physical abuse than urban women.

Table 5.3 shows overall analogous associations with emotional violence. Women married to relatives had significantly lower rates of emotional abuse than those married to nonrelatives, but the relation was statistically significant only in Jordan. Education, age at first marriage, marital duration, and wealth index were statistically significantly associated with emotional IPV in both countries. Women with higher educational attainment were less likely to report emotional abuse than their counterparts with lower education. The association between emotional abuse and age at first marriage was linear in Egypt but not in Jordan. Nonetheless, in both countries, women who were married at the age of 23 or older were significantly less likely to report emotional abuse than those women who married at younger ages.

The effect of duration of marriage on emotional abuse was statistically significant in both countries but the pattern of association was slightly different. In Jordan, the association was clearly positive: women who have been married for a longer time were more likely to experience emotional abuse. In contrast, in Egypt, the risk of emotional abuse was higher among those who have been married for 5–19 years. In both countries, women who lived in poorer households were significantly more likely to report emotional abuse than those in richer households. The data in Table 5.3 also show that nonworking women were more at risk of being emotionally abused only in Jordan. In contrast, rural women were more likely than urban women to report experiencing emotional violence in the past year only in Egypt.

Table 5.4 indicates that consanguinity was not associated with sexual abuse in both countries unlike for physical and emotional violence. Younger age, lower education, shorter marital duration, and lower wealth were associated with sexual abuse in both countries. Rural residence and unemployment were significantly associated with sexual abuse in Egypt but not in Jordan.

Table 5.5 displays adjusted associations between the three forms of violence and background variables. The results of the multivariate model indicate that consanguineous marriages are protective of abuse across types, but the association is only statistically significant for emotional abuse in both countries. Women married to relatives were about 1.5 times less at risk for emotional violence in both countries. This association is marginally significant for physical and sexual abuse. Interestingly, being younger and married at a younger age was no longer statistically significantly associated with IPV in the multivariate models. On the other hand, low educational level was significantly associated with both physical and emotional violence even after controlling for other factors. Women who have less than secondary education were twice more at risk for physical and emotional violence in Jordan and about four times in Egypt. Women with secondary education were also more vulnerable to physical and emotional violence than women with higher than secondary education,

Table 5.3 Prevalence of emotional violence during past year by selected background variables, Jordan (2007) and Egypt (2005)

Variable	Jordan		Egypt	
	N (%)	P-values*	N (%)	P-values*
Consanguinity				
Relative	113 (8.6)	0.007	178 (9.6)	0.242
Nonrelative	241 (11.5)		396 (10.6)	
Age				
15–29	106 (9.3)	0.249	221 (10.4)	0.076
30–39	141 (10.4)		211 (11.2)	
40–49	107 (11.6)		144 (8.9)	
Education				
Less than secondary	58 (17.2)	0.000	381 (13.5)	0.000
Secondary	224 (11.0)		177 (8.1)	
Higher than secondary	72 (7.0)		17 (2.7)	
Employment				
Not working	325 (10.9)	0.022	441 (10.1)	0.509
Working	30 (7.2)		134 (10.7)	
Age at first marriage				
<16	24 (9.9)	0.017	131 (14.8)	0.000
16–19	156 (12.3)		250 (11.7)	
20–22	96 (10.1)		102 (7.2)	
23+	78 (8.2)		93 (8.0)	
Marital duration				
<5	52 (7.1)	0.000	80 (6.8)	0.000
5–19	194 (10.3)		344 (12.2)	
20+	108 (13.5)		152 (9.4)	
Place of residence				
Urban	304 (10.5)	0.759	200 (8.6)	0.000
Rural	50 (10.0)		375 (11.5)	
Wealth index				
Poorest	87 (13.7)	0.003	160 (15.3)	0.000
Poorer	90 (11.9)		129 (12.7)	
Middle	53 (7.6)		129 (11.4)	
Richer	64 (9.2)		95 (7.7)	
Richest	61 (9.9)		62 (5.2)	
Total	354 (100.0)		575 (100.0)	

*P-values of chi-square statistics

but this association is significant only for Egypt. Education was not significant for sexual abuse, owing perhaps to small sample size.

Overall, longer marital duration (i.e., 5–19 years of marriage) was associated with IPV. This association, after controlling for other factors, was significant only for emotional violence in Egypt. Women married for 5–19 years were twice more

Table 5.4 Prevalence of sexual violence during past year by selected background variables, Jordan (2007) and Egypt (2005)

	Jordan		Egypt	
Variable	N (%)	P-values*	N (%)	P-values*
Consanguinity				
Relative	71 (5.4)	0.603	65 (3.5)	0.321
Nonrelative	122 (5.8)		151 (4.0)	
Age				
15–29	76 (6.7)	0.008	86 (4.1)	0.010
30–39	83 (6.1)		88 (4.7)	
40–49	35 (3.7)		44 (2.7)	
Education				
Less than secondary	27 (8.0)	0.023	122 (4.3)	0.003
Secondary	121 (5.9)		86 (4.0)	
Higher than secondary	44 (4.2)		9 (1.4)	
Employment				
Not working	173 (5.8)	0.412	184 (4.2)	0.016
Working	20 (4.8)		34 (2.7)	
Age at first marriage				
<16	15 (6.1)	0.758	43 (4.8)	0.056
16–19	75 (5.9)		90 (4.2)	
20–22	47 (5.0)		54 (3.8)	
23+	56 (5.9)		31 (2.7)	
Marital duration				
<5	45 (6.2)	0.018	39 (3.3)	0.001
5–19	118 (6.2)		136 (4.8)	
20+	29 (3.6)		42 (2.6)	
Place of residence				
Urban	156 (5.3)	0.067	66 (2.8)	0.001
Rural	37 (7.4)		151 (4.6)	
Wealth index				
Poorest	45 (7.0)	0.000	46 (4.4)	0.000
Poorer	43 (5.7)		51 (5.0)	
Middle	54 (7.7)		55 (4.9)	
Richer	33 (4.7)		48 (3.9)	
Richest	16 (2.6)		18 (1.5)	
Total	193 (100.0)		218 (100.0)	

*P-values of chi-square statistics

likely to report having experienced emotional violence in Egypt. On the other hand, 20 years of marriage or more was associated with a decrease in physical and sexual violence, although these associations were not statistically significant. Exception was observed for women who had been married for 20 years or more in Jordan, they were three times more at risk of being emotionally abused than women married for

Table 5.5 Adjusted odds ratios from logistic regression of physical, emotional, and sexual violence, Jordan (2007) and Egypt (2005)

Variable	Physical violence Jordan	Egypt	Emotional violence Jordan	Egypt	Sexual violence Jordan	Egypt
Consanguinity						
Relative (ref.)	1.000	1.000	1.000	1.000	1.000	1.000
Nonrelative	1.309	1.107	1.591**	1.371*	1.094	1.403
Age						
15–29	1.089	1.481	1.576	1.172	1.665	0.656
30–39	0.932	1.213	1.371	1.057	1.479	0.883
40–49 (ref.)	1.000	1.000	1.000	1.000	1.000	1.000
Education						
<Secondary	2.130*	3.909***	2.107*	4.197***	2.047	1.435
Secondary	1.497	2.468***	1.433	2.699**	1.357	1.433
Higher (ref.)	1.000	1.000	1.000	1.000	1.000	1.000
Employment						
Not working	0.810	0.977	1.900	0.792	1.028	1.505
Working (ref.)	1.000	1.000	1.000	1.000	1.000	1.000
Age first marriage						
<16	1.192	0.864	0.726	1.225	0.878	1.793
16–19	0.901	1.037	1.117	1.073	0.845	1.431
20–22	0.724	0.870	1.110	0.767	0.777	1.353
23+ (ref.)	1.000	1.000	1.000	1.000	1.000	1.000
Marital duration						
<5 years (ref.)	1.000	1.000	1.000	1.000	1.000	1.000
5–19	1.098	1.337*	1.831	1.705**	1.131	1.242
20+	0.683	0.863	3.289*	1.038	0.855	0.463
Place of residence						
Urban (ref.)	1.000	1.000	1.000	1.000	1.000	1.000
Rural	0.887	0.974	0.840	0.820	1.236	1.227
Wealth index						
Poorest	1.349	1.424	1.373	2.055**	1.978	2.332*
Poorer	1.323	1.487*	1.254	1.828*	1.752	2.574*
Middle	0.899	1.396	0.740	1.724*	2.601	2.642*
Richer	1.332	1.176	0.988	1.180	1.776	2.167*
Richest (ref.)	1.000	1.000	1.000	1.000	1.000	1.000

ref. reference category
*** $P \leq 0.001$; ** $P \leq 0.01$; * $P \leq 0.05$

less than 5 years. After adjusting for other variables, residing in rural areas in Egypt was no more associated with IPV.

Finally, lower wealth was significantly associated with emotional, sexual, and physical violence in Egypt, but not in Jordan. In fact, poorer women were about 2–3 times at higher risk for emotional and sexual abuse, and 1.5 times higher for physical violence, in Egypt.

Discussion and Conclusion

The data from the Jordan and Egypt DHS survey indicate that more than one-third of Egyptian and Jordanian women have been exposed to any form of emotional, physical, and/or sexual violence during their lifetime. It should be noted that the current research analyzes past year experiences with IPV, which are generally lower than the lifetime experiences with IPV. Nonetheless, past year assessment might be a more accurate measure of IPV because it reduces recall bias (Xu et al. 2005) and provides a better insight into the problem.

Our results show that the prevalence of physical, sexual, and emotional intimate partner violence during the past year in Jordan and Egypt is relatively high, with higher rates reported from Egypt. IPV prevalence varies tremendously from one country to another as shown in the multi-country population-based household surveys carried out by the World Health Organization (WHO), where the prevalence of physical or sexual partner violence or both during past year fluctuates between as low as 4 % in Japan to 54 % in Ethiopia (Garcia-Moreno et al. 2006). The rates are also comparable to the ones observed in large population-based studies conducted in primary care settings with a prevalence of past year IPV of 6–21 % (Laanpere et al. 2012; Xu et al. 2005).

Our findings reveal that physical violence was the most common type of violence reported in Jordan and Egypt followed by emotional and sexual to a much lesser extent. This is not in line with a cross-sectional study conducted in Alexandria in 2009 among 3,271 ever-married women, which showed that emotional abuse was the most common form of IPV (Mamdouh et al. 2012). Similar findings were reported in the USA, where 28 % of women in health care setting were found to be emotionally abused, 12 % were physically abused, and 4 % were sexually abused during the past year (Kramer et al. 2004). In another general practice-based prevalence study carried out in Melbourne, Australia, more than 25 % of women were exposed to physical or emotional abuse from their partner in the previous year and 13 % experienced rape or attempted rape (Mazza et al. 1996). These findings show that the prevalence and patterns of IPV are not strictly comparable in various and quite different cultures.

Several contributing factors to IPV emerged in bivariate analyses of these two demographic and health surveys; however, in the multivariate models only few remained significant. Many of these factors were studied in the literature and are discussed below.

Education was found to correlate strongly but negatively with physical and emotional intimate partner violence in both countries. Women with less than secondary education were significantly twice more at risk for physical and emotional violence in Jordan and four times for physical and emotional violence in Egypt after controlling for other variables. Furthermore, in Egypt, women with secondary education were also found more vulnerable to physical and emotional abuse than women with higher than secondary education. This contradicts the finding from another Arab country (Saudi Arabia) where illiterate women had decreased risk for physical abuse and husbands with higher education had more risk of having an abusive behavior toward their wives (Tashkandi and Rasheed 2010).

However, the above-mentioned relation of education to IPV is consistent with research from other parts of the world where the women's and the husband's higher educational levels correlated with lower IPV (Mamdouh et al. 2012; Abramsky et al. 2011). Moreover, population-based surveys conducted by the WHO between 2000 and 2003 in several countries revealed that the lowest level of IPV occurred when husbands and wives had completed the same level of education (Abramsky et al. 2011). It is possible to speculate that husbands who have undergone similar years of schooling would share similar norms of gender equality. Yet, our research could not look at differences in education between husbands and wives as it included ever-married women and hence information on husbands would be missing for some.

It is interesting that education was associated with sexual violence in bivariate analysis for both countries, but lost its significance in logistic regression models. Although education is considered a strong predictor of women's empowerment, autonomy, and gender equality and hence expected to decrease the risk of violence among couples, it didn't seem to affect the sexual violence within IPV in the Arab world. As it is secondary data analysis, some factors that could have played a role in counter affecting the role of education were not measured. For example, alcohol and drug use has shown in many studies to be strongly associated with domestic violence (Hamzeh et al. 2008; Worden and Carlson 2005; Abramsky et al. 2011). Moreover, the general concept prevailing in the Arab world, even among women, that sexual intercourse is considered the husband's right, so a man can engage sexually with his wife when he pleases, could also explain this relation. Marital rape is not considered a crime in all Arab states.

Five to 19 years of marital years tend to increase the odds of physical, emotional, and sexual violence in Jordan and Egypt. However, after 20 years of marriage and over, there is a fall in physical and sexual violence in both countries and in emotional violence in Egypt. Similar to the findings of the study conducted among Saudi women, a significant decline of physical abuse has been observed after 20 years of marriage. Several explanations could be provided for this finding: after lengthy years of marriage, factors such as the presence of grown-up children or husbands' maturity toward their own abusive conduct might influence a decrease in IPV (Tashkandi and Rasheed 2010); or women could also become more tolerant to their husbands' acts of violence. In fact, one study showed that women who have 15 years of marriage or more were more likely to justify their husbands beating them (Yount 2005). In our study, the surprising finding of positive association between emotional violence in Jordan (but not in Egypt) and marital duration of 20 years and more, which increased the odds three times, needs to be explained. This may be attributed to place of residence, as the Jordan sample included more women residing in urban areas and could be more exposed to awareness campaigns on violence and women's rights. After several years of marriage, wives may be less tolerant to their husband's abusive behavior and more prone to disclose the emotional abuse to which they are subjected.

Residence in rural areas is significantly associated with physical abuse, emotional violence, and sexual violence in Egypt. This finding is similar to two studies conducted in Iran (Vakili et al. 2010; Faramarzi et al. 2005) and China (Xu et al. 2005), where women from rural areas were more exposed to IPV. However, the association lost its significance when we controlled for education in the multivariate analysis, showing that education, and not residence, is actually a more important determinant of abuse.

Wealth index, measure of household income and poverty, was associated with IPV in Jordan and Egypt. However, poverty seems to be a stronger predictor for violence in Egypt since this association remained significant in the multivariate model only for Egypt. Women from poorer households were twice more at risk for emotional and sexual violence than richer women in Egypt. This confirms the findings of a household survey carried out in Minya, Egypt, where household wealth was found to protect women from wife beating (Yount 2005). Poverty and its resultant stress were shown in many studies to impact the risk for IPV and wealth in the contrary to buffer this risk (Koenig et al. 2003; Abramsky et al. 2011). The absence of this correlation in Jordan warrants further investigation.

Our findings did not show correlation between employment and physical IPV in the multivariate model for all types of IPV in both countries, although there were some indications that nonworking women could be at risk for emotional abuse in Jordan and sexual abuse in Egypt. The relation of employment to IPV has been controversial in the literature. In Iran, for example, housewives were at greater risk for any type of IPV (Vakili et al. 2010). In the Minya study, the socioeconomic dependence of wives has been found to impact positively physical abuse regardless of household wealth (Yount 2005). However, in Lebanon, more working women reported exposure to violence (Usta et al. 2007) and in Saudi Arabia, women having a personal income were more at risk for physical abuse (Tashkandi and Rasheed 2010). Moreover, in the same study, women married to an unemployed husband were more exposed to physical abuse. This was attributed to the effect of poverty. It seems that more autonomous and income-earning women living in traditional settings are more exposed to risk of violence. Yet, autonomy did not seem to have an effect on violence in less conservative areas (Koenig et al. 2003).

Age and age at first marriage did not correlate with exposure to different types of IPV in our study, similar to the findings by Tashkandi and Rasheed (2010). The lack of age effect on physical abuse was attributed to inherent personality characteristics that would precipitate physical violence rather than the age of wives or husbands (Tashkandi and Rasheed 2010). A better measure of the influence of age could be the age difference between husbands and wives, which had a strong effect on physical abuse in the study conducted in Syria (Maziak and Asfar 2003).

Consanguinity emerges as a protective factor for intimate partner violence in Jordan and Egypt as well. After controlling for other factors, the association remained significant for emotional violence only. Being married to a nonrelative increased the odds for emotional violence in Jordan and Egypt. Similar to the study among Saudi women, physical abuse has been significantly lower among consanguineous marriages (16.8 %) than marriages with nonrelatives (25.1 %) (Tashkandi and Rasheed 2010). However, this association lost its significance in the multivariate model. It seems that social factors have a major influence on the risk of IPV exposure.

Actually, one of the suggested hypotheses for preference of consanguinity in the Middle East is the assumption of better adaptability and acceptability of the female in her new environment and more stability within the family (Bittles 2008). In the study by Tashkandi and Rasheed, when women and husbands originated from the same region in Saudi Arabia, the risk for physical abuse decreased (Tashkandi and Rasheed 2010). Being married to a relative in the context of traditional and patriarchal Middle Eastern and Arabic family structure appears to buffer marital conflicts and protect against domestic violence. It is possible that with the influence of Western modernization and the change in social structure, having a spouse who shares similar family and cultural background and therefore gender role perceptions would decrease the potential for conflicts. Indeed, unmet role expectations of the spouse were highlighted in a study conducted among low-income Lebanese families as a reason for family conflict (Keenan et al. 1998).

Moreover, as identified by Keenan and colleagues, consanguineous wives may use better suited coping strategies such as negotiation and taking initiative (Keenan et al. 1998). Additionally, they may benefit from the support of their extended family members, as the probability is higher for her to be living closer to her family, being married to a relative. In the Minya household survey, women experienced more physical abuse when they were deprived from the presence and support of biological family living next to their homes (Yount 2005). In fact, the perceived quality of social support in Iran played a major role in affecting IPV than the number of people providing the support (Mozdeh et al. 2012). In India, having the support from the wife's family was associated with lower rates of IPV (Rao 1997). Finally, women in consanguineous marriages might be more tolerant to abuse and find IPV socially acceptable and may not report these acts. In the study conducted in Minya, Egypt, women involved in endogamous marriages were more likely to accept and justify their husbands' beating attitudes (Yount 2005).

The study recognizes the effect of consanguinity on IPV. In the context of the countries under study, where women's autonomy is generally low, poverty high, and women are frequently unemployed, consanguinity seems to protect even after controlling for the other factors. Further qualitative research is needed to fully understand the reasons behind the protective role of consanguinity in a patriarchal family structure. The contribution of family and social resources, the power dynamics between husbands and wives, conflict management strategies, and family support need to be further investigated.

Limitations

The study adds to the exiting body of literature on IPV in general, and in the Arab world in particular where consanguineous marriages are quite frequent. It is a large-scale study using DHS and FHS data. However, the cross-sectional design of the study may be a limitation in gaining understanding of the causal associations of the identified factors with IPV. A possible second limitation is that the surveys relied on self-reports of violence which may be associated with underreporting. IPV is a sensitive issue and some women may be reluctant to reveal abuse from their husbands. Finally, because it is a secondary data analysis, other potential risk factors that could affect IPV were not accounted for in this study such as women's autonomy index, number of wives (monogamy vs. polygamy), family status (nuclear vs. extended), and husband's substance abuse.

Disclaimer The views expressed herein are those of the authors and do not necessarily reflect the views of the United Nations.

References

Abramsky, T., Watts, C. H., Garcia-Moreno, C., Devries, K., Kiss, L., Ellsberg, M., Jansen, H., & Heise, L. (2011). What factors are associated with recent intimate partner violence? Findings from the WHO multi-country study on women's health and domestic violence. *BioMed Central Public Health, 11,* 109.

Al-Gazali, L. I., Bener, A., Abdulrazzaq, Y. M., Micallef, R., al-Khayat, A. I., & Gaber, T. (1997). Consanguineous marriages in the United Arab Emirates. *Journal of Biosocial Science, 29*(4), 491–497.

Al-Salem, M., & Rawashdeh, N. (1993). Consanguinity in north Jordan: Prevalence and pattern. *Journal of Biosocial Science, 25*(4), 553–556.

Assaf, S., & Khawaja, M. (2009). Consanguinity trends and correlates in the Palestinian Territories. *Journal of Biosocial Science, 41*(1), 107–124.

Barbour, B., & Salameh, P. (2009). Consanguinity in Lebanon: Prevalence, distribution and determinants. *Journal of Biosocial Science, 41*(4), 505–517.

Bener, A., & Alali, K. A. (2006). Consanguineous marriage in a newly developed country: The Qatari population. *Journal of Biosocial Science, 38*(2), 239–246.

Bener, A., Ayoubi, H. R., Ali, A. I., Al-Kubaisi, A., & Al-Sulaiti, H. (2010). Does consanguinity lead to decreased incidence of breast cancer? *Cancer Epidemiology, 34*(4), 413–418.

Bener, A., El Ayoubi, H. R., Chouchane, L., Ali, A. I., Al-Kubaisi, A., Al-Sulaiti, H., et al. (2009). Impact of consanguinity on cancer in a highly endogamous population. *Asian Pacific Journal of Cancer Prevention, 10*(1), 35–40.

Bittles, A. H. (2008). A community genetics perspective on consanguineous marriage. *Community Genetics, 11*(6), 324–330.

Bittles, A. H., & Black, M. L. (2010). Evolution in health and medicine Sackler colloquium: Consanguinity, human evolution, and complex diseases. *Proceedings of the National Academy of Sciences of the United States of America, 107*(Suppl 1), 1779–1786.

Bras, H., Van Poppel, F., & Mandemakers, K. (2009). Relatives as spouses: Preferences and opportunities for kin marriage in a Western society. *American Journal of Human Biology, 21*(6), 793–804.

Clark, C. J., Hill, A., Jabbar, K., & Silverman, J. G. (2009). Violence during pregnancy in Jordan: Its prevalence and associated risk and protective factors. *Violence Against Women, 15*(6), 720–735.

Denic, S., Bener, A., Sabri, S., Khatib, F., & Milenkovic, J. (2005). Parental consanguinity and risk of breast cancer: A population-based case-control study. *Medical Science Monitor, 11*(9), CR415–CR419.

Department of Statistics [Jordan] and Macro International Inc. (2008). *Jordan Population and Family Health Survey 2007.* Calverton, MD: Department of Statistics and Macro International Inc.

El-Hazmi, M. A., al-Swailem, A. R., Warsy, A. S., al-Swailem, A. M., Sulaimani, R., & al-Meshari, A. A. (1995). Consanguinity among the Saudi Arabian population. *Journal of Medical Genetics, 32*(8), 623–626.

El-Mouzan, M. I., Al-Salloum, A. A., Al-Herbish, A. S., Qurachi, M. M., & Al-Omar, A. A. (2007). Regional variations in the prevalence of consanguinity in Saudi Arabia. *Saudi Medical Journal, 28*(12), 1881–1884.

El-Zanaty, F., & Way, A. (2006). *Egypt demographic and health survey 2005*. Cairo: Ministry of Health and Population [Egypt], National Population Council, El-Zanaty and Associates, and ORC Macro.

Faramarzi, M., Esmailzadeh, S., & Mosavi, S. (2005). Prevalence and determinants of intimate partner violence in Babol City, Islamic Republic of Iran. *Eastern Mediterranean Health Journal, 11*(5–6), 870–879.

Fikree, F. F., Jafarey, S. N., Korejo, R., Afshan, A., & Durocher, J. M. (2006). Intimate partner violence before and during pregnancy: Experiences of postpartum women in Karachi, Pakistan. *Journal of the Pakistan Medical Association, 56*(6), 252–557.

Freire-Maia, N. (1968). Inbreeding levels in American and Canadian populations: A comparison with Latin America. *Eugenics Quarterly, 15*(1), 22–33.

Garcia-Moreno, C., Jansen, H. A., Ellsberg, M., Heise, L., & Watts, C. H. (2006). Prevalence of intimate partner violence: Findings from the WHO multi-country study on women's health and domestic violence. *Lancet, 368*, 1260–1269.

Gunaid, A. A., Hummad, N. A., & Tamim, K. A. (2004). Consanguineous marriage in the capital city Sana'a, Yemen. *Journal of Biosocial Science, 36*(1), 111–121.

Hafez, M., El-Tahan, H., Awadalla, M., El-Khayat, H., Abdel-Gafar, A., & Ghoneim, M. (1983). Consanguineous matings in the Egyptian population. *Journal of Medical Genetics, 20*(1), 58–60.

Hamamy, H., Antonarakis, S. E., Cavalli-Sforza, L. L., Temtamy, S., Romeo, G., Kate, L. P., et al. (2011). Consanguineous marriages, pearls and perils: Geneva International Consanguinity Workshop Report. *Genetics in Medicine, 13*(9), 841–847.

Hamamy, H., Jamhawi, L., Al-Darawsheh, J., & Ajlouni, K. (2005). Consanguineous marriages in Jordan: Why is the rate changing with time? *Clinical Genetics, 67*(6), 511–516.

Hamzeh, B., Farshi, M. G., & Laflamme, L. (2008). Opinions of married women about potential causes and triggers of intimate partner violence against women. A cross-sectional investigation in an Iranian city. *BioMed Central Public Health, 8*, 209.

Jaber, L., Halpern, G. J., & Shohat, T. (2000). Trends in the frequencies of consanguineous marriages in the Israeli Arab community. *Clinical Genetics, 58*(2), 106–110.

Jurdi, R., & Saxena, P. C. (2003). The prevalence and correlates of consanguineous marriages in Yemen: Similarities and contrasts with other Arab countries. *Journal of Biosocial Science, 35*(1), 1–13.

Kanaan, Z. M., Mahfouz, R., & Tamim, H. (2008). The prevalence of consanguineous marriages in an underserved area in Lebanon and its association with congenital anomalies. *Genetic Testing, 12*(3), 367–372.

Keenan, C. K., El-Hadad, A., & Balian, S. A. (1998). Factors associated with domestic violence in low-income Lebanese families. *The Journal of Nursing Scholarship, 30*(4), 357–362.

Khawaja, M., & Hammoury, N. (2008). Coerced sexual intercourse within marriage: A clinic-based study of pregnant Palestinian refugees in Lebanon. *Journal of Midwifery & Women's Health, 53*(2), 150–154.

Khlat, M. (1988). Consanguineous marriages in Beirut: Time trends, spatial distribution. *Social Biology, 35*(3–4), 324–330.

Khoury, S. A., & Massad, D. (1992). Consanguineous marriage in Jordan. *American Journal of Medical Genetics, 43*(5), 769–775.

Koenig, M. A., Ahmed, S., Hossain, M. B., & Mozumder, K. A. A. B. (2003). Women's status and domestic violence in rural Bangladesh: Individual-and community level effects. *Demography, 40*(2), 269–288.

Kramer, A., Lorenzon, D., & Mueller, G. (2004). Prevalence of intimate partner violence and health implications for women using emergency departments and primary care clinics. *Women's Health Issues, 14*(1), 19–29.

Laanpere, M., Ringmets, I., Part, K., & Karro, H. (2012). Intimate partner violence and sexual health outcomes: A population-based study among 16-44 year old women in Estonia. *European Journal of Public Health, 23*(4), 688–693.

Mamdouh, H. M., Ismail, H. M., Kharboush, I. F., Tawfik, M. M., El Sharkawy, O. G., Abdel-Baky, M., et al. (2012). Prevalence and risk factors for spousal violence among women attending health care centres in Alexandria, Egypt. *Eastern Mediterranean Health Journal, 18*(11), 1118–1126.

Maziak, W., & Asfar, T. (2003). Physical abuse in low-income women in Aleppo, Syria. *Health Care Women International, 24*(4), 313–326.

Mazza, D., Dennenrstein, L., & Ryan, V. (1996). Physical, sexual and emotional violence against women: A general practice-based prevalence study. *Medical Journal of Australia, 164*(1), 14–17.

Mozdeh, N. L. A., Ghazinour, M., Nojomi, M., & Richter, J. (2012). The buffering effect of social support between domestic violence and self-esteem in pregnant women in Teheran, Iran. *Journal of Family Violence, 27*, 225–231.

Othman, H., & Saadat, M. (2009). Prevalence of consanguineous marriages in Syria. *Journal of Biosocial Science, 41*(5), 685–692.

Pedersen, J. (2002). The influence of consanguineous marriage on infant and child mortality among Palestinians in the West Bank and Gaza, Jordan, Lebanon and Syria. *Community Genetics, 5*(3), 178–181.

Radovanovic, Z., Shah, N., & Behbehani, J. (1999). Prevalence and social correlates to consanguinity in Kuwait. *Annals of Saudi Medicine, 19*(3), 206–210.

Rao, V. (1997). Wife-beating in rural south India: A qualitative and econometric analysis. *Social Science and Medicine, 44*, 1169–1180.

Saadat, M., & Vakili-Ghartavol, R. (2010). Parental consanguinity and susceptibility to drug abuse among offspring, a case-control study. *Psychiatry Research, 180*(1), 57–59.

Sharkia, R., Zaid, M., Athamna, A., Cohen, D., Azem, A., & Zalan, A. (2008). The changing pattern of consanguinity in a selected region of the Israeli Arab community. *American Journal of Human Biology, 20*(1), 72–77.

Stoltenberg, C., Magnus, P., Lie, R. T., Daltveit, A. K., & Irgens, L. M. (1998). Influence of consanguinity and maternal education on risk of stillbirth and infant death in Norway, 1967–1993. *American Journal of Epidemiology, 148*(5), 452–459.

Straus, M. A., Hamby, S. L., Buncy-McCoy, S., & Sugarman, D. B. (1996). The revised Conflict Tactics Scales (CTS2): Development and preliminary psychometric data. *Journal of Family Issues, 17*(3), 283–316.

Tadmouri, G. O., Nair, P., Obeid, T., Al Ali, M. T., Al Khaja, N., & Hamamy, H. A. (2009). Consanguinity and reproductive health among Arabs. *Reproductive Health, 6*, 17. doi:10.1186/1742-4755-6-17.

Tashkandi, A. A. W., & Rasheed, P. (2010). Physical wife abuse: A study among Saudi women attending primary health care centers. *Journal of the Bahrain Medical Society, 22*(1), 23–30.

Usta, J., Farver, J. A., & Pashayan, N. (2007). Domestic violence: The Lebanese experience. *Public Health, 121*, 208–219.

Vakili, M., Nadrian, H., Fathipoor, M., Boniadi, F., & Morowatisharifabad, M. A. (2010). Prevalence and determinants of intimate partner violence against women in Kazeroon, Islamic Republic of Iran. *Violence and Victims, 25*(1), 116–127.

Vardi-Saliternik, R., Friedlander, Y., & Cohen, T. (2002). Consanguinity in a population sample of Israeli Muslim Arabs, Christian Arabs and Druze. *Annals of Human Biology, 29*(4), 422–431.

Worden, A., & Carlson, B. (2005). Attitudes and beliefs about domestic violence: Results of a public opinion survey: II. Beliefs about causes. *Journal of Interpersonal Violence, 20*(10), 1219–1243.

Xu, X., Zhu, F., O'Campo, P., Koenig, M. A., Mock, V., & Campbell, J. (2005). Prevalence and risk factors for intimate partner violence in China. *American Journal of Public Health, 95*(1), 78–85.

Yount, K. M. (2005). Resources, family organization, and domestic violence against married women in Minya, Egypt. *Journal of Marriage and Family, 67*(3), 579–596.

Chapter 6
Women and Health in Refugee Settings: The Case of Displaced Syrian Women in Lebanon

Jinan Usta and Amelia Reese Masterson

Abstract The current conflict and humanitarian crisis in Syria continue to displace thousands of Syrians to neighboring countries, including Lebanon. This chapter examines the relation between refugee status, reproductive health outcomes, and domestic violence. We conducted a rapid needs assessment from June to August 2012 in Lebanon to collect information on Syrian women's current reproductive health status; their reproductive history before the conflict; their need for services; their experience with sexual and gender-based violence; and their help-seeking behaviors. We interviewed 452 displaced Syrian women aged 18–45 who have been in Lebanon for an average of 5.1 (±3.7) months. Additionally, 29 women participated in three focus group discussions. Of the 452 women surveyed, 74 were pregnant during the conflict, and several of them were pregnant more than once since the beginning of the conflict. Preterm delivery was highly reported (27 %), as well as pregnancy-related problems, including anemia, abdominal pain, and bleeding. As for reproductive health, menstrual irregularity, dysmenorrhea, and symptoms of reproductive tract infections were common. Moreover, 31 % of women had personal experience of violence (physical, sexual, or psychological), and many reported currently experiencing intimate partner violence. A conceptual framework is proposed to show how multiple factors may interplay to affect the reproductive health of women and their exposure to violence, with stress and mental distress being the main mitigating factors. Provision of psychological support within humanitarian aid is proposed to alleviate the effect of war and displacement.

Keywords Syrian women • Refugee • Reproductive health • Domestic violence • Sexual and gender-based violence

---

This chapter draws on previously published work written by the authors: Reese Masterson A., Usta J., Gupta J., Ettinger A.S. (2014). Assessment of reproductive health and violence against women among displaced Syrian in Lebanon. *BMC Women's Health,* 14:25.

J. Usta (✉) • A. Reese Masterson
American University of Beirut, Family Medicine Department, Beirut, Lebanon
e-mail: ju00@aub.edu.lb; areesemasterson@gmail.com

© Springer International Publishing Switzerland 2015   119
Y.K. Djamba, S.R. Kimuna (eds.), *Gender-Based Violence,*
DOI 10.1007/978-3-319-16670-4_6

Introduction

Wars have deleterious effects on the health and well-being of individuals, families, and communities causing tremendous mortality and disability, reduction in material and human capital, as well as disruption of the social and economic fabric of nations. The consequences of war last long after the conflict is over and may include not only death, but also endemic poverty, malnutrition, disability, socioeconomic decline, and psychosocial illnesses. Women, because of their vulnerability, bear a substantial proportion of war's effects.

Gender-Based Violence During Wartime

Studies have revealed that women, during armed conflicts and in refugee settings, become more susceptible to sexual and gender-based violence (SGBV) both as a weapon of war and in the form of intimate partner violence (McGinn 2000). Acts of war-related SGBV include forced sex and resulting pregnancy, abduction, rape, sexual slavery, and forced prostitution (Depoortere et al. 2004; Hynes et al. 2004; Van Herp et al. 2003).

A growing body of research suggests a link between exposure to violence by armed groups and domestic violence (Catani et al. 2008; Gupta et al. 2009), particularly in refugee settings (Pittaway 2004; Usta et al. 2008; Stark and Ager 2011), with women often facing just as much danger in the home as outside the home (El-Jack 2003). High levels of domestic violence have been reported in postwar and refugee settings around the world, as highlighted in United Nations (UN) agency and nongovernmental organization (NGO) reports from the West Bank and Gaza (Human Rights Watch 2006), refugee settings in Tanzania (Human Rights Watch 2000), Nepal (Human Rights Watch 2003), postwar Peru (Gallegos and Gutierrez 2011), and Sri Lanka (Rajasingham-Senanayake 2004). Additionally, refugee crises were found to affect domestic violence even in host communities (Nikolic-Ristanovic 2000).

For several reasons, researching violence to which women are exposed during war is difficult. To begin with, survivors of violence are more likely to suffer in silence because of fear of shame and stigmatization (Zimmerman 1995). The breakdown of law and order associated with war makes it even more difficult for survivors to report violence through formal mechanisms (World Health Organization 2007; Byrne 1996). In addition, structures needed to cope with and monitor domestic violence are impaired in times of war (Farnsworth et al. 2012), making data collection quite challenging. Yet, findings suggest a relationship between war violence and family violence, which is reflected in high levels of spousal beatings in refugee and resettlement communities (Pittaway 2004).

Several studies in Lebanon have addressed the issue of domestic violence in refugee settings. A household survey among Palestinian refugee couples reveals that 22–29.5 % reported domestic violence to have ever occurred, while 10 %

reported an episode of domestic violence in the previous year (Khawaja and Tewtel-Salem 2004). Another study in Lebanon among 310 women displaced by the 2006 war found that 39 % reported at least one encounter with violence perpetrated by soldiers, while 27 % reported at least one incident of domestic abuse during the conflict, and 13 % reported at least one incident perpetrated by their husbands or other family members after the conflict (Usta et al. 2008).

Reproductive Health During Conflict and Displacement

Research also shows that conflict and displacement can affect women's reproductive health through both individual and environmental or social mechanisms. A review of the literature on refugee women identified five categories of reproductive health issues—fertility, sexually transmitted infections, SGBV, pregnancy and childbirth, and health service access—that can be affected by conditions of displacement (Gagnon et al. 2002; McGinn 2000).

Findings on migration's effect on fertility rates are mixed, but it is clear that decision making surrounding family planning is affected by displacement, with some women or couples opting to delay pregnancy because of instability and uncertainty, while others seek to replace deceased family members (Gagnon et al. 2002; McGinn 2000). Research has shown that risk of sexually transmitted infection increases during wartime due to various factors such as displacement or migration, military movement, widespread SGBV, psychological stress, and economic disruption (Gagnon et al. 2002; McGinn 2000). Additionally, risk of reproductive tract infections (non-sexually transmitted) may increase in refugee settings. Pregnancy and childbirth outcomes in such settings vary depending on the nature of the refugee situation (stable, camp setting vs. informal or urban housing), and level of access to services such as antenatal care and delivery (IAWG 2010; Gagnon et al. 2002; McGinn 2000; Jamieson et al. 2000; Lederman 1995).

Syrian Refugee Situation

The current Syrian refugee crisis provides a unique setting to study reproductive health and gender-based violence in conflict situations; with conflict beginning in March 2011 and continuing to displace Syrians today, a relatively long duration of follow-up is available. There is a wide variety in displacement living conditions, with refugees in both informal and formal camps, rural and urban settings, and many constantly on the move.

At the beginning of data collection for this study in 2012 there were approximately 48,000 displaced Syrians in Lebanon (UNHCR 2014a). By May 2014, the number of Syrian refugees in Lebanon was estimated to be slightly over one million (UNHCR 2014a) and approaching two million according to local reports.

Further, approximately 25 % of Syrian refugees in Lebanon are women between the ages of 18 and 45 years. The mountainous border region of North Lebanon (in the areas of Akkar and Wadi Khaled) and the Bekaa Valley along Lebanon's eastern border continue to host the majority of Syrian refugees in Lebanon, and the two locations are the study site for this research.

Numerous agency reports and media accounts describe violence (including SGBV) and reproductive healthcare shortages surrounding the Syrian conflict (El-Masri et al. 2013; MSF 2012; Tuysuz 2011; Amnesty International 2012; Human Rights Watch 2012; International Rescue Committee 2012). Thus, measurement of these issues is critical. Syrian women and girls are at increased risk of SGBV, deteriorating mental health, and maternal and newborn complications, as well as facing daily struggles meeting basic needs for themselves and their families. Around 25 % of refugee households in Lebanon are now female headed, and there has been a shift in gender roles due to unemployment among males, changing household structures, and women's lack of access to the resources and services that were once available to them in Syria (UNHCR 2014b; El-Masri et al. 2013) (Fig. 6.1).

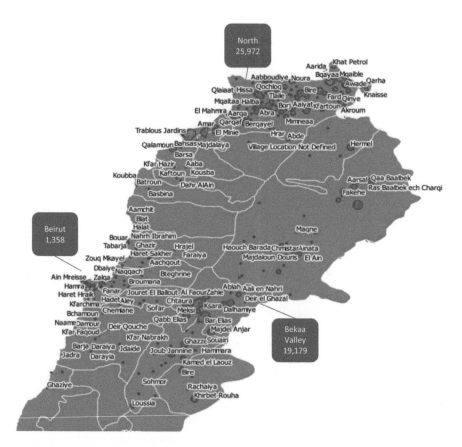

Fig. 6.1 Map of Syrian refugee distribution in Lebanon at the time of study (UNHCR, September 2012)

Study Aims

In addition to contributing to the larger body of literature on SGBV and reproductive health in conflict settings, this study builds on local understanding of SGBV and reproductive health needs among Syrian refugee women for the purpose of informing humanitarian response. The goals of this study align with research priorities set by the Interagency-Working Group (IAWG) on Reproductive Health in Crisis (CDC 2011), including understanding how to strengthen comprehensive GBV prevention and response services in refugee settings, improving access to delivery care and emergency obstetric services for refugee women, and understanding how conflict affects fertility and pregnancy-related decisions.

The overall goals of this study are to understand the reproductive health and GBV-related outcomes of displaced Syrian women living in Lebanon and to inform humanitarian programs and services aimed at supporting Syrian women. The specific aims of the research are to (a) describe the current reproductive status and needs of displaced Syrian women living in Lebanon; (b) explore factors that may be associated with poor reproductive outcomes, including health service access and experiences of violence; (c) describe the type and characteristics of violence, including SGBV experienced by Syrian women; and (d) identify the coping strategies and behaviors of Syrian women survivors of violence.

Methodology

Study Setting

This study was carried out as a needs assessment under the auspices of and with support from the United Nations Population Fund (UNFPA) in Lebanon between June and August 2012, 1 year after the conflict erupted in Syria, and as refugee numbers were rapidly escalating. A cross-sectional survey was carried out in six primary health clinics in North Lebanon and the Bekaa Valley, areas with the highest concentration of Syrian refugees. Three clinics were supported by a private foundation, two were jointly run by the Lebanese Ministry of Public Health (MOPH) and a private foundation, and one clinic was run solely by the MOPH. This study was approved by the Human Subjects Committee at Yale School of Public Health (YSPH) and by the United Nations Population Fund (UNFPA), Lebanon.

Three focus group discussions (FGDs) were carried out in different community centers—Baalbek, Arsal (Bekaa Valley), and Wadi Khaled (North Lebanon). The focus groups provided the perspectives of Syrian women outside of primary healthcare clinics and explored the issue of intimate partner violence (which was not a part of the survey).

Study Sample

For the survey component, clinics were selected based on the number of displaced Syrian women attending per month (at least 100) and the provision of comprehensive reproductive health services. We chose clinics supported by both government and nongovernment organizations in order to minimize bias. All clinics were receiving some type of support from UNFPA and its partners. We used a proportional sampling method, based on the number of Syrian women attending each clinic during the month prior to the study with the aim of recruiting at least 400 displaced Syrian women that fit the eligibility criteria, who were attending the selected clinics for any reason. The data collection started in July and ended in August when the desired sample size was reached. All displaced Syrian women attending the six clinics were approached for recruitment, screened for eligibility, and asked if they would like to participate in the study. This process was followed until the target number was reached. Eligibility criteria included (1) ability to speak Arabic, (2) identity as a Syrian national, (3) having come to Lebanon since the conflict in Syria began in March 2011, and (4) age between 18 and 45 (inclusive). Once screened, women were escorted into a separate room where an IRB-approved consent form was explained and signed prior to questionnaire administration.

FGD participants were recruited by local NGOs in areas where there was the highest concentration of Syrian refugees. Each FGD included 8–12 women aged between 18 and 45 years, who speak Arabic, and were present in Lebanon for over a month.

Measurement and Data Collection

The interviewer-administered questionnaire used in this study was adapted from the "Gender-based Violence Tools Manual - For Assessment & Program Design, Monitoring & Evaluation in Conflict-Affected Settings" (RHRC 2004) and the "Reproductive Health Assessment Toolkit for Conflict-Affected Women" (CDC 2007). The questionnaire was designed in English, discussed with the various stakeholders, translated into Arabic and pilot tested among Syrians in Lebanon, and administered in Arabic by trained research assistants. It included six sections addressing the following topics: (1) individual characteristics and displacement history; (2) general health status; (3) reproductive history and current status; (4) exposure to violence, including SGBV; (5) coping strategies and stress; and (6) pregnancy-related information (among a subset of those who were pregnant at any time during the conflict).

The discussion in the focus groups followed a guide adapted from the *Reproductive Health Response in Crisis Consortium* (RHRC), which is part of the *Women's Commission for Refugee Women and Children* and covered topics related to living conditions, reproductive and general health issues, violence, including both domestic violence and conflict-related violence, and coping strategies.

All participants received a UNFPA "dignity kit" containing basic sanitation supplies and clothing to compensate for their time, and were also given telephone numbers for agencies providing protection, health, and psychosocial resources for survivors of violence.

Data Analysis

Using survey data, bivariate associations were estimated using Pearson's correlations and X^2 test. Risk factors associated with outcomes of interest and covariates associated with both risk factors and outcomes (at the level of $p < 0.05$) were retained in multivariate models. Multivariate logistic regression was used to examine the relationships between independent variables (exposure to conflict violence and stress score) and health outcomes (gynecologic conditions, self-rated health, and access to reproductive health services). Stress was also examined as a mediating variable between conflict violence and health outcomes.

Conflict violence was coded as a binary variable, which was measured by a positive response ("1–2 times" or "frequently") to any of the indicators of violence from an armed person since the conflict began, including being slapped or hit; choked; beaten or kicked; threatened with a weapon; shot at or stabbed; detained against will; intentionally deprived of food, water, or sleep; emotional abuse or humiliation; deprived of money; or subjected to improper sexual behavior. Stress was assessed using a 6-question subscale previously used in UNFPA surveys in Lebanon and adapted to include a question about child beating as a response to stress, based on qualitative findings. The subscale included the following: feeling constantly tense, sick or tired, worried or concerned, irritable or in a bad mood, suffering from loss of sleep or sleep disorders, reduced ability to complete normal tasks, and beating or taking anger out on children. Principal component analysis was used to create a stress score variable based on participant responses.

The following variables were examined as potential confounders in the relationship between violence, stress, and reproductive health outcomes using bivariate analysis; and those with biological plausibility were included in multivariate models: age, education, marital status, region in Lebanon, clinic and clinic type (government funded or not), place of origin (urban versus rural), months in Lebanon, food insecurity indicators, cigarette smoking, anemia, and hypertension. Data were analyzed using Statistical Analysis Software (SAS) v 9.2, and principal component analysis was carried out in IBM SPSS Statistics 21 due to ease of use.

For the qualitative component, the three FGD audio-recordings were transcribed verbatim in Arabic, translated into English, and reviewed by two researchers to identify major themes. Researchers then manually coded each transcript for the presence of themes and differences of opinion were discussed and resolved.

Results

Sample Characteristics

Of the 489 Syrian women approached to participate, 9 did not meet eligibility criteria, 28 declined to participate, and 452 (92.4 %) completed the interviews. Of these, 251 lived in North Lebanon and 201 in the Bekaa Valley (Table 6.1). Demographic characteristics were similar across regions, with several exceptions in statistical significance: those in the Bekaa Valley were slightly younger ($p=0.03$) and less likely to have been married ($p=0.01$). More women were living in formal housing in North Lebanon (91.6 %) than in the Bekaa Valley (80.0 %) ($p=0.0004$); women in North Lebanon had been in Lebanon longer on average (6 months) than those in the Bekaa Valley (4.5 months) ($p=0.001$); and those in the North Lebanon were more likely to receive humanitarian services than those in Bekaa Valley (88.6 % and 62.9 %, respectively, at $p<0.0001$).

The focus group participants were 29 women who had lived in Lebanon for about 4 months, most were married, and 3 were pregnant at the time that the FGDs were conducted. Some of the women were staying in informal dwellings accommodating several families, and others in shared rented houses or apartments.

Table 6.1 Characteristics of the sample by region[a]

	North Lebanon ($n=251$) N (%) or mean (±SD)	Bekaa ($n=201$) N (%) or mean (±SD)	p-Value
Age			
18–24	53 (21.4)	64 (31.8)	0.03
25–34	111 (44.8)	83 (41.3)	
35–45	84 (33.9)	54 (26.9)	
Ever-married	232 (92.4)	166 (82.6)	0.01
Living in formal housing	229 (91.6)	160 (80.0)	0.0004
Avg. months in Lebanon	6±3.9	4.5±3.4	0.001
Have received humanitarian services	220 (88.6)	126 (62.9)	<.0001
From urban area in Syria	124 (49.6)	97 (48.7)	0.86
Education			
No education	37 (14.8)	26 (13.1)	0.75
Less than high school	154 (61.6)	127 (64.1)	
High school	43 (17.2)	29 (14.7)	
Greater than high school	16 (6.4)	16 (8.1)	

[a]Numbers may not sum up to total due to missing data; percentages may not sum up to 100 % due to rounding or multiple-response questions. Column percent is reported

Living Conditions and General Health

Respondents reported lack of access to amenities for basic hygiene, including piped drinking water (31.9 %), feminine hygiene products (27.7 %), washing water (25.9 %), soap (26.3 %), and bathing facilities (20.8 %). Focus group participants echoed these gaps in service provision, giving a picture of difference between their lives before the conflict and their lives now. Several needs came to the forefront of the discussion. All spoke of water shortages resulting in inability to bathe, wash the children, and do laundry. One of the FGD respondents noted, "In Syria, it was better even during the conflict. We had water, so if the kids want to play they can wash." Some had to travel long distances to a well to get water for daily use and buy bottled water to drink but lamented the price of water, as one woman from the focus groups stated, "One plastic water bottle here is 1,000 Lebanese Liras (0.66 U.S. dollars); this is expensive."

Survey results found crowded conditions with 12.8 % of women living with more than five children and five adults in a single dwelling (i.e., not group housing). Focus group results highlighted the issue of crowding, and lack of activities for children that led to stress. One FGD participant reported, "We are all living in a tin house. We are six families with 13 children playing around and we are not able to control them. There are no toys, games, or playing groups."

The majority of survey respondents agreed with all three indicators of food insecurity. Women in focus groups talked about food deficiency and the lack of storage for food, given the hot and crowded conditions in which they lived: "We need fridge; we need a place to keep the food away from insects." In general, women reported that the cost of living in Lebanon was much higher than in Syria, which was worrisome to the well-being of the family. In addition, lack of registration as a refugee with UNHCR contributed to limiting their access to basic services. Needs such as money for rent, healthcare services, activities for children, and water seemed to take precedence over the need for food aid for some women. "We don't want food, we need health care. We wish you can secure healthcare for us and help us."

When asked in the survey, "How would you rate your overall health: excellent, good, acceptable, poor, or very poor?" most participants rated their overall health as acceptable (38.9 %) and 17.7 % rated their health as poor or very poor. The majority (79.7 %) reported never smoking cigarettes or water pipe (85.2 %). Anemia was the most commonly reported condition with an overall reported prevalence of 27.4 %. Current medication use was reported by 39.4 %, most commonly for cardiovascular conditions (6.9 %), mental health conditions (5.3 %), and gynecologic infections (4.4 %) (Table 6.2).

Women spoke at great length in focus groups about mental health needs, both among their children and themselves. They identified several major sources of stress in their lives: fear for family members back in Syria, boring routine, lack of distracting activities, safety concerns in Lebanon, and helplessness at seeing their children suffer from psychological distress. A woman from the focus groups said,

Table 6.2 Individual characteristics, displacement characteristics, and general health status of Syrian refugee women in Lebanon (N=452)[a]

	N (%) or mean (±SD)
Individual characteristics	
Region of current residence	
North Lebanon	251 (55.5)
Bekaa Valley	201 (44.5)
Age	
18–24	117 (25.9)
25–34	194 (42.9)
35–45	138 (30.5)
Education	
No education	63 (13.9)
Less than high school	129 (28.5)
High school	152 (33.6)
Greater than high school	104 (23.0)
Marital status	
Married	381 (84.3)
Widowed	11 (2.4)
Divorced/separated	6 (1.3)
Never married	54 (12.0)
Consanguineous marriage[b]	172 (38.1)
Age at first marriage[b]	19.0±4.0
Currently employed	11 (2.4)
Primary source(s) of income	
No income	153 (33.9)
Husband	171 (37.8)
Family	61 (13.5)
Self	14 (3.1)
Charity/assistance	98 (21.7)
Displacement characteristics	
From a city in Syria (not a village)	221 (48.9)
Reasons for leaving	
Security concerns/fear	445 (98.5)
Lack of daily necessities	306 (67.7)
Lack of health care	279 (61.7)
Other	13 (2.9)
Living situation in Lebanon	
Residing in informal housing (tent, shop, school, etc.)	61 (13.5)
Months in current place of residence	4.6±3.6
Months in Lebanon	5.1±3.7
No. of children (<18) in residence	3.8±2.8
No. of adults (>18) in residence	3.7±3.7

(continued)

Table 6.2 (continued)

	N (%) or mean ($\pm$SD)
Food insecurity	
Worry about having enough food (sometimes/often)	284 (62.8)
Eat non-preferred food (sometimes/often)	264 (58.4)
Skip meals (sometimes/often)	249 (55.1)
General health status	
Self-rated overall health	
Excellent	37 (8.2)
Good	157 (34.7)
Acceptable/fair	176 (38.9)
Poor	64 (14.2)
Very poor	16 (3.5)
Cigarette smoker (some days/every day)	90 (19.9)
Chronic conditions	
Anemia	124 (27.4)
Hypertension	55 (12.2)
Diabetes	14 (3.1)
Others[c]	120 (26.6)
Currently on medication for any condition	178 (39.4)

(*Table reference*: Adapted from Reese Masterson et al. 2014)
[a]Numbers may not sum to total due to missing data
[b]Denominator is ever-married women ($n=398$)
[c]Others: Musculoskeletal issues, cardiovascular issues, abdominal issues, mental health and psychosomatic issues, vaginal infections, and urinary-tract infections

"My son is 4 years; he got scared from the first shelling that struck nearby. His jaw was broken. I take him to the doctor every three months for treatment, I pay for it."

At the end of the survey interview, women were asked to identify their three "biggest health concerns." These were grouped into loose categories and listed in Table 6.3 according to the frequency with which they were cited. Concerns related to reproductive health were the most common. Additionally, 26 women raised issues related to pregnancy or breastfeeding, with delivery costs and services highlighted as most important issues to address.

Reproductive Health

Table 6.4 below shows the reproductive history and current status and use of health services. Of the 452 women interviewed, the majority reported gynecologic problems experienced during the conflict, including menstrual irregularity (53.5 %), symptoms of reproductive tract infection (53.3 %), and severe pelvic pain or

Table 6.3 Syrian refugee women's top health concerns

Health concern	Description	# Times cited
Reproductive health needs	Genital infections, infertility, pelvic pain, OB/GYN services, contraception	58
Musculoskeletal issues	Injuries and musculoskeletal pain	37
Needs of children	Milk, diapers, doctor's visit	40
General relief services	Range of daily items needed for survival	30
Pregnancy issues	Delivery, pregnancy complications and concerns, breastfeeding	26
Cardiovascular issues		24
Abdominal issues		24
Headaches and general pain	Issues for which women are taking basic painkillers	20
Access to care and medication		17
Nutritional issues		12
Mental health	Depression, anxiety, psychological issues	12
Urinary issues	UTI, kidney stones, renal problems	11
Medical testing/surgery		11
Psychosomatic issues	Stress, fatigue, dizziness, loss of appetite, repeated vomiting, need for sedatives, sleeping issues	9
Anemia	Self-reported iron deficiency	8

dysmenorrhea (51.6 %). Additionally, 37.8 % reported having all three conditions. Of the 26.1 % who visited a gynecologist in the past 6 months, 27.2 % were diagnosed with a reproductive tract infection. Similarly, women in the FGDs disclosed having gynecological problems, including irregular menstruation. For instance one woman noted, "When they took my husband, my menses stopped." Also, the women reported heavier menstruation than normal and symptoms of reproductive tract infection including itchiness, long-standing abnormal vaginal discharge, and infection.

When asked about access to reproductive health services, only 32.3 % thought that these services were easily accessible, while 37.8 % reported that these services were unavailable and 16.8 % answered that they did not know if these services existed. Women reported cost (49.7 %), distance or transport (25.4 %), and fear of mistreatment (7.9 %) as the primary barriers to accessing reproductive health care. Other barriers included security concerns, shame, unavailability of a female doctor, and insufficient provision of services. The majority (59.7 %) reported that they had not visited a gynecologist except when they were pregnant. Although 69.3 % of women knew about contraception, only 34.5 % were using some method of contraception, which is below that reported among the general population in pre-conflict Syria (58.3 %) (UNICEF 2008). The most commonly used method of contraception was the intrauterine device (IUD) (19.0 %), followed by oral contraceptives (8.6 %) and the rhythm method (3.5 %). This was consistent with Syrian national statistics (UNICEF 2008). Similar to barriers to accessing care, women reported that cost,

Table 6.4 Reproductive history, current reproductive status, and use of services among 452 Syrian refugee women in Lebanon[a]

	N (%) or mean (±SD)
Reproductive history	
Age at menarche	15.4±11.1
Age at first pregnancy	19.9±4.4
Number of pregnancies	4.7±3.5
At least one miscarriage	126 (27.9)
At least one abortion (induced)	11 (2.4)
At least one cesarean section	111 (24.6)
At least one child death	80 (17.7)
Current reproductive status	
Pregnant at some point during the conflict	74 (16.4)
Currently pregnant	43 (9.5)
Reported gynecologic issues during conflict	
Menstrual irregularities	242 (53.5)
Severe pelvic pain/dysmenorrhea	233 (51.6)
Symptoms of reproductive tract infection	241 (53.3)
Perception and use of reproductive health services	
Perception of RH service availability	
Available	202 (44.7)
Unavailable	171 (37.8)
Don't know	76 (16.8)
Perception of RH service accessibility	
Easily accessible	146 (32.3)
Inaccessible/difficult to access	177 (39.2)
Don't know	47 (10.4)
Perceived barriers to access (n=177)	
Price	88 (49.7)
Distance/transport	45 (25.4)
Fear of mistreatment	14 (7.9)
Security concerns	11 (6.2)
Shame/embarrassment	11 (6.2)
Other	8 (4.5)
Use of RH services during past 6 months	
Visited OB/GYN doctor for any reason	118 (26.1)
Diagnosed with reproductive tract infection	123 (27.2)
Use of Family Planning Method/Contraception	
None	296 (65.5)
IUD	86 (19.0)
Birth control pill	39 (8.6)
Rhythm method	16 (3.5)
Surgical method	11 (2.4)
Condoms	8 (1.8)
Injection	1 (0.2)

(*Table reference*: Adapted from Reese Masterson et al. 2014)
[a]Numbers may not sum to total due to missing data

distance or transportation, and unavailability were the primary barriers to contraceptive use. Additionally, some reported fear of using contraceptives, and others reported that they simply had not acquired contraceptives.

Of the entire sample, 65.9 % had ever been pregnant and 16.4 % reported being pregnant at some point during the conflict (see Table 6.5). Among this pregnancy subset of 74 women, 73.0 % had attended at least one antenatal care visit. The most commonly reported barriers to antenatal care use were unavailability of a reproductive health clinician (18.9 %), cost (9.5 %), and distance or transportation (6.8 %). Thirty-eight women delivered or had an abortion (spontaneous or induced) during the conflict, with the majority occurring in a hospital (71.1 %), though some were reported to have taken place at home (23.7 %). Among those who completed a pregnancy since the conflict began, there were nine preterm births (23.7 %), four spontaneous and induced abortions (10.5 %), four low-birth-weight term infants

Table 6.5 Characteristics of 74 Syrian refugee women who were pregnant at some time during the conflict[a]

	N (%)
Pregnancy status[a]	
Currently pregnant	43 (9.5)
Delivered	34 (7.5)
Aborted fetus	4 (0.9)
Primiparous	16 (21.6)
At least one antenatal care visit	54 (73.0)
Pregnancy complications among currently pregnant (n = 43)	
Feeling unusually weak/tired	11 (25.6)
Severe abdominal pain	7 (16.3)
Vaginal bleeding	4 (9.3)
Fever	2 (4.7)
Swelling of hands and face	2 (4.7)
Others (vaginal infection, blurred vision, preeclampsia)	3 (7.0)
Delivery/abortion complications (n = 38)	
Hemorrhage	11 (29.0)
Abnormal vaginal discharge	3 (7.9)
Others (convulsions, fever, hypertension, fetal heart problem, vaginal tearing)	5 (13.2)
Place of delivery/abortion (n = 38)	
Home	9 (23.7)
Hospital	27 (71.1)
Clinic or doctor's office	2 (5.3)
Birth outcomes among those who delivered (n = 34)	
Preterm birth	9 (26.5)
Low birth weight[b]	4 (10.5)
Infant death	1 (2.9)

(*Table reference*: Adapted from Reese Masterson et al. 2014)
[a]Numbers may not sum to total due to missing data
[b]Infant birth weight not known (n=3)

(10.5 %), and one infant death. The most common complications during labor, delivery, or abortion were cited by 36.8% of women, with hemorrhage being the most commonly reported (29.0 %).

Of the 33 live births, 52 % reported that their infant experienced some type of complication within the first 40 days of birth, including sickness and abdominal pain, respiratory distress and infections, injury, disability, malnutrition, umbilical hernia, and issues related to preterm birth requiring a stay in the intensive care unit. Only 48.5 % of these reported any breastfeeding, citing the inability to breastfeed, illness, and constant displacement as reasons for not breastfeeding. Most of the 43 women pregnant at the time of the survey were pregnant upon arrival to Lebanon while 32.6 % became pregnant after displacement. Pregnancy problems were reported by 39.5 % including feeling abnormally weak and tired (25.6 %), severe abdominal pain (16.3 %), vaginal bleeding (9.3 %), and fever (4.7 %). Of those currently pregnant, 69.8 % had at least one antenatal care visit; however, the majority had not accessed antenatal care since arriving in Lebanon.

Focus group participants corroborated survey findings, highlighting anemia, decreased access to antenatal care, and negative effects of stress on the pregnancy. Focus group findings elucidate barriers to accessing antenatal care, with women expressing their frustration at visiting the local clinic, but continually finding that the reproductive health doctor had traveled, was booked with other patients, or was otherwise unavailable when needed. There was also worry about paying for antenatal services and delivery. One woman noted, "I went to Hariri clinic but it was 2000 L.L. [$2.32] for services for pregnant women there." This price is unaffordable for some Syrian women. One woman expressed that she and her husband are intentionally delaying pregnancy due to the high cost of delivery. Others expressed problems identifying a hospital in their vicinity with free delivery services. One other woman even said that she planned to use her Lebanese relative's identity to deliver her baby in order to gain access to reduced price delivery services.

Violence

Survey results showed that almost one-third of women ($N=139$, 30.8 %) reported exposure to conflict violence and more than a quarter ($N=125$, 27.7 %) reported exposure to more than one type of conflict violence. Almost all women (95.7 %) identified the perpetrator as an armed person, and 14 women (3.1 %) disclosed sexual violence perpetrated against them by an armed person in Syria. Of those who experienced violence, 27.7 % suffered physical injury and 67.7 % suffered psychological difficulties. Of those who experienced violence, 15 women were pregnant at some point during the conflict. Direct physical violence—such as hitting, slapping, or choking—was reported only among three pregnant women. One woman who was pregnant during the conflict said that she had been detained. The relationship between pregnancy complications and violence could not be assessed given the small number of pregnant women with direct exposure to violence.

In bivariate analyses, experience of conflict-violence had a strong positive association with menstrual irregularity ($p<0.001$), severe pelvic pain ($p<0.001$), reproductive tract infection (RTI) symptoms ($p<0.001$) among nonpregnant women, and self-rated health ($p=0.01$) among the entire sample (data not reported). Conflict violence was not associated with accessing obstetric/gynecology services ($p=0.20$). In multivariate models, among nonpregnant women, experience of conflict violence was significantly associated with all gynecologic outcomes, except self-rated health.

When asked to rate stress-related symptoms over the past month, relative to normal or usual levels, over 75 % of women reported having all seven stress-related symptoms more than usual. Based on principal component analysis, we created a "stress score" variable including all questions from the original 7-item stress scale, except for the question about feeling worried or concerned as it had a low loading in this analysis (0.43). Beating children, as an indicator of stress, had a high loading (0.7) on the stress construct and was therefore retained. Almost 76 % (75.8 %) of women reported beating their children more than usual. Only 16 % of women said that they never beat their children.

Looking at stress scores (Table 6.6), those who experienced conflict violence had a significantly higher mean stress score than those who did not ($p<0.0001$). In bivariate analysis, stress score was found to be associated with menstrual irregularity ($p<0.001$), severe pelvic pain ($p=0.02$), and RTI symptoms ($p=0.04$) among nonpregnant women, but not associated with accessing obstetric/gynecology services ($p=0.81$). In multivariate models, nonpregnant women were more likely to have menstrual irregularity with increasing stress levels ($p<0.01$) (Table 6.6). Stress

Table 6.6 Exposure to violence and stress score[a] with various health outcomes among Syrian women

Variable	N (%) or mean (range)	Menstrual irregularity ($n=409$) β (SE)	Severe pelvic pain ($n=409$) β (SE)	RTI symptoms ($n=409$) β (SE)	Self-rated health ($n=452$) β (SE)
Exposure to any conflict violence[b]	139 (30.8 %)	0.58 (0.27)*	0.68 (0.26)**	0.53 (0.25)*	0.08 (0.23)
Stress score[c]	0[a] (−3.28, 0.94)	0.32 (0.11)**	0.17 (0.11)	0.12 (0.11)	0.30 (0.11)**

(*Table reference*: Adapted from Reese Masterson et al. 2014)
*$p<0.05$, **$p<0.01$
[a]Stress score created using Anderson-Rubin method in SPSS, which gives a variable with mean 0 and SD 1
[b]Models are adjusted for region, age, education, marital status, and anemia; menstrual irregularity model is additionally adjusted for food insecurity; RTI model is additionally adjusted for months in Lebanon; self-rated health is additionally adjusted for food insecurity, hypertension, and cigarette smoking
[c]Models are adjusted for region, age, education, and marital status; model of self-rated health is additionally adjusted for food insecurity, cigarette smoking, and anemia

score, however, was not a significant predictor of other gynecologic conditions. Among the entire sample, women with higher levels of stress were more likely to have poor self-rated health ($p<0.01$). Stress score was found to mediate the relationship between experience of violence and self-rated health.

Focus group discussions moved beyond conflict violence to ask about all types of violence experienced by women since the conflict began. Women reported exposure to sexual violence outside the household and violence from their spouse and community. One woman reported having a neck problem at the beginning of the discussion. When the topic of violence came up, she admitted that her neck problem was due to a beating from her husband. No other women reported physical injuries. They seemed open to talk about this issue, and they referred to the spousal abuse as their husbands "letting go on us" or "letting go of the stress on us." Some participants told stories of sexual verbal harassment like experiencing sexual propositions in a shop, in a taxi, or when walking on the street.

Women pointed to the lack of work and inability to provide for the family as a major factor contributing to stress among men. Some men were sick or injured and could not work. Some had daily work or returned to Syria to work, but are not able to make enough to cover the high cost of living in Lebanon. Unstable housing and having to move the family from place to place were also considered by women as contributing to the tension in the home. "We were thrown out of the house because the landlord had his eye on a relative of mine, and we were all living in a house together. When the wife of the landlord found out, she threw us all out of the house."

Coping Strategies

The survey explored coping mechanisms that women used as a response to violence; however, these results are limited by a low response rate to the stress questionnaire. Of those who responded, the majority said that they have not yet coped with their experience. The others mentioned the following ways of coping: talking to someone (friend or relative), using mental health services, and trying to forget or sleep. Of note, although 71 % of those who experienced violence reported suffering from psychological difficulties, only 9 % reported receiving mental health assistance.

Women who experienced violence reported varying help-seeking behaviors: 41.5 % did not find a way to cope, 50.8 % did not speak with anyone, 24.6 % spoke with their husbands, and the remaining spoke with others in the community. When we asked those who chose not to tell anyone about their experience of violence and why this was the case, most responded that they "thought nothing could be done," and others said that they did not trust anyone or they felt ashamed or stigmatized. Of those exposed to violence, the majority (64.6 %) sought no medical care after their experience due to insufficient funds, lack of knowledge, unavailability, embarrassment, and other reasons. Only 9.2 % reported accessing any mental health or psychosocial assistance.

In focus groups, women were found to justify violence and accepted it as a natural result of the stress that their husbands are facing: "My husband works day and night and earns 5000 L.L. a day. We can't pay rent. We understand that this makes them stressed. They have to support us." Some showed helplessness: "There is nothing to do, we have to accept." Others wondered where to seek help: "Where do we go in case of violence?" or used avoidance: "We can't do anything to distract our mind or vent. We just cover ourselves and sleep." Most women confessed to beating their children to "let go of their stress."

One major positive coping factor that women mentioned was the feeling of solidarity brought by spending time with members of the community. Syrian women said that in some way the experience of displacement had brought them closer to each other. Friends, neighbors, and relatives are helping each other through the difficult times, lending each other kitchen utensils, sharing experiences, and providing solutions to each other's problems. One woman said, "All Syrians help each other. We are a group. Everyone helps everyone." Some women spoke also of supportive neighbors who help them with basic necessities.

Discussion

Our findings indicate that Syrian women displaced to Lebanon during the current crisis experience poor reproductive health—including gynecologic conditions, pregnancy and delivery complications, and poor birth outcomes—and that there is interplay between violence, stress, and poor health, including reproductive health. High rates of menstrual irregularity, severe pelvic pain, and reproductive tract infections among our sample are commensurate with results from prior research studying gynecologic outcomes in settings of conflict and displacement (Gagnon et al. 2002; Campbell 2002). Campbell's (2002) study on the impact of intimate partner violence showed that the most consistent difference between battered and non-battered women is gynecologic problems, including vaginal bleeding or infection, genital irritation, pain on intercourse, chronic pelvic pain, and urinary-tract infections. Similarly, our findings within a population affected by conflict-related violence seem to suggest that gynecologic problems can be women's nonspecific reactions to violence regardless of the origin of violence.

Previous studies of low birth weight among refugee women show mixed results, with some finding an increase in low birth weight among refugee populations and others finding no change or even an actual improvement in birth weight among refugees compared to non-refugees (McGinn 2000; Gagnon et al. 2002; Hynes et al. 2002). Improvements cited in the literature may be due to having comparatively better reproductive health services in refugee camps than in the general population, especially in resource-poor settings (Hynes et al. 2002). Preterm birth was highly reported within pregnant women in our sample, with a prevalence of around 27 %. These findings, however, should be interpreted with caution as they are based on self-reports. Syrian refugee women could be at greater risk for preterm birth for a number of reasons related to their status as refugees, such as inadequate antenatal care (Hamad et al. 2007) or economic hardship (Kramer et al. 2000).

In previous studies, anemia and hypertension were associated with complications surrounding pregnancy and delivery (Yanit et al. 2012; Scholl et al. 1992; Garn et al. 1981). In our study, many women reported feeling abnormally weak and tired during their pregnancy, which could be symptomatic of anemia (CDC 2007), as well as having high blood pressure. Food insecurity, identified among more than half of the respondents, may contribute to anemia prevalence, although anemia from multiple causes is common among women in the Eastern Mediterranean region under normal conditions (De Benoist et al. 2008).

Exposure to violence, abuse, and/or SGBV was reported by over a quarter of Syrian refugee women. Many women experienced multiple types of violence during the current conflict. While several cases of sexual violence were reported, all allegedly perpetrated by armed people in Syria, this number may be much higher based on systematic underreporting of sexual violence due to shame or stigmatization. In focus group discussions, the issue of intimate partner violence was raised repeatedly, with beating, throwing/breaking things, and verbal abuse cited. Syrian women justified intimate partner violence primarily as a result of stress and tension in the home, frustration among unemployed or emasculated men, and general worry or anger about the situation back home in Syria. Among the coping strategies women employed to deal with such violence, many chose to keep quiet or avoid the issue and accepted it as a result of the increased pressure on male partners to provide for their families.

Researchers have explored several theories to explain domestic violence during wartime and in refugee settings (Loue 2001). Domestic violence has been found to increase in post-conflict settings, partially due to the transformation that war can produce in societies and households. A recent report on changing gender roles among Syrian refugees in Lebanon demonstrates the ways that war can reshape household dynamics through increased female-headed households, absent or unemployed males, crowding and multifamily households, which can result in the destruction of what some women consider their primary domain, and more females joining the workforce (El-Masri et al. 2013). Additionally, a survey among Iraqi refugees in Syria revealed a potential relationship between domestic violence and household financial distress (Tappis et al. 2012). Sexual violence has been found to increase among refugees, including both domestic violence and violence outside the home. This can be explained by the increase in levels of frustration in refugee settings, and the tendency to take out such frustration on "the weak" (Skjelsbaek 2001). Participant stories in our study highlight the relationship between limited resources, stress, tension, and violence in the home, providing support to this explanation.

Availability of and access to reproductive health services and services for survivors of violence were limited among this refugee population. Humanitarian services, including support for healthcare and reproductive services, are available to Syrian refugees registered with the United Nations. Some clinics are supported by aid agencies and able to offer discounted medications and clinic visits to Syrian refugees. For example, at the time of our study prices at one of the study sites in the north of Lebanon were the same for Syrians and Lebanese. However, due to the exchange rate, Syrians were at a disadvantage coming from a system of free primary health care to an extremely expensive, highly privatized healthcare setting in Lebanon. During our study, clinic costs in this particular clinic were as follows: a consultation was 5000 L.L. ($3.30), an ultrasound was 10,000 L.L. ($6.60), and an IUD insertion was 15,000 L.L. ($9.90). Although UNHCR and partners have begun covering increased primary healthcare costs for Syrian refugees, the cost is still a major barrier to accessing sufficient health care for Syrians in Lebanon.

Gagnon et al. (2002) explain that limited access or delayed entrance to antenatal care is one of the key determinants of pregnancy outcomes in refugee populations. There are often significant disparities in access to and use of antenatal care among refugee populations compared to non-refugee populations (Carolan 2010). Our study supports this finding and contributes to the literature on access to reproductive health care in refugee settings by identifying perceived barriers to access among a conservative population in the Middle East. The majority of Syrian refugee women had never visited an obstetrician-gynecologist except for pregnancy care, indicating low baseline rates of gynecological exams in this population. While costs and long distances were the primary barriers to accessing gynecologic care, one unique barrier reported in our survey was lack of availability of a female doctor.

Finally, cost, distance to service delivery, and discrimination were cited as barriers to accessing basic services. Participants in both the survey and focus group discussions clearly indicated that they are suffering from a lack of basic services and daily necessities (e.g., housing, food, water, hygiene supplies, blankets). Refugees living in organized camps or group housing supported by a relief agency or religious entities often received more direct aid. With limited or no income, lack of access to water and sanitation, crowding, and food insecurity, Syrian women are at a higher risk for a variety of health problems, including poor reproductive health. Focus group participants highlighted this lack of coverage for basic needs and discrimination in aid distribution as a source of daily stress, leading to worse health outcome.

In summary, a conceptual model is proposed in Fig. 6.2 to illustrate the interplay of the factors mentioned above (as well as other factors identified in the literature)

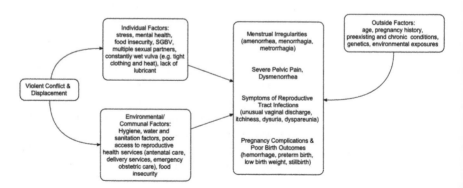

Fig. 6.2 Conceptual model of potential links between violent conflict/displacement and reproductive health

and their effect on the reproductive health of women displaced by conflict. War and displacement cause significant changes in the environment of individuals, characterized by decreased resources, crowding, unstable living conditions, food insecurity, limited water, and poor hygiene. These factors may be particularly important in communities, such as Syrian refugees, who wear conservative clothing most of the time, even in hot weather, and have limited access to hygiene. Settings of conflict and displacement can increase the level of stress and may lead to reproductive health issues and SGBV, which in turn may increase reproductive morbidity.

Limitations

This study has several limitations. For the quantitative component, although we selected a proportionally representative sample, results cannot be generalized to all Syrian refugee women in Lebanon, particularly to those without access to health clinic services. Additionally, due to the ongoing nature of the Syrian crisis, with the number of Syrian refugees changing on monthly and sometime daily basis, it is possible that newly arrived refugees have different characteristics from those described in this study. Such changes are inevitable in research conducted in emergency settings and this study provides essential baseline data to assess the rapidly changing situation.

It should also be noted that we relied on self-reports, which may be subject to under- or overreporting—particularly of key reproductive health or sexual violence outcomes, and particularly in settings of political or religious discrimination or fear of discrimination. To address this issue, we took steps to ensure privacy during interviews and followed WHO-recommended practices for interviewing survivors of violence (World Health Organization 2007). Sexual violence questions were not asked using "event-based" items (e.g., forced to engage in a sexual act when participant did not want to), which may have increased underreporting (Garcia-Moreno et al. 2005). Finally, the choice of survey location at primary healthcare centers poses a limitation on generalizability of the results, as women attending these centers may differ from the general population with respect to knowledge about health services or health behaviors.

With regard to the focus group discussions, the qualitative nature of this portion of the study means that information collected cannot be generalized to the rest of Syrian refugee women in Lebanon. Rather, results serve to help us better understand their situation.

Despite these limitations, this study provides important information about a vulnerable population that is growing in number as the current humanitarian crisis shows no signs of abating. In addition, information gained from this study may help inform programs offered for Syrian refugees and assist in planning for future humanitarian crises of a similar nature.

Conclusions

The picture emerging from Syrian women's stories and survey responses clearly demonstrates a shortage of essential services for women in conflict settings. It is clear that increased access to conventional reproductive health and SGBV response services for refugee women is a priority. Additionally, there is a need for adapting existing approaches that take into account the particular barriers to care faced by a largely conservative, Middle Eastern population whose traditional gender roles in the household and community have been disrupted by conflict and displacement. Sexual violence is highly stigmatized in this population and designing services that reach those affected requires local knowledge and cultural understanding. Humanitarian program models developed in other countries and contexts need to be modified to the local setting.

This study finding of a statistically significant relationship between conflict-related violence and poor health outcomes, with stress as a potential mediator, points to a need to integrate psychological and mental health services into health services for refugee women. In order to address poor reproductive health, both medical and psychological needs should be considered. While some services are in place for survivors of violence, our findings reveal a need for greater provision of such services, and increased awareness raising in the community about existing services, while simultaneously addressing barriers preventing displaced populations from accessing them.

Acknowledgements This study was carried out with the support of the Okvuran Fellowship for International Support (Yale School of Public Health) and the United Nations Population Fund (UNFPA). We acknowledge Dr. Adrienne Ettinger and Dr. Jhumka Gupta (Yale School of Public Health) for their input on this study. We would also like to acknowledge cooperating organizations in Lebanon: The Lebanese Ministry of Public Health (MOPH), International Medical Corps (IMC), the Danish Refugee Council (DRC), the Makassed Communal Healthcare Bureau, the Rafik Hariri Foundation, Jassor Al-Noor, Association Success & Happiness, and the Sawa Group. We would also like to acknowledge the Syrian women who agreed to participate in this research and who are facing immense challenges with bravery.

References

Amnesty International. (2012). *I wanted to die: Syria's torture survivors speak out*. London, UK: Amnesty International Ltd. Retrieved March 14, 2013, from http://www.amnestyusa.org/research/reports/i-wanted-to-die-syria-s-torture-survivors-speak-out
Byrne, B. (1996). Towards a gendered understanding of conflict. *IDS Bulletin, 27*, 31–40.
Campbell, J. C. (2002). Health consequences of intimate partner violence. *Lancet, 359*, 1331–1336.
Carolan, M. (2010). Pregnancy health status of sub-Saharan refugee women who have resettled in developed countries: A review of the literature. *Midwifery, 26*, 407–414.
Catani, C., Jacob, N., Schauer, E., Kohila, M., & Neuner, F. (2008). Family violence, war, and natural disasters: A study of the effect of extreme stress on children's mental health in Sri Lanka. *BMC Psychiatry, 8*(1), 33.

Center for Disease Control (CDC). (2011). *Technical workshop on setting research priorities for reproductive health in crisis settings: Summary of proceedings*. Inter-agency Working Group on Reproductive Health in Crisis (IAWG). Atlanta, GA: Center for Global Health, Division of Global Disease Detection and Emergency Response.

Centers for Disease Control (CDC). (2007). *Reproductive health assessment toolkit for conflict-affected women*. Atlanta, GA: Centers for Disease Control and Prevention. Retrieved March 14, 2013, from http://www.cdc.gov/reproductivehealth/Global/CrisisSituations.htm

De Benoist, B., McLean, E., & Cogswell, M. (Eds.). (2008). *Worldwide prevalence of anaemia 1993-2005: WHO database on anaemia*. Geneva: World Health Organization.

Depoortere, E., Checci, F., Broillet, F., Gerstl, S., Minetti, A., Gayraud, O., et al. (2004). Violence and mortality in West Darfur, Sudan (2003-2004): Epidemiological evidence from four surveys. *Lancet, 364*, 1315–1320.

El-Jack, A. (2003). *Gender and armed conflict*. Brighton, England: University of Sussex.

El-Masri, R., Harvey, C., & Garwood, R. (2013). *Shifting sands: Changing gender roles among refugees in Lebanon*. Joint Research Report. Oxfam GB and ABAAD-Resource Center for Gender Equality.

Farnsworth, N., Qosaj-Mustafa, A., Ekonomi, M., Shima, A., & Dauti-Kadriu, D. (2012). *At what cost? Budgeting for the implementation of the legal framework against domestic violence in Kosovo*. United Nations Development Programme. ISBN 978-9951-498-07-4.

Gagnon, A. J., Merry, L., & Robinson, C. (2002). A systematic review of refugee women's reproductive health. *Refuge, 21*(1).

Gallegos, J. V., & Gutierrez I. A. (2011). The Effect of civil conflict on domestic violence: The case of Peru. *SSRN Working Paper Series*, 1–29.

Garcia-Moreno, C., Jansen, H. A. F. M., Ellsberg, M., Heise, L., & Watts, C. (2005). *WHO multi-country study on women's health and domestic violence against women: Initial results on prevalence, health outcomes and women's responses*. Geneva: World Health Organization (WHO).

Garn, S. M., Keating, M. T., & Falkner, F. (1981). Hematologic status and pregnancy outcomes. *American Journal of Clinical Nutrition, 34*, 115–117.

Gupta, J., Acevedo-Garcia, D., Hemenway, D., Decker, M. R., Raj, A., & Silverman, J. G. (2009). Premigration exposure to political violence and perpetration of intimate partner violence among immigrant men in Boston. *American Journal of Public Health, 99*(3), 462.

Hamad, K. A., Abed, Y., & Hamad, B. A. (2007). Risk factors associated with preterm birth in the Gaza Strip: Hospital-based case-control study. *Revue de Santé de la Méditerranée orientale, 13*(5), 1,132–1,141.

Human Rights Watch. (2000). *Seeking protection: Addressing sexual and domestic violence in tanzania's refugee camps*. http://www.hrw.org/reports/2000/tanzania

Human Rights Watch. (2003). Trapped by inequality: Bhutanse refugee women in Nepal. *Human Rights Watch*. Retrieved September 14, 2014, from http://www.hrw.org/sites/default/files/reports/nepal0903full.pdf

Human Rights Watch. (2006). A question of security: Violence against Palestinian women and Girls. November 2006, Vol 18, No. 7(E). *Human Rights Watch*. Retrieved September 14, 2014, from http://www.hrw.org/reports/2006/opt1106/opt1106web.pdf

Human Rights Watch. (2012). Syria: Sexual assault in detention. *Human Rights Watch*. Retrieved April 23, 2013, from http://www.hrw.org/news/2012/06/15/syria-sexual-assault-detention

Hynes, M., Robertson, K., Ward, J., & Crouse, C. (2004). A determination of the prevalence of gender-based violence among conflict-affected populations in East Timor. *Disasters, 28*, 294–321.

Hynes, M., Sheik, M., Wilson, H. G., & Spiegel, P. (2002). Reproductive health indicators and outcomes among refugee and internally displaced person in postemergency phase camps. *JAMA, 288*(5), 595–603.

Inter-agency Working Group on Reproductive Health in Crisis (IAWG). (2010). Inter-agency field manual on reproductive health in humanitarian settings (Revision to Field Review). *IAWG*.

International Rescue Committee. (2012). *Syrian women and girls: Fleeing death, facing ongoing threats and humiliation, a gender-based violence rapid assessment.* Retrieved April 23, 2012, from http://www.eldis.org/go/display&type=Document&id=63829#.UXk4DL_Ad8E

Jamieson, D. J., Meikle, S. F., Hillis, S. D., Mtsuki, D., Mawji, S., & Duerr, A. (2000). An evaluation of poor pregnancy outcomes among Burundian refugees in Tanzania. *JAMA, 283*(3).

Khawaja, M., & Tewtel-Salem, M. (2004). Agreement between husband and wife reports of domestic violence: Evidence from poor refugee communities in Lebanon. *International Journal of Epidemiology, 33*, 526–533.

Kramer, M. S., Seguin, L., Lydon, J., & Goulet, L. (2000). Socio-economic disparities in pregnancy outcome: Why do the poor fare so poorly? *Paediatric and Perinatal Epidemiology, 14*, 194–210.

Lederman, R. P. (1995). Relationship of anxiety, stress, and psychosocial development to reproductive health. *Behavioral Medicine, 21*(3), 101–112.

Loue, S. (2001). *Intimate partner violence: Societal, medical, legal and individual responses.* New York, NY: Kluwer Academic/Plenium Publishers.

McGinn, T. (2000). Reproductive health of war-affected populations: What do we know? *International Family Planning Perspectives, 26*(4), 174–180.

Medecins Sans Frontiers (MSF). (2012). Misery beyond the war zone: Life for Syrian refugees and displaced populations in Lebanon. *Medecins Sans Frontiers.*

Nikolic-Ristanovic, V. (2000). *Women, violence and war: Wartime victimization of refugees in the Balkans.* Budapest: Central European University Press.

Pittaway, E. (2004). *The ultimate betrayal: An examination of the experiences of domestic and family violence in refugee communities.* Occasional Paper Center for Refugee Research, UNSW.

Rajasingham-Senanayake, D. (2004). Between reality and representation: Women's agency in war and post-conflict Sri Lanka. *Cultural Dynamics, 16*(2–3), 141–168.

Reese Masterson, A., Usta, J., Gupta, J., & Ettinger, A. S. (2014). Assessment of reproductive health and violence against women among displaced Syrian in Lebanon. *BMC Women's Health, 14*, 25.

Reproductive Health Response in Conflict Consortium (RHRC). (2004). Gender-based violence tools manual—For assessment & program design, monitoring & evaluation in conflict-affected settings. *RHRC.* Accessed on March 14, 2013..

Scholl, T. O., Hediger, M. L., Fischer, R. L., & Shearer, J. W. (1992). Anemia vs iron deficiency: Increased risk of preterm delivery in a prospective study. *American Journal of Clinical Nutrition, 55*, 985–988.

Skjelsbaek, I. (2001). Sexual violence in times of war: a new challenge for peace operations? In L. Olsson & T. L. Tryggestad (Eds.), *Women and International Peacekeeping* (pp. 69–84). Portland, OR: Frank Cass Publishers.

Stark, L., & Ager, A. (2011). A systematic review of prevalence studies of gender based violence in complex emergencies. *Trauma, Violence & Abuse, 12*, 127–134.

Tappis, H., Biermann, E., Glass, N., Tileva, M., & Doocy, S. (2012). Domestic violence among Iraqi refugees in Syria. *Health Care for Women International, 33*(3), 285–297.

Tuysuz, G. (2011). Syrian men promise to marry women who were raped. *Washington Post.* Retrieved September 8, 2014, from http://www.washingtonpost.com/world/middle-east/syrian-men-promise-to-marry-women-who-were-raped/2011/06/20/AG6sO1cH_story.html

United Nations Children's Fund (UNICEF). (2008). *Multiple Indicator Cluster Survey 3 (MICS 3) in the Syrian Arab Republic.* Retrieved September 14, 2014, from http://www.childinfo.org/files/MICS3_Syria_FinalReport_2006_Eng.pdf

United Nations High Commissioner for Refugees (UNHCR). (2012). *Syria refugee response portal.* Retrieved September 8, 2014, from http://data.unhcr.org/syrianrefugees/regional.php

United Nations High Commissioner for Refugees (UNHCR). (2014a). *Syria refugee response portal.* Retrieved September 8, 2014, from http://data.unhcr.org/syrianrefugees/regional.php

United Nations High Commissioner for Refugees (UNHCR). (2014b). *Woman alone: The fight for survival by Syria's refugee women.* UNHCR.

Usta, J., Farver, J. A. M., & Zein, L. (2008). Women, war, and violence: Surviving the experience. *Journal of Women's Health, 17*(5), 793–804.

Van Herp, M., Parque, V., Rackley, E., & Ford, N. (2003). Mortality, violence, and lack of access to health care in the Democratic Republic of Congo. *Disasters, 27*(2), 141–153.

World Health Organization (2007). *Ethical and safety recommendations for researching, documenting and monitoring sexual violence in emergencies.* Geneva: WHO. Retrieved from http://www.who.int/gender/documents/EthicsSafety_web.pdf

Yanit, K. E., Snowden, J. M., Cheng, Y. W., & Caughey, A. B. (2012). The impact of chronic hypertension and pregestational diabetes on pregnancy. *American Journal of Obstetrics and Gynecology, 207*(4), 333.e1–333.e6.

Zimmerman, K. (1995). *Plates in a basket will rattle: Domestic violence in Cambodia. A summary.* Phnom Penh, Cambodia: Project against Domestic Violence.

Chapter 7
Gender Dynamics in Palestinian Society: Domestic and Political Violence

Sarah Memmi

Abstract Several studies have shown how political conflict can lead to the "normalization" of violence within a society, at the same time increasing domestic violence against women. I use the 2006 Palestinian Family Health Survey data to assess the levels and determinants of domestic violence in Palestinian society. The analysis explores the extent to which patriarchy and Israeli occupation are associated with domestic violence. The results show that the probability of accepting violent behavior is significantly related to the experience that women have of domestic violence. Women who have experienced violence from their spouses are more likely to report that domestic violence is acceptable. Moreover, the probability of accepting domestic violence and of reporting acts of violence is significantly associated with exposure to political violence: women who live in the areas most affected by political violence and mobility restrictions are more likely to report having experienced violence and to accepting it; their households also suffer from economic insecurity. Thus, the violence experienced by society as a whole seems to legitimize and increase violence in the couple.

Keywords Political conflict • Acceptance of domestic violence • Women • Palestine

Introduction

The Israeli policy of separation, implemented after the first *Intifada* (1987–1993), has resulted in recurring roadblocks and the establishment of checkpoints and circulation permits. These changes have entailed major mobility restrictions for Palestinians (Hass 2002; Hanieh 2006; Handel 2009). Since the second *Intifada* (2000–2006), Israel has adjusted its occupation regime to secure its policy and hegemony in the long term. This has led to a tightening of bureaucratic and administrative measures to control the Palestinian population (Latte Abdallah and

S. Memmi (✉)
CEPED—Paris Descartes Sorbonne University, Paris, France
e-mail: sarah.memmi@ceped.org

© Springer International Publishing Switzerland 2015   145
Y.K. Djamba, S.R. Kimuna (eds.), *Gender-Based Violence*,
DOI 10.1007/978-3-319-16670-4_7

Parizot 2011), including the construction of the separation barrier in 2002 (Arieli and Sfard 2008) and a blockade of the Gaza Strip after its takeover by Hamas in 2006 (Legrain 2007).

Israel's separation policy has political, social, and economic effects (Latte Abdallah and Parizot 2011)—for example, access to employment. Many Palestinians who worked in Israel can no longer travel there because of mobility restrictions. Unemployment has soared, particularly among men (Farsakh 2005; Kuttab 2006), and Palestinian households have been "pauperized" (Hilal 2010). The Palestinian population is living amid heavy sociopolitical instability and pervasive constraints that generate much real or symbolic violence.

Several Palestinian studies have sought to show the degree to which a conflict can lead to the "normalization" of violence in a society. Some authors have noted the resurgence of violence among young Palestinians (Haj-Yahia and Abdo-Kaloti 2003; Al-Krenawi et al. 2007; Lev-Wiesel et al. 2007). Qualitative studies have examined the effects of the sociopolitical context on violence in Nablus (Yaish unpublished) and the Gaza Strip (Hammami 2009; Muhanna 2010). More recently, a study has shown that political violence was significantly linked to an increase of physical and sexual abuse in intimate partnerships (Clark et al. 2010).

This chapter follows up directly on those studies. It considers male violence as a social mechanism that results from women's subordination to men and helps to perpetuate it. Moreover, such violence ties in with a context of conflict. I argue that this situation contributes substantially to the use of violence. Accordingly, this chapter sets out to examine the determinants of domestic violence in a society subjected to a combination of two constraints that heavily shape married life: patriarchy and the Israeli separation policy. Far from separating these two factors, I look for connections between them. First, I analyze the level and determinants of domestic violence in the Palestinian territories.[1] Next, I explore the representations of domestic violence by spouses and study the process leading to the occurrence of violent behavior. This analysis of domestic violence offers an illustration of the social consequences of Israeli occupation policy on the very core of marital intimacy.

Method

This research combines two complementary approaches: (1) a secondary analysis of the Palestinian Family Health Survey (PFHS) modeled on the Demographic and Health Survey (DHS), to provide a quantitative measure of the levels and determinants of domestic violence in Palestine, and (2) the analysis of in-depth interviews of married men and women. The interviews provide insights into the issues that generate confrontation between spouses. They also make it possible to capture each partner's attitude toward domestic violence.

---

[1] "Palestinian territories" is the term used in international law to designate East Jerusalem, the West Bank, and the Gaza Strip.

The PFHS was conducted in 2006 by the Palestinian Central Bureau of Statistics (PCBS)[2] and the Pan Arab Project for Family Health (PAPFAM), using a multistage sample. A total of 13,238 households participated out of the 15,044 households that were sampled, giving a response rate of 88.0 %. Of the total, 8,781 were living in the West Bank and 4,457 in the Gaza Strip. The section of the survey on sexual and reproductive health was administered exclusively to women of reproductive age (15–54 years). Only those who were married at the time of the survey ($N = 5,266$) were selected for this study.

Two indicators were selected as dependent variables: the reporting of acts of violence[3] and the attitude expressed toward domestic violence.[4] The independent variables are divided into three categories: socio-demographic variables (age, education, and employment status), contextual variables (socioeconomic status, place of residence, region, and exposure to occupation), and gender relation variables (employment status of the couple, age at first marriage, women's autonomy, and opinion about female employment). Bivariate analysis was conducted to examine the relationship between each independent variable and levels of violence. Then, the net effect of each of the independent variables on the dependent variable was determined in logistic regression models. The only variables introduced into the logistic regression model are those displaying significance at the 10 % level.

Data from in-depth semi-directed interviews conducted by the author between January and December 2011 among married men (20) and women (22) were also used. The interviewees exhibited diverse socio-demographic characteristics and were selected using the "snowball" model.[5] The interviews covered life histories, focusing on partnership formation, type of partnership, distribution of roles in the couple, and reproductive behavior. All interviews were audio-recorded and transcribed. I obtained the respondents' consent and anonymized all interviews. Whenever possible, I carried out the interviews in English. For interviews in Arabic, I relied on a professional translator.

Results

Sample Characteristics

In the Palestinian Family Health Survey, among the sample of married Palestinian women, 16.5 % were aged 15–24, 37.4 % were 25–34, 29.8 % were 35–44, and 16.4 % were 45 and older (Table 7.1). More than six women over ten get married

---

[2] The PCBS is the Statistical Institute of the Palestinian Authority.

[3] The question was worded as follows: "Were you exposed to any domestic violence in the last 6 months."

[4] The question was worded as follows: "Now I would like to talk to you about domestic violence. Sometimes the husband feels annoyed or angry for things that his wife does. In your opinion, is it justified for the husband to beat or hit his wife?" Answer: "yes/no."

[5] For more information on this method, see Lamont and White (2008).

Table 7.1 Distribution of survey respondents across categories of independent variables, Palestinian territories, 2006 PFHS

	Distribution of the sample	
	N	%
Socio-demographic characteristics		
Women's age		
15–24	871	16.5
25–34	1,971	37.4
35–44	1,568	29.8
45+	856	16.4
Men's age		
15–34	1,784	34.0
35–44	1,920	36.6
45+	1,543	29.4
Women's educational attainment		
Basic	1,779	33.8
Primary	1,803	34.2
Secondary	1,065	20.2
High	619	11.8
Men's educational attainment		
Basic	1,789	34.2
Primary	1,492	28.5
Secondary	964	18.4
High	983	18.8
Women's work status		
Employed	517	10.0
Unemployed	163	3.2
Housewife	4,475	86.8
Men's work status		
Employed	3,647	70.4
Unemployed	1,235	23.8
Househusband	303	5.8
Contextual variables		
Socioeconomic status		
Low	992	18.8
Middle	3,258	61.9
High	1,016	19.3
Type of place of residence		
Urban	2,813	53.4
Rural	1,546	29.4
Refugee camp	907	17.2
Region of residence		

(continued)

Table 7.1 (continued)

	Distribution of the sample	
	N	%
West Bank	2,677	50.9
East Jerusalem	542	10.3
Gaza Strip	2,047	38.8
Facing mobility restrictions for women		
Yes	3,800	85.9
No	1,466	14.1
Gender relation variables		
Work status within couple		
Both work	416	8.2
Husband works, wife doesn't work	3,154	62.1
Wife works, husband doesn't work	90	1.8
Both don't work	1,417	27.9
Age at first marriage for women		
Less than 20 years	3,301	62.7
20–24	1,537	29.2
25+	428	8.1
Women's autonomy—to make purchases		
Is an obstacle	2,340	44.5
Is not an obstacle	2,924	55.5
Women's autonomy—to go out		
Is an obstacle	4,573	86.9
Is not an obstacle	689	13.1
Women's attitude about future employment		
Doesn't work and doesn't want a paid job in future	2,579	50.5
Doesn't work and want a paid job in future	2,063	39.6
Works	624	10.0
Reporting domestic violence		
Yes	494	9.4
No	4,772	90.6
Accepting violent behavior by the husband		
Yes	408	7.7
No	4,858	92.3
Total	5,266	100.0

before 20 (62.7 %). Around 34 % of the respondents had a basic level of education and only 11.8 % went beyond high school. Results for their husbands show that 34.2 % had a basic educational level and 18.8 % had more than a high school education. In more than a half of the couples, the husbands worked but the wives did not (62.1 %) and more than a half of jobless women (unemployed or housewives) did not want a paid job in the future. For nearly nine women over ten, autonomy to go out[6] is an obstacle (86.9 %). A majority of the married women in the sample were living in West Bank (50.9 %), more than a third in Gaza Strip (38.8 %), and others in East Jerusalem (10.3 %). Mobility restrictions concern more than eight women over ten (85.9 %). Most of them are living in the urban area (53.4 %) whereas refugee camp represented a slightly smaller proportion (17.2 %) and rural area nearly a third of the sample (29.4 %).

Measure of Domestic Violence

In the survey, 9.4 % of Palestinian women reported having been subjected to violence from their husbands in the 6 months before the survey and 7.7 % stated that such violence was justified (Table 7.1). It is worth mentioning that the Palestinian Family Health Survey measured the levels of violence with a single question to the female respondent to determine whether they have already been exposed to violence or not. Some women, however, do not talk about their experience of violence until they have established a relationship of trust with the interviewer (Browning and Dutton 1986). As such the levels of violence reported here may be lower than the actual episodes of wife abuse in the society.

In sum, violence is hard to measure, especially in societies where gender norms are very strong. Under such circumstances, underreporting of domestic violence can be significant. In addition, in these societies, many women do not consider most insults and humiliations as acts of violence. This lack of precision also prevents an analysis of violence in its multiple dimensions, as the United Nations recommends.

> [Violence against women] is any act of gender-based violence that results in, or is likely to result in, physical, sexual or mental harm or suffering to women, including threats of such acts, coercion or arbitrary deprivation of liberty, whether occurring in public or in private life.[7]

---

[6] We do not have direct data to measure the autonomy of Palestinian women. We have therefore used as a proxy an autonomy indicator for access to health services. The question was worded as follows: "Many factors may prevent women from seeking medical care or treatment for themselves. When you are ill and need to get medical care or treatment, does getting permission to go act as a major barrier for you or not?" (yes/no). We also regard women's educational attainment as an indirect indicator of female autonomy.

[7] Definition of violence adopted by the UN in 1993.

So, these results should be interpreted with caution. But despite underreporting and definition bias, the PFHS data are valuable for this study because it is the only survey covering the full set of individual, partnership-related, and contextual factors linked to domestic violence in Palestine.

Bivariate Analysis

Reporting domestic violence was associated with men's age, with a greater proportion of 15–34 years old (10.6 %) than of men aged 35–44 (8.9 %) or 45 and older (8.5 %) who used violence against their wife (Table 7.2). This phenomenon was more prevalent among the less educated women and less educated husbands. Use of domestic violence was also higher if the woman was unemployed (14 %) or her husband was unemployed (13.1 %). Considering gender relation variables, we can see that reporting domestic violence is higher when the wife worked and husband did not (12.9 %) than when both did not work (11.1 %). The last finding suggests that financial instability and imbalance between partners increase, probably, the risk for domestic violence. The use of violence is also more important when women didn't work but want a paid job in the future.

Accepting violent behavior was associated with women's and men's educational attainment: it is higher among less educated people. This phenomenon was most prevalent among women whose partners were unemployed (10.0 %) and those who had a low socioeconomic. However, it was lower if the wife worked and the husband did not (3.3 %). Reports of domestic violence and accepting violent behaviors were also higher in Gaza Strip and among women who face mobility restrictions. Women's age is not statistically correlated with the prevalence of domestic violence ($P=0.559$ for reporting violence and $P=0.124$ for accepting violence).

Determinants of Domestic Violence Reporting

In Table 7.3, in the first logistic regression model, which controlled for the probability to report domestic violence for all the study's variables, the risk was highest among less educated women and less educated partners (odd ratios 4.28 and 2.11, respectively, for those with basic education). In terms of age, younger men were significantly more likely to use domestic violence against their wives than older men. As for region or residence, women living in the Gaza Strip were significantly more likely to report being victims of domestic violence as compared to those living in the West Bank. Women who faced mobility restrictions were also more likely to report domestic violence than those who were free to move. Moreover, women who reported they had autonomy to go out were less likely than the others to report domestic violence. This phenomenon was also highest among couples whose wives

Table 7.2 Bivariate analysis of reporting domestic violence in 6 months prior to survey and accepting violence by husband, Palestinian territories, 2006 PFHS

		Reporting domestic violence		Accepting violent behavior by the husband		
	N	%	P-value*	N	%	P-value*
Socio-demographic characteristics						
Women's age			0.559			0.124
15–24	82	9.4		80	9.2	
25–34	193	9.8		148	7.5	
35–44	148	9.4		106	6.7	
45+	70	8.1		74	8.5	
Men's age			0.008			0.575
15–34	190	10.6		146	8.2	
35–44	171	8.9		140	7.3	
45+	132	8.5		121	7.8	
Women's educational attainment			<0.001			0.052
Basic	245	13.7		170	9.5	
Primary	145	8.0		139	7.7	
Secondary	81	7.6		79	7.4	
High	22	3.5		20	3.2	
Men's educational attainment			0.020			0.054
Basic	231	12.9		170	9.5	
Primary	134	9.0		105	7.0	
Secondary	75	7.8		79	8.2	
High	43	4.4		51	5.2	
Women's work status			0.030			<0.001
Employed	38	7.3		18	3.4	
Unemployed	23	14.0		11	6.7	
Housewife	428	9.5		374	8.3	
Men's work status			<0.001			0.003
Employed	286	7.8		257	7.1	
Unemployed	162	13.1		124	10.0	
Househusband	31	10.2		23	7.6	
Contextual variables						
Socioeconomic status			0.678			<0.001
Low	136	13.5		102	10.1	
Middle	308	9.4		271	8.3	
High	49	4.8		35	3.5	
Type of place of residence			0.017			<0.001
Urban	290	10.3		276	9.8	
Rural	119	7.7		73	4.7	
Refugee camp	85	9.4		59	6.5	
Region of residence			<0.001			<0.001
West Bank	215	8.0		165	6.1	

(continued)

Table 7.2 (continued)

	Reporting domestic violence			Accepting violent behavior by the husband		
	N	%	P-value*	N	%	P-value*
East Jerusalem	21	3.9		13	2.4	
Gaza Strip	257	12.5		230	11.2	
Facing mobility restrictions for women			0.006			0.003
Yes	379	10.5		317	8.9	
No	115	6.3		91	4.8	
Gender relation variables						
Work status within couple			0.023			0.045
Both work	25	6.0		13	3.1	
Husband works, wife doesn't work	256	8.1		240	7.6	
Wife works, husband doesn't work	15	12.9		3	3.3	
Both don't work	183	11.1		143	10.1	
Age at first marriage for women			0.093			0.007
Less than 20 years	330	10.0		284	8.6	
20–24	131	8.5		108	7.0	
25+	32	7.4		14	3.3	
Women's autonomy—to go out			<0.020			0.010
Is an obstacle	112	16.3		71	10.3	
Is not an obstacle	380	8.3		406	7.3	
Women's attitude about future employment			<0.001			0.190
Doesn't work and doesn't want a paid job in future	192	7.8		195	7.9	
Doesn't work and want a paid job in future	240	12.2		176	9.0	
Works	38	7.3		30	3.4	
Experienced domestic violence						<0.001
No				340	7.1	
Yes				66	13.4	
Total	494	9.4		408	7.7	

*P-values of chi square

worked and the husbands did not (2.23), and if the women did not work but wanted paid work in the future (1.79). In contrast, there was no significant difference in reporting domestic violence by type of place of residence.

In the second logistic regression model which controlled for the probability to accept violence behaviors for all the study's variables, the risk was greater among less educated women and men (1.96 and 1.10, respectively, among those with basic education). Compared to West Bank residents, women living in East Jerusalem

Table 7.3 Adjusted odds ratios (AOR) from logistic regression analysis of factors influencing the probability of reporting domestic violence in 6 months prior to survey and the probability of accepting violence by the husband, Palestinian territories, 2006 PFHS

	Reporting domestic violence			Accepting violent behavior by the husband		
	A.O.R.		[95 % CI]	A.O.R.		[95 % CI]
Socio-demographic characteristics						
Women's age						
15–24	NA			NA		
25–34	NA			NA		
35–44	NA			NA		
45+	NA			NA		
Men's age						
15–34	1.452	*	[1.093–1.928]	NA		
35–44	1.171	+	[0.901–1.542]	NA		
45+ (ref)	1.000					
Women's educational attainment						
Basic	4.284	***	[2.205–8.347]	1.965	**	[1.142–3.367]
Primary	2.611	**	[1.357–5.031]	1.667		[0.972–2.847]
Secondary	2.712	***	[1.411–5.220]	1.568		[0.901–2.710]
High (ref)	1.000			1.000		
Men's educational attainment						
Basic	2.113		[1.391–3.199]	1.100	*	[0.990–1.368]
Primary	1.645		[1.083–2.502]	1.040		[0.712–1.522]
Secondary	1.467		[0.945–2.702]	1.070		[0.675–1.075]
High (ref)	1.000			1.000		
Women's work status						
Employed	NA			NA		
Unemployed	NA			NA		

Variable	OR		CI	OR		CI
Housewife	NA			NA		
Men's work status						
Employed	NA			NA		
Unemployed	NA			NA		
Househusband	NA			NA		
Contextual variables						
Socioeconomic status						
Low	NA			2.443	***	[1.591–3.745]
Middle	NA			2.091	***	[1.442–3.053]
High (ref)	NA			1.000		
Type of place of residence						
Urban	1.451		[0.871–1.781]	1.322		[0.809–1.432]
Rural	0.882		[0.773–1.030]	0.901		[0.850–1.090]
Refugee camp (ref)	1.000			1.000		
Region of residence						
West Bank (ref)	1.000			1.000		
East Jerusalem	0.652		[0.40–1.05]	0.410	**	[0.232–0.733]
Gaza Strip	1.811	**	[1.42–2.32]	1.610	*	[1.261–2.042]
Facing mobility restrictions for women						
Yes	1.120	*	[1.00–1.98]	1.050	*	[1.013–1.872]
No (ref)	1.000			1.000		
Gender relation variables						
Work status within couple						
Both work (ref)	1.000			1.000		
Husband works, wife doesn't work	0.946		[0.22–4.06]	1.487		[0.811–2.715]
Wife works, husband doesn't work	2.231	**	[1.341–3.403]	0.753		[0.201–2.690]

(continued)

Table 7.3 (continued)

	Reporting domestic violence			Accepting violent behavior by the husband		
	A.O.R.		[95 % CI]	A.O.R.		[95 % CI]
Both don't work	0.787		[0.201–3.771]	1.541	+	[0.991–1.456]
Age at first marriage for women						
Less than 20 years	NA			2.570	***	[1.391–4.517]
20–24	NA			2.512	***	[1.414–4.686]
25+ (ref)	NA			1.000		
Women's autonomy—to go out						
Is an obstacle	1.892	**	[1.460–2.461]	1.452	**	[1.093–1.944]
Is not an obstacle (ref)	1.000			1.000		
Women's attitude about future employment						
Doesn't work and doesn't want a paid job in future (ref)	1.000			NA		
Doesn't work and want a paid job in future	1.790	**	[1.354–2.397]	NA		
Works	0.572	*	[0.431–0.881]	NA		
Experienced domestic violence						
No (ref)	NA			1.000		
Yes	NA			1.485	*	[1.101–1.996]

ref reference category

***$P \leq 0.001$; **$P \leq 0.01$; *$P \leq 0.05$; +$P \leq 0.10$

NA: "not applicable" is used if the variable was no significant in bivariate analysis (e.g., women's age), if the variable was collinear (e.g., women's work status is collinear with work status within couple)

were significantly less likely to accept violent behaviors (odds ratio = 0.41), whereas those in the Gaza Strip were significantly more likely to accept such acts (odds ratio = 1.61). The acceptance of domestic violence was also significantly associated with socioeconomic status with women of lower socioeconomic status being more favorable to such behaviors.

The association between gender relation variables and acceptance of violent behaviors was important. Indeed, if both partners didn't work, the women were more likely to accept violent behaviors (odds ratio = 1.54), compared to couples whose spouses worked. The effect of age at first marriage is statistically significant. All women who were married at younger ages (before age 25) were more likely to accept violent behaviors by the husband than their counterparts who married at older ages (25+). Likewise, women who reported mobility restrictions were more likely to accept domestic violence (odds ratio = 1.45) compared to those who said that such mobility was not a problem for them. Finally, Palestinian women who have been exposed to domestic violence are more likely than others to justify the use of violence (1.48).

These findings show that domestic violence is not specific to one category of the population and it is not disappearing. The risk of exposure to violence is also greater for women if their husbands are young. Financial, residential, and mobility-related difficulties often force young Palestinian couples to live with the husband's parents after the partnership is formed (Mitchell 2010). This situation greatly restricts marital intimacy and may aggravate tension between spouses. Moreover, as emphasized in a study of Palestinian refugees in Jordan, young people are often more likely to justify domestic violence as a means of settling disputes (Khawaja et al. 2008).

The prevalence of domestic violence is higher among the Palestinian women most exposed to male dominance. As other studies conducted in the Middle East indicate (Haj-Yahia 2000; Maziak and Asfar 2003; Usta et al. 2007; Khawaja et al. 2008; Hammoury et al. 2009), violence mainly affects the least educated women (or their spouses) and those who marry early. By contrast, autonomous women are less exposed to violence. An opinion analysis of Palestinian refugees in Jordan underscores the fact that men who support female autonomy oppose domestic violence (Khawaja et al. 2008). In other words, the evidence suggests that the representations and practices that promote female autonomy reduce the risk of violence.

However, the determination of Palestinian women to circumvent certain norms or to change their social status increases the risk of violence. In response to these various situations, some men apparently seek to reassert their dominance, if need be through violence—as emphasized by other studies conducted in Egypt (Ambrosetti et al. 2013) and among Israeli Arabs (Haj-Yahia 2000).

Our results also point to a link between the experience of violence and attitudes to violence, as is the case in other countries of the region (Khawaja et al. 2008; Ambrosetti et al. 2013). Finally, the conditions in the place of residence are associated with domestic violence, which is consistent with previous research on violence in unstable contexts (Haj-Yahia and Abdo-Kaloti 2003; Hammami 2009; Muhanna 2010; Clark et al. 2010; Yaish unpublished).

The results below suggest multiple determinants for Palestinian domestic violence, linked to specific personal characteristics, the marital relationship, and the residential context.

Domestic Violence by Spouses

Using the interviews of married men and women, I examined the relationship between observed behavior in terms of domestic violence and the accounts of such behavior by the spouses. This qualitative information allows us to see what is at stake in conflicts between spouses. In this qualitative sample, the average age was 38.4 years old for women and 40.5 for men. Slightly more than a third (38 %) of interviewees stopped school before finishing their *Tawjihi*[8]; 43 % were living in a rural area, 38 % in an urban area, and 19 % in refugee camps.

Legitimation of Domestic Violence by Men: When Women Do Not Comply with Certain Norms

The first reason given by men to justify domestic violence is that women do not conform to their gender-determined role. Disagreements largely focus on the nurturing and maternal role expected of women. Some of our female interviewees, for example, were exposed to abuse when the meal was not ready "on time" or was "too" hot or "too" cold. This happened to Sylvia (F, 50, Christian, employee, city),[9] whose husband engaged in violent behavior (insults, blows, and other abuse) when dinner did not go as he wished. Yet Sylvia believes that she has always done her best to satisfy him. Other women were punished by their husbands for not being "good mothers." Oum Shadi (F, 55, Muslim, housewife, refugee camp)[10] had suffered abuse for the first time when she was pregnant; her husband was furious that she had taken medication for a headache. He struck her in the face but also several times in the belly, putting her pregnancy at risk.

Men also justify domestic violence if they feel that their wives are challenging their authority. There is an inherent contradiction in marital arrangements: women are in charge of managing the household, but it is the man who generally embodies authority. The frontier can therefore be thin and shifting between what constitutes an acceptable female decision and what does not. Our interviewees cited several causes of conflict involving wives who disobeyed or took on undue prerogatives. Abu Ahmad (M, 46, Muslim, employee, village)[11] beat his wife just after she had

[8] The *Tawjihi* is the last examination in the last year of high school.
[9] Interview: 20/09/11 in Ramallah.
[10] Interview: 10/05/11 in Al Amary camp.
[11] Interview: 11/2011 in Nablus.

bought beds for their children. He believes that she was not entitled to decide by herself to spend such a large sum of money. Furthermore, the purchase required her to save for several months a part of the daily allowance that he gave her for shopping. For Abu Ahmad, financial management did not fall within his wife's decision-making power.

Another argument often invoked to justify violence concerns women going out without permission. Ibrahim (M, 29, Muslim, employee, village)[12] is often away from home for several days because of his work. When he is absent, he doesn't want his wife to go out, except for domestic obligations. When he hears that she has disobeyed him, he beats her. If he refuses to let her go out, "it's for her sake," and "it's to protect her"—but also because he's afraid of gossip about his ability to "keep his wife under control." The arguments he uses to justify his acts revolve around the issue of honor and reputation.[13]

Exogenous Origin of Domestic Violence

The justifications for domestic violence in the Palestinian territories appear to be rooted in patriarchal patterns as in other countries. Men legitimize violence to preserve a patriarchal order when their wives—so they argue—fail to stay within the bounds of their assigned role.

Nevertheless, we need to understand this interpretation by looking at domestic violence in the context of the sociopolitical violence and tensions experienced by Palestinians daily. In this interpretative scenario, the context contributes to the toxic climate between spouses and "normalizes" the use of violence in the home. The reasons cited earlier become "pretexts" for the expression of a violence whose causes lie outside the conjugal unit.

Tighter restrictions on mobility have caused a sharp rise in unemployment among Palestinians—from 18.2 % in 1995 to 26.3 % in 2008 for all Palestinian territories (Khawaja and Omari 2009) with wide gaps between the Gaza Strip (44.8 %) and the West Bank (19.8 %) (Naqib 2009). The weakening of the job market considerably undermines the position of men. They are finding it harder to earn enough to have housing of their own, marry, and start a family (Mitchell 2010). Men's exposure to economic instability makes their families more vulnerable and jeopardizes male power.

Most of the men we surveyed cite the capacity to provide financial support for the household as one of the main attributes of masculinity.[14] Many of them had worked several years in Israel and were earning more at the time than they were

---

[12] Interview: 10/2011 in *Abu Dis*.

[13] This refers to what Stephanie Latte Abdallah (2006) has observed among Palestinian refugees in Jordan. He argues that their failure to defend their land has contributed to their determination to defend women's honor.

[14] We asked our respondents "how do you define a successful man?," "what makes you a man/a head of household?," or "what makes you especially proud in your daily life?"

earning when they were interviewed. Despite this deteriorating situation, it is vital for men to play their role as providers, regardless of the major sacrifices this requires, such as accepting a succession of precarious job contracts, combining several small jobs, commuting long hours, and risking prison by entering Israel illegally. These men notice a huge gap between their accounts of masculinity and their actual situation. The discrepancy fuels a feeling of powerlessness, and all the men say that they need to assert their superiority—if need be, through violence.

Nasser (M, 33, Muslim, employee, city), who lives in Al-Azarieh, a near suburb of Jerusalem, lost his job after the second *Intifada* (2000–2006). Until the early 2000s, the inhabitants of Al-Azarieh could travel to East Jerusalem to attend school, and access health services or work (BADIL 2006). Nasser was employed as an IT worker in an Israeli telecoms firm. His salary allowed him to save enough to marry. A few months after his marriage, he was banned from traveling to East Jerusalem. He failed to obtain a work permit in Israel and lost his job. A long unemployment spell followed, during which he had moved back to his parents' home to live with his wife. Deeply affected by this situation, Nasser now recognizes that his wife showed great patience:

> I had the impression I was a child again. It was making me crazy. She said it didn't bother her, and actually I think that made me even madder. Yes, there were times when I yelled at her [...] twice I even slapped her, but I regret it. She was very patient all that time, and she gave me lots of support.[15]

Fadil (M, 41, Muslim, employee, city) had experienced several unemployment spells, which he attributes to two causes. First, he was placed under house arrest in Nablus for several years because of his militant activity in Fatah. Second, his imprisonment and torture during the first *Intifada* left him with a constant trembling and an impaired left arm. He still carries a large scar on his forearm, which he showed us proudly.[16] His inability to act as financial provider explains his present feeling of diminishment and loss of status. After his day in the limelight as an activist during the *Intifada*, when the time came to "settle down," go back to a stable life, and take on the role of head of household, he explains:

> I was very nervous at home. I never beat my wife but I often yelled at her. I regret having acted like that with her. It's not good to take it out on her. It wasn't her fault. But I felt totally useless. It was terrible for me.[17]

---

[15] Interview: 01/2011, Al-Azarieh.

[16] During the first *Intifada*, masculinity rested on the capacity of Palestinian men to resist occupation, and to support the violence and injustice inflicted by the occupying power. The Israeli army would beat men in public in an attempt to weaken them. But instead of making Palestinian men feel more humiliated, Julie Peteet (1994) explained that this bodily ordeal ultimately served to strengthen their sense of honor, virility, and moral superiority. It acted as what she calls the "rites of passage of masculinity."

[17] Interview: 11/2011 Nablus.

To cope with their husbands' financial hardship, some Palestinian women have started to seek work. They can also try to receive aid from humanitarian organizations, as has been documented in the Gaza Strip after Israel imposed a blockade in 2006 (Muhanna 2010). Other women already in employment found themselves having to cover a large share of household expenses.

All these developments have led to a shift in responsibilities and gender-specific roles between spouses. That is what happened to Shuruk (F, 38, Muslim, 38, employee, city).[18] For many years, her husband was a construction worker in Israel. For the past few years, he has been alternating unemployment spells and short-term jobs in East Jerusalem. Shuruk attributes this situation to the growing inequality affecting Palestinians in East Jerusalem, who are not regarded as full-fledged citizens (Sibany 2007; Dembik and Marteu 2009). She says that she is very distressed to see her husband so undermined by being out of work. She endures his daily insults to preserve family stability, protect their children, and avoid aggravating tension.

Another less common but certainly significant example concerns couples who do not enjoy the same residential status and hence the same mobility.[19] For these reasons, some are forced to leave their jobs. Sheerine (F, 39, Christian, employee, city)[20] met her husband in East Jerusalem when both were working for the United Nations. They applied for family reunification so that her husband from the West Bank could come to live with her in Jerusalem. Pending completion of the procedure, he was no longer able to commute to Jerusalem and so lost his job. He has since been working in Ramallah and his earnings have fallen sharply,[21] making Sheerine the household's chief financial provider. Moreover, her husband's daily commute is highly time consuming—the round trip takes an average of 3 h—and uncertain, because it requires crossing the *Qalandya* checkpoint. Sheerine's husband is thus the daily victim of symbolic violence and of humiliations inflicted by the Israeli army. In this couple, economic instability, tension, and humiliation have compounded the marital instability due to family reunification policy. This situation has substantially aggravated the tension between partners—her husband often yells at her and insults her—despite the fact that they were very much in love and considerate toward each other before the onset of all these events.

According to several studies, women who work and earn a living are more often involved in domestic decisions than economically inactive women (Bowlus and Seitz 2005). They would thus appear to be protected from an adverse conjugal environment. By contrast, when they have no earnings of their own, women are financially dependent on their partners and are more easily exposed to domestic violence (Gartner 1990). However, our results show that the relationship between employment and domestic violence is not one-way: the category most exposed to violence consists of working Palestinian women with unemployed husbands (Table 7.2).

---

[18] Interview: 09/2011, East Jerusalem.

[19] For more detail on this subject see Conte (2005), Bourmaud (2012), and Memmi (in press).

[20] Interview: 10/2011 East Jerusalem.

[21] Wages are lower in the West Bank than in East Jerusalem.

It should be noted that this role reversal is, in most cases, involuntary, for it is due to the political context and fragile economic conditions. Male unemployment and/ or the difficulties encountered by men in meeting the household's financial needs can lead to a paradoxical situation: the man has the authority but lacks the resources to back it up. He therefore uses violence to reassert his authority by force.

In other words, as MacMillan and Gartner explain (1999), a woman's participation in the labor force reduces the risk of violence only when her husband has a job as well. In contrast, the risk is greater if her male partner is out of work.[22] This observation is consistent with the theory of marital incompatibility, which holds that violence results from an unbalanced distribution of resources between spouses (Yick 2001). We must therefore qualify the notion that a greater economic contribution by women is a form of gender equality and suffices to reduce domestic violence (Zuhur 2003). To produce a deeper change in gender relations, female participation in the economic sphere must go hand in hand with a challenge to patriarchal norms, a change in the status of women in the family and in the couple, and a greater involvement of women in decision making.

Conclusion

From this analysis, we can draw an initial conclusion. In the Palestinian territories, the patriarchal characteristics of society alone cannot explain the domestic power relationship. Similarly, the argument that domestic violence is the result of the political context and the pressure exerted by Israel is too reductionist. On the contrary, we need to take into account the Palestinians' social, historical, as well as political environment. We must do so to understand how power is exercised in the couple and how a certain form of violence can emerge. The violence can be physical but also, and most often, symbolic. To grasp the power relationship and outbreaks of violence in Palestinian couples, we must therefore view them in a broader context.

Our findings show that Palestinian domestic violence is linked to the dominance relationship in the couple, as has been documented in many developing countries (Hindin 2003; Hollander 2003; Kishor 2005; Kishor and Johnson 2006). The risk of exposure to violence is thus higher among women who seek change by renegotiating the dominance relationship.

However, justifications for the use of violence can also have exogenous causes, that is to say, outside the conjugal unit. This chapter confirms that conflict can contribute to the "normalization" of violence in a society. Violence remains a pervasive problem, which mainly concerns young Palestinians. A study conducted in Nablus after the second *Intifada* (2000–2006) revealed that young unemployed men are more frustrated and worried about their future than their elders (Yaish unpublished).

---

[22] We also have seen in the quantitative analysis that the probability of reporting domestic violence is higher when the woman works and the husband doesn't work (adjusted OR = 2.231).

The study suggests that they adopt more violent behavior toward their wives and families. For women as well, the acceptance of domestic violence varies according to their personal experience of violence. The probability for a woman to accept violence is higher if the financial situation of her husband has deteriorated and if he is subjected to daily humiliation by Israeli soldiers. Most wives do not seek confrontation with their spouses. On the contrary, they are very understanding and want their husbands to regain their dignity. Female acceptance of violence, it is argued, is a form of "passive resistance."[23] For example, although domestic violence is a punishable offence in East Jerusalem,[24] few complaints are filed by Palestinian women (Amnesty International 2005). They refuse to have the Israeli police intervene in their private life and, at the same time, they do not want their husbands to be confronted with such interference.

Lastly, the study sees both female consent and use of violence by men as "a sign of a struggle for the maintenance of certain fantasies of identity and power" (Moore 1994:70). In this sense, they converge toward a common interest: the preservation of the symbolic image of masculinity.

Our analysis implicitly raises the issue of individual construction. As the philosopher Alex Honneth explains, the individual is constructed from three distinct spheres (Honneth 2005): the sphere of family relations, which promotes emotional construction; the sphere of law, which allows people to see themselves as political subjects; and the social sphere, which helps to promote specific personal values such as work. The construction of the individual from these three spheres implies the occurrence of violence (symbolic or physical) if recognition is inadequate or altogether denied. The Palestinians are subjected to this "denial of recognition" in social, legal, and political terms. Consequently, the marital relationship could be viewed as a space for compensation. Within that space, physical and verbal violence against women serves as an outlet for the political and social violence endured by men. In this particularly coercive context, one cannot combat the determinants of domestic violence without understanding and acting on the actual and symbolic violence endured by Palestinians daily.

---

[23] Here, the phrase echoes the Palestinian term *sumud*, which has often been associated with Palestinian women's daily struggle to preserve a degree of normality in family and community life.

[24] The Palestinian legal system reflects territorial fragmentation. In the West Bank, it is derived from Jordanian law; in the Gaza Strip, it is based on Egyptian law; in East Jerusalem, it has been determined by Israeli law since 1976. In East Jerusalem, domestic violence is punishable under a 1998 amendment to the Israeli penal code, which calls for a 4-year minimum jail sentence. The Family Violence Prevention Act stipulates that an Israeli court can issue a protection order for anyone who has suffered physical, psychological, or sexual abuse. See Article 3 of the Act, available at http://www.knesset.gov.il/review/data/eng/law/kns12_familyviolence_eng.pdf

References

Al-Krenawi, A., Graham, J. R., & Sehwail, M. A. (2007). Tomorrow's players under occupation: An analysis of the association of political violence with psychological functioning and domestic violence among Palestinian youth. *American Journal of Orthopsychiatry, 77*, 427–433.

Ambrosetti, E., Abu Amara, N., & Condon, S. (2013). Gender-based violence in Egypt: Analyzing impacts of political reforms, social, and demographic change. *Violence Against Women, 19*, 400–421.

Amnesty International. (2005). *Israel—Briefing to the Committee on the Elimination of Discrimination Against Women*. MDE 15/037/2005, Amnesty International, 42.

Arieli, S., & Sfard, M. (2008). *'Homa vemehdal', Sfarey alyat hagag*. Tel Aviv, Israel: Yediot Aharonot, Sfarey Hemed.

BADIL. (2006). *Displaced by the wall: Forced displacement as a result of the West Bank wall and its associated regime* (p. 69). Bethléem et Genève: Badil Resource Center for Palestinian Residency and Refugee Rights.

Bourmaud, P. (2012). Santé et territorialité: L'assurance maladie et l' "expulsion silencieuse" des familles palestiniennes. In IISMM (Ed.), *Les Palestiniens entre Etat et diaspora* (pp. 119–148). Paris, France: Le temps des incertitudes.

Bowlus, A. J., & Seitz, S. (2005). *Domestic violence, employment and divorce*. Retrieved May 8, 2012, from http://qed.econ.queensu.ca/pub/faculty/seitz/abuse11.pdf

Browning, J., & Dutton, D. (1986). Assessment of wife assault with the Conflict Tactics Scale: Using couple data to quantify the differential reporting effect. *Journal of Marriage and Family, 48*, 375–379.

Clark, C., Everson-Rose, S., Suglia, S., Btoush, R., Alonso, A., & Haj-Yahia, M. (2010). Association between exposure to political violence and intimate-partner violence in the occupied Palestinian territory: A cross-sectional study. *The Lancet, 375*(9711), 310–316.

Conte, E. (2005). L'autre mur: Mariages bannis et citoyennetés fragmentées en Israël-Palestine. *Études Rurales, 173*(174), 127–152.

Dembik, C., & Marteu, E. (2009). La communauté arabe d'Israël, entre intégration et reconnaissance. *Revue Averroès, 1*, 79–87.

Farsakh, L. (2005). *Palestinian labour migration to Israel: Labour, land and occupation* (The Routledge political economy of the Middle East and North Africa series). New York: Routledge.

Gartner, R. (1990). The victims of homicides: A temporal and cross-national comparison. *American Sociological Review, 55*, 92–106.

Haj-Yahia, M. (2000). The incidence of wife abuse and battering and some sociodemographic correlates as revealed by two national surveys in Palestinian society. *Journal of Family Violence, 15*(4), 347–374.

Haj-Yahia, M., & Abdo-Kaloti, R. (2003). The rates and correlates of the exposure of Palestinian adolescents to family violence: Toward an integrative-holistic approach. *Child Abuse and Neglect, 27*, 781–806.

Hammami, R. (2009). *Voicing the needs of women and men in Gaza: Beyond the aftermath of the 23-day Israeli military operations*. Ramallah Territoires, Palestiniens: UNIFEM.

Hammoury, N., Khawaja, M., Mahfoud, Z., Afifi, R. A., & Madi, H. (2009). Domestic violence against women during pregnancy: The case of Palestinian refugees attending an antenatal clinic in Lebanon. *Journal of Women's Health, 18*(3), 337–345.

Handel, A. (2009). Where, where to and when in the occupied territories? An introduction to geography of disaster. In M. Givoni (Ed.), *Occupation: Israeli technologies of rule and governance in Palestine*. New York: Zone Books.

Hanieh, A. (2006). The politics of curfew in the occupied territories. In J. Beinin & R. L. Stein (Eds.), *The struggle for sovereignty: Palestine and Israel 1993–2005* (pp. 324–337). Stanford, CA: Stanford University Press.

Hass, A. (2002). *Les bouclages imposés par Israël sont en train de provoquer l'effondrement de l'économie palestinienne*. Retrieved October 9, 2014, from http://www.lapaixmaintenant.org/article940

Hilal, J. (2010). The pauperization of Palestinian women, men and children in the West Bank and Gaza Strip. In J. Hilal (Ed.), *A dangerous decade: The 2nd gender profile of the occupied West Bank and Gaza* (pp. 2000–2010). Birzeit, Palestine: Institute for Women's Studies, Birzeit University.

Hindin, M. (2003). Understanding women's attitudes towards wife beating in Zimbabwe. *Bulletin of the World Health Organization, 81*(7), 501–508.

Hollander, D. (2003). In Zimbabwe, substantial minorities of women are accepting of wife-beating. *International Family Planning Perspectives, 29*(4), 194.

Honneth, A. (2005). Invisibilité: Sur l'épistémologie de la reconnaissance. *Réseaux, 1*(129–130), 39–57. Retrieved January 27, 2014, from http://www.cairn.info/revue-reseaux-2005-1-page-39.htm

Khawaja, M., Linos, N., & El-Roueiheb, Z. (2008). Attitudes of men and women towards wife beating: Findings from Palestinian refugee camps in Jordan. *Family Violence, 23*(3), 211–218.

Khawaja, M., & Omari, M. (2009). *Labour market performance and migration flows in Palestine*. National Background Paper, Robert Schuman Centre for Advanced Studies, European University Institute, Florence, mimeo.

Kishor, S. (2005). Domestic violence measurement in the Demographic and Health Surveys: The history and the challenges. In UN Division for the Advancement of Women (Ed.), *Violence against women: A statistical overview, challenges and gaps in data collection and methodology and approaches for overcoming them*. Geneva, Switzerland: UN Division for the Advancement of Women.

Kishor, S., & Johnson, K. (2006). *Profil de la violence domestique*, OD39, 122. Retrieved May 8, 2012, from http://www.measuredhs.com/publications/publication-OD39-OtherDocuments.cfm

Kuttab, E. (2006). The paradox of women's work: Coping, crisis and family survival. In L. Taraki (Ed.), *Living Palestine: Family survival, resistance and mobility under occupation* (pp. 231–274). Syracuse: Syracuse University Press.

Lamont, M., & White, P. (2008). *Interdisciplinary standards for systematic qualitative research*. Cultural Anthropology, Law and Social Science, Political Science, and Sociology Programs, Supportive Workshop, The National Science Foundation, 180.

Latte Abdallah, S. (2006). Femmes réfugiées palestiniennes. Partage du savoir: PUF et le Monde, 237.

Latte Abdallah, S., & Parizot, C. (2011). A l'ombre du mur: Israéliens et palestiniens entre séparation et occupation. In S. Latte Abdallah & C. Parizot (Eds.), *Etudes méditerranéennes* (p. 334). Paris: Actes Sud/MMSH.

Legrain, J.-F. (2007). La dynamique de la guerre civile en Palestine. *Critique Internationale, 36*, 147–165.

Lev-Wiesel, R., Al-Krenawi, A., & Sehwail, M. A. (2007). Psychological symptomatology among Palestinian male and female adolescents living under political violence 2004–2005. *Community Mental Health Journal, 43*, 49–56.

MacMillian, R., & Gartner, R. (1999). When she brings home the bacon: Labor-force participation and the risk of spousal violence against women. *Journal of Marriage and the Family, 61*(4), 947–958.

Maziak, W., & Asfar, T. (2003). Physical abuse in low-income women in Aleppo, Syria. *Health Care for Women International, 24*, 313–326.

Memmi, S. (in press). Les couples palestiniens à l'épreuve de la politique de séparation israélienne. In C. Parizot & S. Latte Abdallah (Eds.), *L'illusion de la séparation: Occupation israélienne et régime du mouvement en Palestine*. Actes Sud.

Mitchell, L. (2010). *Coping, closure and gendered life transitions: Palestinian's response to the erosion of male breadwinning work*. Accessed October 9, 2014, from http://www.fafo.no/pub/rapp/20178/20178.pdf

Moore, H. (1994). *Passion for difference: Essays in anthropology and gender*. Cambridge: Indiana University Press.

Muhanna, A. (2010). Changing family and gender dynamics during the siege against Gaza: Spousal relations and domestic violence. *Review of Women's Studies, 6*, 40–52.

Naqib, F. M. (2009). *Economic & social monitor*. Ramallah: Palestine Economic Policy Research Institute.

Peteet, J. (1994). Male gender and rituals of resistance in the Palestinian Intifada: A cultural politics of violence. *American Ethnologist, 21*(1), 31–49.

Sibany, S. (2007). Les Arabes d'Israël: Une minorité nationale palestinienne? *Hérodote, 1*(124), 79–92.

Usta, J., Farver, J. A., & Pashayan, N. (2007). Domestic violence: The Lebanese experience. *Public Health, 121*(3), 208–219.

Yaish, Z. (Unpublished). *Negotiating authority and masculinity in households living in crisis situation: the case of Palestinian male breadwinners losing jobs*. Faculty of Graduate Studies at Birzeit University, Palestine.

Yick, A. G. (2001). Feminist theory and status inconsistency theory: Application to domestic violence in Chinese immigrant families. *Violence Against Women, 7*(5), 545–562.

Zuhur, S. (2003). Women and empowerment in the Arab world. *Arab Studies Quarterly, 25*(4), 17–38.

Part III
Gender-Based Violence: Perspectives from India

Chapter 8
Examining Nonconsensual Sex and Risk of Reproductive Tract Infections and Sexually Transmitted Infections Among Young Married Women in India

Ajay Kumar Singh, Rabindra Kumar Sinha, and Ruchi Jain

Abstract A young woman's powerlessness and inability to exercise sexual choices in her marital home exacerbate the nonconsensual nature of early sex, particularly forced sexual initiation. Worldwide, at least one woman in three has been beaten, coerced into sex, or otherwise abused in her lifetime. This chapter explores young married women's perception on sexual and reproductive rights, gender roles, and husband's extramarital relationship and its association with the experience of sexual and physical violence and sexual health problems. The study analyzes a cross-sectional data on married women (15–29 years) in Delhi, India, during the years 2007–2008. More than two-thirds of women reported ever experiencing coercive sex by husband in their lifetime. Of this, 55 % ($p < 0.05$) reported coercive sex during the last 12 months of the survey. Among women who ever experienced sexual violence, 44 % had at least one STD symptom during the last 6 months compared to 27 % who did not experience any STD symptoms ($p < 0.05$); and 59 % ($p < 0.05$) of women reported problems during menses.

Keywords Coercive sex • Risk of reproductive tract infections • Sexually transmitted infections • Young women • India

A.K. Singh (✉)
John Snow Research and Training Institute (JSI), New Delhi, India
e-mail: krsajay@yahoo.co.in

R.K. Sinha
Independent Consultant, Mumbai, India
e-mail: rksinha35@gmail.com

R. Jain
National Council for Applied Economic Research, New Delhi, India
e-mail: ruchi_iips@yahoo.co.in

© Springer International Publishing Switzerland 2015   169
Y.K. Djamba, S.R. Kimuna (eds.), *Gender-Based Violence*,
DOI 10.1007/978-3-319-16670-4_8

Background

Evidence suggests that substantial sexual coercion against women occurs within marriage. An analysis of over 50 population-based surveys found that approximately 10–50 % of adult women around the world reported having been physically assaulted by an intimate male partner (including their husbands) at some point in their lives (WHO 2005). Studies that have explored sexual violence have found that sexual abuse is present in approximately one-third to half of the cases of physical abuse by an intimate partner (Heise et al. 1999). In many developing settings, notably South Asia and sub-Saharan Africa, early marriage of girls remains widespread. However, in the context of early marriage from a rights perspective, it has been pointed out that the right to free and full consent to a marriage is recognized in the 1948 Universal Declaration of Human Rights and in several subsequent instruments on human rights (UNICEF 2001).

It is important to note that arranged marriage is not synonymous with forced marriage. Within the rights framework used by UNICEF, for example, a young person of sufficient maturity can give (or refuse) consent to an arranged marriage. In fact, a collection of studies from South Asia found that in many settings, adolescents strongly supported the idea that their parents should decide whom they are to marry (Bott and Jeejebhoy 2003). However, the Universal Declaration of Human Rights argues that consent cannot be "free and full" if at least one partner is very immature, and in many settings, young people—particularly young girls—are often forced to marry and consummate the marriage at a young age in the absence of informed consent (UNICEF 2001). In the Gambia, for example, a study reveals that the prevalence of early marriage of young girls under the age of 15 is 8.6 %, and those under age 18 constitute 46.5 % (Buttaye 2013).

A small body of research has begun to look at the circumstances surrounding the sexual experiences within marriage of girls who marry as young adolescents. Some of these studies highlight the extent to which marital sexual initiation is often characterized by force, fear, and pain. For example, several studies from India, some reporting the retrospective experiences of adult women, reveal that early marital sexual experiences were typically traumatic, distasteful, and painful, and often involved the use of physical force (George and Jaswal 1995 Mumbai study; Khan et al. 1996 Uttar Pradesh study; Sodhi and Verma 2003 New Delhi study).

The World Report on Violence and Health cautions that sexual violence is complicated by the multiple forms it takes and the contexts in which it occurs, and by the fact that risk factors may vary in importance according to the life stage of the victim (WHO 2002). The report cites a number of factors that may increase the vulnerability of women, in particular to sexual violence, namely at young ages, alcohol and drug consumption, previous experiences of abuse, multiple partner relations, and poverty. Some researches have explored the types of structural and environmental factors that put young people at greater risk of sexual coercion, including poverty, patriarchy, societal norms that support sexual violence and gender inequity, early marriage, inadequate educational and health systems, and ineffective laws and policies.

Most available studies have focused on young women's—rather than young men's—experiences and suggest that young people who experience nonconsensual sex are more likely than others to report poor educational attainment, migrant status, residence away from parents, and alcohol and drug use (see for example, Bohmer and Kirumira 1997; Yimin et al. 2001; WHO 2002), although in some cases these may be consequences of rather than risk factors for abuse. Anecdotal evidence points, moreover, to such factors as crowded housing conditions and the lack of adequate or safe housing as additional, yet unexplored, factors. While few studies have directly explored beyond these factors, the context of nonconsensual relations described in these largely qualitative studies offers an insight into the kind of risk factors that make young people more vulnerable to sexual abuse. These factors work at the individual, family, community, and systemic levels. Prominent among these are gender double standards, power imbalances and inadequate negotiation skills, lack of awareness of rights and opportunities for recourse, lack of supportive environments and trusted adults on sexual health matters, unfriendly institutional responses (health, crime, legal), and, perhaps most important, a failure on the part of social and legal institutions in the community to recognize the problem and punish the perpetrators rather than the victims.

Nonconsensual sex within marriage is one of the most common and repugnant forms of masochism in Indian society, which is hidden behind the curtain of marriage. In Uttar Pradesh, India, about two-thirds of 98 respondents reported being forced into sex by their husbands—about one-third of them by being beaten (Khan et al. 1996). In India, marital rape exists de facto but not de jure. Cultural norms and the perceived social stigma attached to rape often discourage the reporting of marital rape.

The World Bank estimates that in industrialized countries, sexual assault and violence take away almost one in five healthy years of life of women aged 15–44 (United Nations Population Fund 1999). In a study conducted in Punjab, India, 81 % of women felt that if their husband opposed the use of contraception, they were obliged to respect his wishes (Population Council 1997). In South Africa, 30 % of young women indicated that their first sex was coerced (Jewkes et al. 2002). Many young women are faced with the challenge of saying no to unprotected sex, especially when dependent economically and socially on their male partners. The fear of violence contributes to the absence of any negotiating position for protected sex (Development Studies 2000). The vital issues to women and their health are nutrition, sanitation, infectious diseases, psychological tension, pregnancy, delivery, and sexual violence. A study in southern India of 451 married young girls (aged 16–22) found high levels of reproductive health problems, including reproductive tract infections (RTIs), where more than 48 % of women reported one or more symptoms of RTIs (Barua and Kurz 2001). Girls are often forced to marry men much older than themselves, leaving them particularly vulnerable to an abusive relationship (UNICEF 1998). A survey of men in selected districts of India showed that a significant percentage of husbands (30.1 %) reported having committed one or more sexual violence against their wives during the preceding year (Koenig et al. 2006).

There are very few studies on the young married women. Most of the available literature generally focuses on young unmarried girls rather than married, despite the fact that in India sex is negotiated and acted mostly under the sanctity of marriage.

This chapter explores the young married women's perception on reproductive and sexual rights and husband's extramarital relationship. It also examines the association of violence, more specifically marital rape, sexual health problems of women, and their vulnerability to STIs and HIV risk.

Data and Methods

The data for this study has been taken from an exploratory study in New Delhi, India, to look at the Reproductive and Sexual Rights of Young Married Women and their Health outcomes in diverse sociocultural and economic settings during the period of December 2007 to January 2008. A total of 300 young married women aged 15–30 years were carefully selected and interviewed using a structured questionnaire. Informed consent was taken from the potential participants. The response rate was high, with 94 % of individuals consenting to participate.

The quantitative data were collected through handheld devices. This method of data collection has been very effective and has been used in various studies (Gravlee 2002; Lal et al. 2000; Grasso and Genest 2001; Fischer et al. 2003; Verma et al. 2008). The research team received intensive training on the use of handheld devices and the software (Perseus) in the classroom and in the field. Systems were developed to download the survey data from the handheld devices to the mainframe computer on a daily basis to ensure that the data were not lost (Verma et al. 2008). Consistency check was run using SPSS v16 to ensure high quality of data. Standardized procedures were established and followed for contacting and interviewing respondents. One-to-one interviews were done confidentially and the identity of respondents was not recorded to ensure anonymity. Twenty in-depth interviews were conducted with purposely selected women to get in-depth understanding of the issues.

Measurements

Reproductive Rights Index

The reproductive rights index was created to measure the degree of women's assertiveness about different dimensions of their rights pertaining to their reproductive life. This index was further used in multivariate analysis as predictors of nonconsensual sex and sexually transmitted disease among women. A composite index of reproductive rights was constructed by giving appropriate weights to a woman's decision on her marital process, decision on contraceptive use with husband, and decision on the number of children with husband. The index also included five statements which determine levels of women's assertiveness to reproductive rights:

1. You should decide on the number of children that you will have
2. You should decide on the spacing of children

3. You should decide on the type of family planning method that best suits you
4. You alone are capable of deciding on spending money on your health needs without husband's consent
5. It is your right whether to keep a pregnancy or to abort it without husband's consent

The responses were recorded as "agree," "somewhat agree," and "do not agree," The most positive response was given a score of 2 and the least positive response was given a score of 0. Thus, the created index weights for these items were 2 for agree, 1 for somewhat agree, and 0 for do not agree. Given this scoring system, a respondent giving the most negative response to all the items received a total score of 0 and a respondent giving the most positive response to all the items received a score of 24. In order to make the results easier to interpret, these scores were categorized as "low" (scores of 0–7), "moderate" (scores of 8–15), and "high" (scores of 16–24). The internal consistency of the items was checked by applying reliability test with a Cronbach alpha value of 0.76.

Sexual Rights Index

The sexual rights index was created to measure the degree of women's control over their body and sexual relationship with their husbands. This index was further used as a predictor of nonconsensual sex and sexually transmitted disease among women. It was also used to explore the association with women's perception about marriage and women's justification of intimate partner violence. A composite index of sexual right was created by allotting higher score to the more positive response. Four items were considered for constructing the sexual rights index, plus a woman's denial of sex and use of condom in the event the husband had extramarital sexual relationship:

1. Refusal of sex when the woman is tired or not in the mood
2. Refusal of sex when the woman has recently given birth
3. Refusal of sex when the woman is aware that her husband has an extramarital relationship
4. Refusal to have sex when she knows that her husband has sexually transmitted disease

The possible response categories were 0, 1, and 2. The resulting index had a minimum value of "0" for the most negative responses and a maximum value of "12" for the most positive responses. For ease of analysis and understanding, the index was further divided into three categories: low (0–3), moderate (4–8), and high (9–12). It was found that most of the women belonged to two different extremes; when it comes to asserting their sexual right, either they were in low category (38 %) or they belonged to high category (47 %). Only 16 % of women fell under the moderate category. The internal consistency of the items was checked using reliability test with the Cronbach alpha score of 0.92.

Autonomy Index

To assess women's autonomy, women in this survey were asked a set of questions concerning their status within the household. The autonomy index was created to assess women's degree of autonomy in decision making at the household level. The autonomy index was further used as a predictor for experiencing violence, reproductive and sexual rights of women, comprehensive knowledge of HIV, and women's risk perception of HIV.

The respondents were asked whether they had any role in making decisions related to purchasing the following items: food, small gifts, jewelry, clothes, or any other expensive items. A score of 0 was assigned if the respondent had no role, 1 if she had some say, and 2 if she had final say. A series of questions were also asked about her freedom in spending money on herself for health purposes, freedom to attend meetings organized by CBOs/NGOs, freedom to limit family size, freedom to visit her native place, etc. A higher score indicates a larger role in decision making related to household purchases. The response categories ranged from 0 to 2 depending upon the intensity of the responses.

A summary index was created and the minimum value was 0 for the least empowered and 22 for the most empowered. The internal consistency of items was done using reliability analysis. The Cronbach alpha score was 0.91. It was further trichotomized as "low autonomy (0–7)," "moderate autonomy (8–14)," and "high autonomy (15–22)."

Results

The mean age of the women selected for the survey was 26.3 years (SD 3.52) and the median years of schooling was 10 years (SD 3.51). The mean age at first marriage was 18.2 years (SD 3.09); however, 27 % of the women were married before the age of 18 years. More than half (54 %) were married for more than 6 years at the time of interview; 21 % were married for 2 years or less. The average household monthly income of the selected sample was 165 USD (Table 8.1).

Table 8.1 Selected socio-demographic characteristics of married women, Delhi, India, 2007–2008

Select background characteristics	$N=300$
Mean age of the women	26.3 years
Median years of schooling	10 years
Mean age at marriage	18.2 years
Average household monthly income	165 USD
Working for money	11 %
Mean marital duration	5.6 years

Table 8.2 Percentage distribution of married women's attitude on different dimensions of reproductive rights, Delhi, India, 2007–2008

	Agree		Partially agree		Do not agree	
Indicator	N	%	N	%	N	%
You should decide upon the number of children that you will have	206	68.7	33	11.0	61	20.3
You should decide upon the spacing of children	233	77.7	18	6.0	49	16.3
You should decide on the type of family planning method that best suits you	185	61.7	44	14.7	71	23.7
You alone are capable of deciding on spending money on your health needs without husband's consent	203	67.7	26	8.7	71	23.7
It is your right whether to keep a pregnancy or to abort it without husband's consent	206	68.7	26	8.7	68	22.7

Perceptions of Women About Sexual and Reproductive Rights

The findings on women's perceptions on sexual and reproductive rights show that about two-thirds of young married women agreed with the statement that they should decide upon the number of children they should have (69 %). About the same percentage agreed on the statements that the wife alone is capable of deciding on spending money on her health needs without husband's consent (68 %) and that it is her right to decide whether to keep a pregnancy or to abort it without husband's consent (69 %). Almost 78 % (77.7 %) of respondents agreed that the women should decide on the spacing of their children and 62 % agreed with the statement that they should decide on the type of family planning method that best suits them (Table 8.2).

Understanding the Sexual Rights of the Women

Women's control over their sexual behavior is a key factor of their sexual well-being. It not only has bearing over their reproductive health, but also has an overarching impact on their mental health and marital life.

In the current study, in order to explore different dimensions of sexual rights of young married women, respondents were asked what their reaction would be, if they found out that their husband was involved in an extramarital sexual relationship. The results in Fig. 8.1 show that over half of the women (59.0 %) reported that they would deny sex and 45.3 % said that they would insist on condom use. Almost 39 % (38.7 %) of women said that they would strongly restrict their husbands from meeting other women, only 9.3 % said that they would go for panchayat or court, 4.0 % said that they would go to CBO/NGOs,

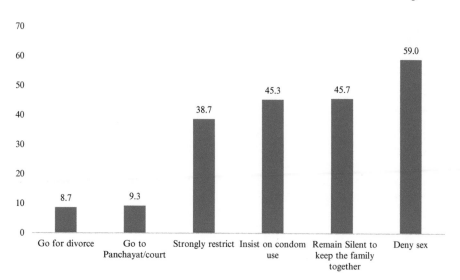

Fig. 8.1 Percentage distribution of women by the type of actions they would take if they found out that their husbands are involved in extramarital sexual relationships (*N*=300)

and only 8.7 % said that they would go for divorce. Very surprisingly, nearly half (45.7 %) of the young married women said that they would remain silent to keep their families together (Fig. 8.1). This clearly shows women's inability to exercise their rights due to social taboos and similarly; dependence on husbands clearly impacts women's autonomy over their sexual life.

Some of the women in in-depth interviews revealed that they were aware of their husbands' extramarital relationships. One of the women said:

> When my children were born, I was in my natal home. He was then involved with some other girl and he did not pay any attention to me or our children … when I came back, I learned that he still keeps meeting that girl and once I caught him red handed with that girl. I beat that girl a lot with my sandal; my husband also scolded me and beat me. Then I told my husband that I will die along with my three children if he does not stop meeting with that girl … and if he wishes to see them alive, he will have to forget that girl… from then on he has never met that girl …
>
> – 29 year old woman, married for 10 years.

Another woman narrated her marital life experience as helpless. Her husband tortures her every day. On extramarital relationship she said:

> … he teases other girls in front of me and when I try to stop him, he starts beating me. I don't understand what to do. I know he had sexual relationship with other women even before marriage but my mother in law does not believe in me. Once he tried to molest my sister, my brother came for her rescue and he beat him … I am living with him only because of the "izzat" (honor) of my in laws or else I would have left him long back.
>
> – 27 year old woman, married for 9 years.

Justification of Violence

Table 8.3 data show that more than half of the women (50.7 %) agreed with the statement that they were justified in refusing sex with their husbands when they are tired or not in the mood, slightly over 56 % (56.3 %) when they have recently given birth, 55 % when a woman knows that her husband has relationships with other women, and also when she knows that her husband has a sexually transmitted disease. However, 32.3 % of women disagreed with all the statements.

There is no significant variation between the age groups on different situations where women agree that they are justified in refusing sex with their husbands. For the age group under 23 years (those aged ≤22 years), the percentage of women who agree that they can refuse to have sex with their husbands under certain circumstances ranges from 45.1 to 52.9 %. The older age group (23 years and above) percent ranges from 51.8 to 57.0. More than two-fifths (44.3 %) of young married women agree to all the four statements about women's justification in refusing sex with their husbands.

No definite pattern emerged from level of educational and women's attitude about such a situation. However, data show that most women with a primary education (64.1–79.5 %) agree with justification for refusing sex with their husbands in different situations. Only 10.3 % of women with a primary education did not agree with any of the situations compared to other levels of education which ranged from 33.0 to 42.1 %.

There are significant differences by religion; for example, nearly 53 % (52.7 %) of Hindu women compared to only 37.5 % of Muslim women agreed that the woman is justified in refusing sex with her husband when she is tired or not in the mood; when she has recently given birth (57.3 % vs. 50.0 %); and when she knows that her husband has extramarital relationships (56.5 % vs. 47.5 %). However, there was no significant difference in women's agreement from half of the women in both religious groups that they are justified in refusing sex when husbands have sexually transmitted diseases. The data in Table 8.3 indicate that 45.8 % of Hindu women agreed with all given situations for refusing sex to husband compared to only 35.0 % of Muslim women. However, close to one-third of the women in both religious groups did not agree with any of the given situations.

Most women from scheduled castes (55.8–68.6 %) said refusing sex was justifiable. Among those in the other backward class the level of agreement for refusing sex ranged between 47.1 and 51.4 %; for other ethnic groups, it was 49.3–52.8 %. "Other backward class (OBC)" is a collective term used by the Government of India to design castes that are educationally and socially disadvantaged. Half of the women belonging to scheduled castes agreed to all the reasons for refusing sex. The corresponding figure for other backward class and other ethnic groups is 41.4 % and 42.4 %, respectively. Close to only one-fourth (24.4 %) of women belonging to scheduled caste did not agree with any of the situations. This figure is much lower than among other groups: 34.3 % among women in the other backward class and 36.1 % for those in other ethnic groups.

The proportion of women who justified refusing sex seems to increase with the duration of marriage. During the initial years of marriage, the justification to refuse

Table 8.3 Socioeconomic and demographic characteristics of young married women by justification of women to refuse sex to their husbands over given situations (%), Delhi, India, 2007–2008

Socioeconomic and demographic characteristics	Percentage of married women who agree that a woman is justified in refusing sex with her husband when				Percentage who agree to all the four reasons	Percentage who do not agree with any of the four reasons
	She is tired or not in the mood	She has recently given a birth	She knows that her husband has sex with other women	She knows that her husband has a sexually transmitted disease		
Age						
≤22	45.1	52.9	52.9	52.9	43.1	39.2
>22	51.8	57	55.8	55.4	44.6	30.9
Education						
Illiterate	43.2	50	46.6	45.5	33	33
Primary 1–7 years	64.1	76.9	69.2	79.5	53.9	10.3
8–9 Years	47.4	55.3	57.9	52.6	44.7	42.1
HS complete	44.4	47.2	52.8	50	36.1	36.1
11–12 Years	54	58.7	58.7	57.1	54	34.9
12+	58.3	55.6	55.6	55.6	52.8	36.1
Religion						
Hindu	52.7	57.3	56.5	55.4	45.8	32.3
Muslim	37.5	50	47.5	52.5	35	32.5
Ethnicity						
Scheduled caste	55.8	68.6	62.8	67.4	50	24.4
Other backward class	47.1	50	51.4	51.4	41.4	34.3
Others	49.3	52.1	52.8	49.3	42.4	36.1
Marital duration						
≤1 year	43.8	43.8	43.8	46.9	43.8	46.9
2 years	43.8	59.4	59.4	56.3	40.6	37.5
3 years	59.1	63.6	63.6	59.1	50	27.3

4 years	55	55	55	65	55	25
5+ years	51.6	57.2	55.7	54.6	43.3	30.4
Working status						
Unemployed/housewife	51.1	55.6	54.5	53.4	44.4	33.2
Daily wage/laborer/maid	46.2	69.2	76.9	76.9	46.2	23.1
Pvt/Govt. salaried	36.4	36.4	36.4	45.5	27.3	36.4
Other	62.5	87.5	75	87.5	62.5	12.5
Number of living children						
0	36.2	36.2	37.7	39.1	34.8	50.7
1	53.4	60.3	60.3	61.6	46.6	27.4
2	53.9	57.7	60.3	53.9	47.4	30.8
3	55.6	66.7	59.3	61.1	44.4	24.1
4+	61.5	73.1	65.4	69.2	53.9	19.2
Husband's occupation						
Pvt. salaried	55.3	64.7	65.3	65.3	51.8	25.3
Daily wage/laborer	50.9	47.2	47.2	47.2	35.9	34.0
Business	43.5	46.4	42.0	40.6	36.2	43.5
Other	12.5	25.0	12.5	12.5	12.5	75.0
Total	50.7	56.3	55.3	55.0	44.3	32.3

sex for all the situations was close to 40 %; during years 3 and 4, that number increased to 55 % and 65 %, respectively, but decreased thereafter. The women who were working in private- and government-salaried jobs were less likely to justify refusing sex as compared to those in other work categories. In contrast, type of husband's occupation did not have any impact on women's beliefs, as close to half of the women did not justify wife refusing sex with her husband irrespective of type of husband's occupation. Finally, the refusal to have sex with the husband is lower among women who have no children and increases with number of children.

Perceived Marital Life and Sexual Right

The analysis in Table 8.4 suggests that the women who scored high on the sexual rights index were significantly more likely to report that their marital life is very happy, compared to those who scored in the low and moderate categories on the sexual rights index.

Women's Autonomy and Sexual Rights

The findings presented in Table 8.5 indicate that women who belonged to moderate and high autonomy categories were more likely to assert their sexual rights. For example, 60.9 % of women who scored moderately on the sexual

Table 8.4 Relationship between perceived married life and sexual rights index, Delhi, India, 2007–2008

Sexual rights index[a]	Perceived married life of women			Number of women
	Very happy	Somewhat happy	Unhappy	
Low	15.9	73.5	10.6	113
Medium	29.8	63.8	6.4	47
High	45.7	52.1	2.1	140
Total	96	186	18	300

[a]All differences in this table are statistically significant at $p < 0.05$ (chi-square test)

Table 8.5 Relationship of women's autonomy index and different dimensions of women's sexual rights, Delhi, India, 2007–2008

	You are justified in refusing sex with your husband when …			
	You are tired or not in the mood	You have recently given a birth	You know that your husband has sex with other women	You know that your husband has a sexually transmitted disease
Autonomy index[a]	% Yes	% Yes	% Yes	% Yes
Low	34.8	34.8	34.8	33.9
Moderate	60.9	72.4	70.1	71.3
High	59.4	66.3	65.3	64.4

[a]All differences in this table are statistically significant at $p < 0.05$ (chi-square test)

autonomy index and 59.4 % of women who scored high on the same index said that they were justified in refusing sex to their husbands when they were tired or not in mood. A similar pattern was observed among all the other dimensions of sexual rights.

Women's Experience of Violence

Previous research in India showed that married women who have experienced both physical and sexual violence by their husbands are nearly four times as likely to be infected with HIV as women who have not experienced either type of intimate partner violence (Silverman et al. 2008). This section deals with various types of violence faced by women and further tries to explore how it impacts women's vulnerability to RTIs and STIs.

Figure 8.2 shows data on the women who experienced physical violence. The results show that one-third of the women reported that they were slapped or pushed by their husbands. Eleven to fourteen percent reported that they were hit by a fist, dragged, chocked, or burnt. According to data on nonphysical violence, three-fifths of women reported that their husbands used to scare them, while one-third were either insulted or humiliated in a public place.

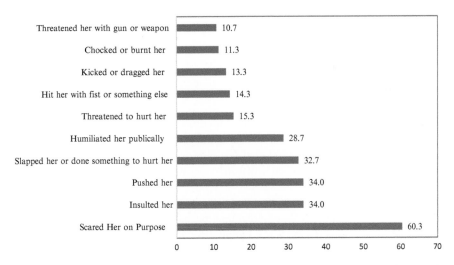

Fig. 8.2 Percent distribution of women by type of physical and nonphysical violence they experienced during their lifetime, Delhi, India, 2007–2008

Experience of Violence by Background Characteristics of Women

The analysis in Table 8.6 suggests that more than three-fourths of women (78.0 %) reported experiencing at least one type of violence. About two-thirds (62.0 %) reported that they have experienced sexual violence during their lifetime and nearly half (44.7 %) percent experienced physical violence. Close to two-thirds of women (63.7 %) reported experiencing nonphysical violence and 41.3 % experienced physical as well as sexual violence from their husbands.

Further, Table 8.6 shows that women 23 years and older were more likely to experience different types of violence than younger women (younger than 23 years of age). For instance, 80.3 % of women older than 23 years of age reported that they had experienced at least one type of violence compared to 66.7 % of women in the younger age group. This age difference was also consistent for sexual violence (64.7 % vs. 49.0 %), physical violence (46.6 % vs. 35.3 %), and nonphysical violence (66.7 % vs. 49.0 %).

Data on the religious category shows the proportion of Muslim women who reported any violence (85.0 %) to be 8 % higher than that of their Hindu counterparts (76.9 %). For sexual violence it was 72.5 % vs. 60.4 % and for physical violence it was 50.0 % vs. 43.9 %.

It was also observed that women with longer marital duration reported more different kinds of violence compared to those who had spent less time in their marital life. Experience of violence also increases with the number of children. More than 96 % of women who had more than four children reported any form of violence; there was however relatively less violence reported by women who had fewer children; it ranged from 68.1 to 90.7 %. A similar pattern was observed with sexual violence, physical violence, and nonphysical violence.

Sexual Coercion by Husband

Under domestic violence, one of the most common forms of violence that is seen in the country and throughout the world is sexual coercion. In this chapter, more than one-third of women (38.4 %) reported that they have been forced by their husbands to have sexual intercourse even when they did not want to (Fig. 8.3). Forty-two percent reported that they had sexual intercourse with their husbands even when they did not want to because they were afraid of what their husbands might do; more than a half of women (51.8 %) said that their husbands forced them to do something sexual that they found degrading or humiliating. Around one-fourth of the married women (23.7 %) reported experiencing all three types of sexual violence. Overall, close to two-thirds of women (62.3 %) experienced at least one form of sexual violence by their husbands.

In-depth interviews suggest that the sexual violence has a detrimental impact on women's overall health. One of the women aged 23 years shares her experiences:

> I have been married for 4 years and blessed with 2 children. My husband beats me regularly and I suffer now from pains in my body, but my worst problem is the way my husband uses

Table 8.6 Distribution of women's experience of violence by socioeconomic and demographic characteristics, Delhi, India, 2007–2008

Socioeconomic and demographic characteristics	Experience of violence			
	Any violence	Sexual violence	Physical violence	Nonphysical, excluding sexual violence
Age				
≤22	66.7	49.0	35.3	49.0
>22	80.3	64.7	46.6	66.7
Education				
Illiterate	88.6	69.3	65.9	81.8
Primary 1–7 years	82.1	61.5	48.7	66.7
8–9 years	71.1	60.5	39.5	57.9
High school complete	66.7	63.9	27.8	52.8
11–12 years	77.8	63.5	36.5	57.1
12+	66.7	41.7	25.0	44.4
Religion				
Hindu	76.9	60.4	43.9	62.3
Muslim	85.0	72.5	50.0	72.5
Ethnicity				
Scheduled caste	77.9	58.1	41.9	74.4
Other backward class	82.9	71.4	52.9	74.3
Others	75.7	59.7	42.4	71.5
Marital duration				
≤1 year	65.6	50.0	31.3	46.9
2 years	71.9	56.3	25.0	46.9
3 years	63.6	50.0	22.7	45.5
4 years	85.0	65.0	45.0	65.0
5+ years	82.0	66.0	52.6	71.1
Working status				
Unemployed/housewife	79.9	63.8	47.0	65.7
Daily wage/laborer/maid	61.5	46.2	30.8	38.5
Pvt/Govt. salaried	45.5	36.4	9.1	36.4
Other	87.5	62.5	37.5	75.0
Number of living children				
0	68.1	55.1	30.4	46.4
1	72.6	56.2	41.1	58.9
2	76.9	64.1	39.7	62.8
3	90.7	70.4	57.4	79.6
4+	96.2	73.1	80.8	92.3
Husband's occupation				
Pvt/Govt. salaried	74.1	56.5	34.1	60.6
Daily wage/laborer	88.7	77.4	69.8	73.6
Business	82.6	66.7	55.1	66.7
Other	50.0	37.5	12.5	37.5
Total	78.0	62.0	44.7	63.7

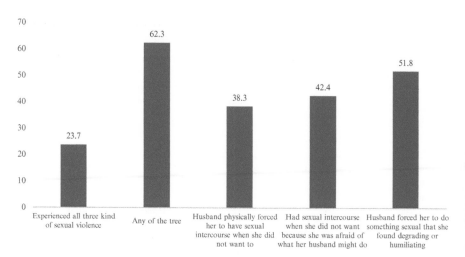

Fig. 8.3 Percent distribution of women by different types of sexual violence they experienced during their lifetime, Delhi, India, 2007–2008

force on me to have sex and this hurts me badly because I suffer from the wounds he causes during forced sex. It is extremely painful, I cannot stop him, he beats me if I do so ...

— 23 year old woman, married for five years.

In one case, men wanted to have sex in her natal home though she did not feel comfortable doing so when her parents and other natal family members were around. She said:

... he always demands sex even if I am in my natal home. That's why I have stopped going to my natal place. He demands sleeping with me even there, I don't like it ... and in the past when I didn't sleep with him ... he beat me up and used foul languages next morning in front of my natal family... it was very insulting and embarrassing ... I cried a lot ...

— 22 year old woman, married for two years.

Violence and Risk Perception of Women

Among the young women who experienced any violence, around 23.7 % reported that their husbands have extramarital sexual relationships compared to only 1.2 % of women who didn't experience any violence (Table 8.7). Likewise, among the women who experienced any violence, almost 20 % (19.5 %) reported that they were worried about being infected with HIV compared to only 4.7 % of women who did not experience any violence.

More specifically, over one-fourth (26.3 %) of women who experienced sexual violence and 30.6 % of those who experienced physical violence felt that their husbands have extramarital relationships. Among those who did not experience such violence, the fear of husbands having extramarital sex was much lower.

Table 8.7 Association between wife abuse and woman's perception of her husband's extramarital relations and her perception of her own HIV infection risk, Delhi, India, 2007–2008

Experienced type of violence[a]	Feel that husband has extramarital sexual relationship	Worried that she can be infected with HIV	Number of women
Sexual violence			
Yes	26.3	21.5	186
No	2.6	5.3	114
Physical violence			
Yes	30.6	24.6	134
No	6.6	7.8	166
Any violence (sexual or physical)			
Yes	23.7	19.5	215
No	1.2	4.7	85
Total %	17.3	15.3	300

[a]All differences in this table are statistically significant at $p < 0.05$ (chi-square test)

More than a fifth (21.5 %) of women who experienced sexual violence and around a fourth (24.6 %) of women who experienced physical violence reported that they could be infected with HIV and AIDS.

Predictors of Sexual Violence by Husband

Two binary logistic regression models were administered to examine the determinants of sexual coercion and RTI/STDs. In the first model, experience of sexual coercion by the husband was the dependent variable. Controlling for age, education, marital duration, religion, and ethnicity, women who reported having some level of spousal communication with their husbands on reproductive and sexual health were 40 % less likely to experience sexual violence (OR 0.6, 95 % CI 0.4, 0.6). Likewise, women who scored higher on the autonomy index were 60–70 % less likely to experience sexual violence. The analyses also suggest that women who scored higher on the reproductive rights index were 40–60 % less likely to have experienced sexual violence. Similarly, women who scored higher on sexual rights index were 20–40 % less likely to have experienced sexual violence. Also, nonworking women and older women (23+ years) were 3.4 times more likely to face violence than working women and younger women (Table 8.8).

Women's Experience of Sexual Coercion and Its Relation to Women's Health Including RTIs, STIs, and Menstruation

Table 8.9 shows that women, who experience sexual coercion, reported more RTI and STI symptoms. For example, among women who experienced unwanted forced sex, around a third (32.8 %) reported having any symptoms of RTI and STIs

Table 8.8 Odds ratios from logistic regression analysis assessing the associations between background characteristics and experience of sexual coercion by husband, Delhi, India, 2007–2008

Background variables	Exp(B)	95 % C.I. for EXP(B)	
		Lower	Upper
Age of women			
≤22 years (ref.)			
>22 years	3.4***	1.2	12.5
Education level of women			
Illiterate (ref.)			
Till class 7	1.3	0.4	4.9
Classes 7–9	2.6	0.7	9.9
Completed high school	2.8	0.6	12.5
Classes 10–12	1.0	0.3	3.0
12+	1.6	0.4	6.4
Religion			
Hindu (ref.)			
Muslim	1.4	0.4	5.0
Ethnic group			
Others (ST and general) (ref.)			
Other backward caste	1.3	0.5	3.8
Scheduled caste	1.0	0.4	2.4
Marital duration			
≤1 year (ref.)			
2 years	2.6	0.5	13.6
3 years	1.9	0.4	9.4
4 years	5.3	0.5	57.6
5+ years	1.5	0.4	6.2
Number of children			
0 (ref.)			
1	1.2	0.4	3.7
2	1.5	0.5	5.1
3	1.8	0.5	7.0
4+	8.1	0.7	8.2
Spousal communication on reproductive and sexual health			
No (ref.)			
Yes	0.6**	0.4	0.6
Working status of women			
Yes (ref.)			
No	3.4***	1.2	10.1
Sexual right of women			
Low (ref.)			
Moderate	0.8*	0.3	0.9
High	0.6***	0.4	0.8

(continued)

Table 8.8   (continued)

Background variables	Exp(B)	95 % C.I. for EXP(B)	
		Lower	Upper
Reproductive rights of the women			
Low (ref.)			
Moderate	0.4***	0.2	0.7
High	0.6***	0.2	0.8
Autonomy index			
Low (ref.)			
Moderate	0.4*	0.4	0.6
High	0.3***	0.3	0.6

***p<0.01; **p<0.05; *p<0.10
Notes: (*ref.*) reference group

compared to 27.2 % of women who did not experience any sexual violence. A little more than a fifth of women (22.0 %) who experienced sexual violence reported experiencing pain during urination. Likewise, among the women who experienced sexual violence, a higher proportion (10.8 %) reported foul-smelling discharge than those who did not experience sexual violence (7.9 %).

Similarly, women who experienced any violence were more likely to report menstruation-related problems. The results in Fig. 8.4 show that 38.5 % of women who experienced any violence experienced menstruation-related problems compared to only 13.6 % of women who did not experience any violence. More specifically menses-related problems were aggravated by the experience of physical violence (44.8 % vs. 23.5 %) and sexual violence (41.4 % vs. 19.3 %).

Predictors of RTIs and STDs Among Women

The results from the logistic regression analyses suggest that the age of the woman, reproductive and sexual rights indices, and husband's alcohol use were strong predictors of RTI and STD symptoms (Table 8.10). The results show that the women belonging to the older age group were two times more likely than their younger counterparts to report the experience of RTIs and STIs (OR 2.3, 95 % CI 1.4, 6.8). Further, it was found that women who experienced sexual violence were 60 % more likely to report any symptoms of RTIs and STDs (OR 1.6, 95 % CI 1.3, 2.2). Women who reported having discussions with their husbands on reproductive and sexual matters were 50 % (OR 0.5, 95 % CI 0.3, 0.8) less likely to have any symptoms of STD. Also, women who reported that they did not have any menstruation-related problems were 87 % (OR 0.13, 95 % CI 0.2, 0.8) less likely to report RTI/STD problems. Among women who reported that their husbands drink alcohol, the likelihood of reporting RTI and STI symptoms increased by 90 % (OR 1.9, 95 % CI 1.1, 4.3). Likewise, women who felt that their husbands have extramarital affairs were significantly more likely to report RTI/STIs than their counterparts with faithful spouses (OR 1.6, 95 % CI 1.2, 3.6).

Table 8.9 Experience of sexual violence and its relationship with STI and RTI symptoms, Delhi, India, 2007–2008

RTI/STI symptoms										
Experienced type of violence	Any symptoms	White discharge	Pain during intercourse	Pain during urination	Some mass coming out during urination	Pain in lower abdomen	Blood in urine	Blisters around genitals	Foul smelling	Number of women
Sexual violence										
Yes	32.8*	24.7	12.9	22.0*	3.8	13.4	4.3	1.1	10.8	186
No	27.2	21.1	17.5	16.7	3.5	16.7	4.4	1.8	7.9	114
Total %	30.7	23.3	14.7	20.0	3.7	14.7	4.3	1.3	9.7	300

*$p < 0.05$, chi-square test

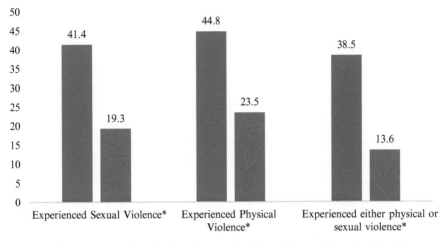

Fig. 8.4 Experience of violence and menstruation-related problems, Delhi, India, 2007–2008. $*p < 0.05$, chi-square test

Table 8.10 Odds ratios from logistic regression analysis assessing the associations between background characteristics and symptoms of RTIs/STIs, Delhi, India, 2007–2008

Characteristics	Exp(B)	95.0 % C.I. for EXP(B)	
		Lower	Upper
Current age of the married women			
≤22 years (ref.)			
>22 years	2.3***	1.4	6.8
Education level of women			
Illiterate (ref.)			
Primary 1–7 years	0.5	0.2	1.3
8–9 years	1.4	0.5	3.8
High school complete	1.8	0.7	4.7
11–12 years	1.1	0.5	2.8
12+	1.2	0.4	3.6
Ethnic group			
Scheduled caste (ref.)			
Others	1.1	0.5	2.3
Other backward class	1.1	0.5	2.4
Religion of women			
Hindu (ref.)			
Muslim	0.5	0.2	1.3
No. of children to the woman			
0 (ref.)			
1	1.3	0.5	3.3
2	1.0	0.4	2.8

(continued)

Table 8.10 (continued)

Characteristics	Exp(B)	95.0 % C.I. for EXP(B)	
		Lower	Upper
3	1.7	0.6	5.2
4+	1.6	0.4	6.2
Marital duration			
≤1 year (ref.)			
2 years	0.7	0.2	2.6
3 years	0.9	0.2	4.0
4 years	0.6	0.1	2.9
5+ years	0.6	0.2	2.0
Working for money			
Yes (ref.)			
No	1.4	0.5	3.6
Spousal communication on reproductive and sexual health			
No (ref.)			
Yes	0.5**	0.3	0.8
Experienced sexual violence			
No (ref.)			
Yes	1.6***	1.3	2.2
Reproductive right index			
Low (ref.)			
Moderate	0.6	0.2	1.3
High	0.4**	1.1	1.9
Sexual rights index			
Low (ref.)			
Moderate	0.8	0.3	1.8
High	0.6*	0.2	0.7
Menses problem			
Yes, have menses problem (ref.)			
No menses-related problem	0.13***	0.2	0.8
Feel that husband has extramarital sexual relations			
No (ref.)			
Yes	1.6*	1.2	3.6
Husband drinks alcohol			
No (ref.)			
Yes	1.9***	1.1	4.3

***$p < 0.01$; **$p < 0.05$; *$p < 0.10$
Notes: (*ref.*) reference group

Violence Experienced for Refusing to Have Sex with Husband

In this study, about a third of women (34 %) reported that they experienced physical violence when they refused sex with their husbands, and about one-fourth (26.3 %) were forced or blackmailed to have sex. Around 5–6 % said that their husbands

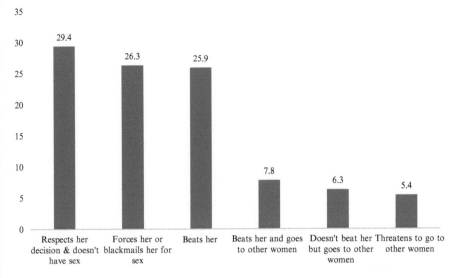

Fig. 8.5 Reaction of husband when his wife refuses to have sex, Delhi, India, 2007–2008

either go to other women or threaten them to go out to some other women. Only 29.4 % of women reported that their husbands respect their decision and don't have sex with them when they don't want to (Fig. 8.5).

Most of the women who participated in in-depth interviews said that they faced physical violence when they refused sex with their husbands. One woman said:

> Whenever he wants it [sex], he must have it. Sometimes I don't feel like doing it [sex] and I tried stop him but he became angry and if I do it again, he beats me and does it [sex] forcefully and that is very painful ...
>
> – 24 year old woman, married for 6 years.

Another woman narrated the similar story:

> I am now married for 10 years but still he keeps insisting me for sex even in front of our children, I refuse it sometime, he becomes impatient and sometimes beats me severely for minor issues. It is impossible to tell him no ...
>
> – 29 year old woman, married for 10 years.

Summary and Conclusion

This study is one of the first efforts to explore the linkages between coercive sex within marriage and women's reproductive health in India. The data provide evidence that coercive sex can significantly compromise a person's reproductive and sexual health. The findings underscore the need for reproductive health programs to consider patterns of coercive sex when addressing the reproductive health and other needs of young people, particularly those needs that are tailored for married women. Even though many women are aware of their sexual and reproductive rights, a considerable number of these women are battered and are sexually coerced by their husbands. It is disheartening to see that many women who experience violence also justify violence. This study clearly shows that women who have experienced sexual and other forms of violence are significantly more likely to perceive themselves at high risk of HIV.

A number of obstacles inhibit young married women from protecting themselves from nonconsensual sexual relations and from taking action against their partners or withdrawing from a coercive relationship. Social/familial taboo attached to reporting marital rape restricts women from taking legal action and forces them to suffer alone making them vulnerable to serious health problems including STDs and HIV. Gender double standards and expectations of women and men in the sexual arena dominate these obstacles. Moreover, communication and negotiations on sexual matters tend to be difficult and are often replaced by actions that include force and violence to resolve differences.

The lack of a supportive environment and trusted adults and peers to consult on sexual health matters may also increase young women's vulnerability to coercive sexual relations. Perceptions of institutional indifference—at the community, school, and legal, and health sector levels—can hinder help seeking of both victims and others who may wish to seek counseling on how to confront a potentially threatening situation. The dearth of data on this issue advocates for more research on incidence, forms, and context of sexual coercion among married young women in different settings. Marital rape should be recognized by the Parliament as an offence under the Indian Penal Code. It will also be pertinent to build capacity of local support structures to provide married women who suffer from forced sexual relations easy access to legal services of their choice that are also sensitive to their needs.

References

Barua, A., & Kurz, K. (2001). Reproductive health-seeking by married adolescent girls in Maharashtra, India. *Reproductive Health Matters, 9*(17), 53–62.

Bohmer L., & Kirumira, E. (1997) *Access to reproductive health services: participatory research with Ugandan adolescents*. Final report and working paper. Makerere University, Child Health and Development Centre and Pacific Institute for Women's Health.

Bott, S., & Jejeebhoy, S. J. (2003). Adolescent sexual and reproductive health in South Asia: An overview of findings from the 2000 Mumbai Conference. In S. Bott, S. J. Jejeebhoy, I. Shah, & C. Puri (Eds.), *Towards adulthood: Exploring the sexual and reproductive health of adolescents in South Asia* (pp. 3–30). Geneva: World Health Organization.

Buttaye, I. (2013). Women and girls in The Gambia are victims of gender-based violence. Front Page International. Retrieved November 10, 2014, from http://frontpageinternational.wordpress.com/2013/12/10/women-and-girls-in-the-gambia-are-victims-of-gender-based-violence/

Development Studies Network. (2000). Conflict and peacemaking in the Pacific: social and gender perspectives. *Development Bulletin, 53*.

Fischer, S., Stewart, T. E., Mehta, S., Wax, R., & Lapinsky, S. E. (2003). Handheld computing in medicine. *Journal of American Medical Information Association, 10*(2), 139–149.

George, A., & Jaswal, J. (1995). *Understanding sexuality: an ethnographic study of poor women in Bombay, India* (Women and AIDS research program report series). Washington, DC: International Centre for Research on Women.

Grasso, B. C., & Genest, R. (2001). Use of a personal digital assistant in reducing medication error rates. *Psychiatric Services, 52*(7), 883–884. 886.

Gravlee, C. (2002). Mobile computer-assisted personal interviewing (MCAPI) with handheld computers: the Entryware™ system 3.0. *Field Methods, 14*(3), 322–336.

Heise, L., Ellsberg, M., & Goettemoeller, M. (1999). Ending violence against women. *Population Reports Series L, 11*, 1–43.

Jewkes, R., Levin, J., Mbananga, N., & Bradshaw, D. (2002). Rape of girls in South Africa. *Lancet, 359*, 319–320.

Khan, M. E., Townsend, J. W., Sinha, R., & Lakhanpal, S. (1996). Sexual violence within marriage. New Delhi, India: Population Council. Retrieved November 10, 2014, from http://www.popcouncil.net/uploads/pdfs/frontiers/OR_TA/Asia/india_VAW.pdf

Koenig, M. A., Stephenson, R., Ahmed, S., Jejeebhoy, S. J., & Campbell, J. (2006). Individual and contextual determinants of domestic violence in North India. *American Journal of Public Health, 96*(1), 132–138.

Lal, S. O., Smith, F. W., Davis, J. P., Castro, H. Y., Smith, D. W., Chinkes, D. L., et al. (2000). Palm computer demonstrates a fast and accurate means of burn data collection. *Journal of Burn Care and Rehabilitation, 21*(6), 559–561.

Population Council. (1997). *The gap between reproductive intentions and behaviour: a study of Punjabi men and women.* Islamabad: Population Council.

Silverman, J. G., Michele, R. D., Niranjan, S., Balaiah, D., & Raj, A. (2008). Intimate partner violence and HIV infection among married Indian women. *JAMA, 300*(6), 703–710.

Sodhi, G., & Verma, M. (2003). Sexual coercion amongst unmarried adolescents of an urban slum in India. In S. Bott et al. (Eds.), *Towards adulthood: Exploring the sexual and reproductive health of adolescents in South Asia* (pp. 91–94). Geneva: World Health Organization.

UNICEF. (1998). *The progress of nations.* New York: UNICEF.

UNICEF. (2001). *Early marriage, child spouses. Innocenti digest* (7th ed.). Florence: UNICEF Innocent Research Centre.

United Nations Population Fund. (1999). *Violence against girls and women.* New York: UNFPA.

Verma, R., Pulerwitz, J., Mahendra, V. S., Khandekar, S., Singh, A. K., Das, S. S., et al. (2008). *Promoting gender equity as a strategy to reduce HIV risk and gender-based violence among young men in India. Horizons final report.* Washington, DC: Population Council.

WHO. (2002). *World report on violence and health.* Geneva: World Health Organization.

WHO. (2005). WHO multi-country study on women's health and domestic violence against women: initial results on prevalence, health outcomes and women's responses. Geneva: World Health Organization. Retrieved October 28, 2014, from, http://www.who.int/gender/violence/who_multicountry_study/summary_report/summary_report_English2.pdf

Yimin, C., Baohua, K., Tieyan, W., Xuejun, H., Huan, S., Yuren, L., et al. (2001). Case-controlled study on relevant factors of adolescent sexual coercion in China. *Contraception, 64*(2), 77–80.

Chapter 9
Questioning Gender Norms to Promote Sexual Reproductive Health Among Early Adolescents: Evidence from a School Program in Mumbai, India

Pranita Achyut, Nandita Bhatla, and Ravi Verma

Abstract Early adolescent interventions are expected to prepare grounds for positive sexual and reproductive health (SRH) outcomes at later ages. If girls and boys are socialized into believing in and practicing gender equitable norms and attitudes, they would be more likely to change their behaviors, which would lead to making informed choices and engaging in less risky SRH behaviors. This chapter presents one such intervention called Gender Equity Movement in Schools (GEMS) carried out in Mumbai schools among early adolescent girls and boys of ages 12–14 years. Interventions promoting gender equality included structured group education activities (GEA) and school-based campaigns with students of grades VI and VII over 2 years. Girls and boys exposed to the interventions showed much greater improvement in self-reported measures of sexual and reproductive health than those with no interventions. Domain specific analysis of gender attitudes however showed that some areas of gender relations were less likely to change than others. Findings suggest that the gender-focused initiatives must engage children at early ages and also pay special attention to the areas that are difficult to change.

Keywords Sexual and reproductive health • Early adolescents • Gender equity movement in schools • India

Introduction

For most people, the concepts of sexuality and health are grounded in the formation of notions of gender, beliefs about masculinity and femininity, attitudes toward the opposite sex, and validation of the use of violence to resolve conflicts. Inequitable gender norms affect the health and lives of boys, girls, men, and women around

P. Achyut (✉) • N. Bhatla • R. Verma
International Center for Research on Women, New Delhi, India
e-mail: pachyut@icrw.org; nbhatla@icrw.org; rverma@icrw.org

© Springer International Publishing Switzerland 2015
Y.K. Djamba, S.R. Kimuna (eds.), *Gender-Based Violence,*
DOI 10.1007/978-3-319-16670-4_9

the world and at all levels of society through multiple pathways. In particular, gender norms shape expectations regarding individual behaviors of men and women and also the interactions between and among men and women. Not only do these norms reflect traditional values about the worth of girls compared to boys and appropriate roles and responsibilities for men and women (Sen and Ostlin 2007), they also affect access to resources such as education, employment and income, healthcare, and the distribution of power both in the home and in society more broadly (Krishnan et al. 2008; Sen and Ostlin 2007).

Inequitable gender norms that curtail women's autonomy while expanding men's decision-making authority and control over women tend to condone or justify intimate partner violence (IPV), which has been linked to a number of adverse sexual and reproductive health (SRH) outcomes. Several studies from different settings, including India, show that young men reporting less equitable gender attitudes[1] were more likely than men with more equitable attitudes to have higher numbers of sexual partners, lower rates of condom use, more symptoms of sexually transmitted infections (STIs), drug or alcohol use, and perpetration of IPV (Barker et al. 2007, 2011; Haberland and Rogow 2007; Karim et al. 2003; Pulerwitz et al. 2006; Verma et al. 2008). Similarly, research from diverse samples in the U.S. shows that men with more "traditional" gender role ideologies report more sexual infidelity, casual sex partners, unprotected sex, negative attitudes toward condoms, and more sexual coercion and relationship violence (Santana et al. 2006). Prevailing norms of masculinity that expect men to be more knowledgeable and experienced about sex can also prevent men and boys from seeking information or admitting their lack of knowledge about sex or protection, and can lead them to experiment with sex in unsafe ways and at a young age in order to prove their manhood (UNAIDS 1999).

At the same time, gender norms and expectations related to femininity undermine women's and girl's decision-making power and increase their vulnerability to negative SRH outcomes and violence. In Ghana, women reporting less egalitarian attitudes were less likely to use condoms consistently compared to women reporting more egalitarian attitudes (Karim et al. 2003). In South Africa, a qualitative study reported that adolescent women's perception of men's entitlement to violence and sex within romantic relationships—perceptions that were reinforced by their peers—limited their capacity to protect themselves against coercive sex, unwanted pregnancy, and STIs (Wood et al. 1998). Similar dynamics were reported in India. In one study, both men and women emphasized the importance of women's submissiveness to their husbands, notions of women's purity, and acceptance of extramarital relationships for men, resulting in unprotected sex (Go et al. 2003).

As socialization of expected and accepted behaviors of boys and girls, and men and women begins early, it is important to start the process of creating a strong foundation of equitable attitudes and behaviors at a younger age. It is also critical to engage in the process key stakeholders and institutions that shape young people's gender role socialization. The education system is one such institution that influences

---

[1] Measured as attitudes across various domains including appropriateness of partner violence, equal participation in decision-making, and distribution of domestic chores.

and shapes children's thought processes and understanding of gender stereotypes and roles. Global research has highlighted the importance of addressing gender issues, including gender-based violence within the school setting and among school-going children (Dunne et al. 2005; Pinheiro 2006). Despite high-level acknowledgment of schools' potential to shape norms and behaviors, the evidence reveals that educational institutions more often than not reinforce gender stereotypes and perpetuate patterns of violence (Barker 2006; Mathur et al. 2001; Patel and Andrew 2001; Rigby 2003; Sharp et al. 2000).

In South Asia, particularly in India, studies with children on how they construct gender identities, their notions of sexuality, and violence and its effect on reproductive and sexual health are limited. During 2008–2011, the International Center for Research on Women implemented an intervention project called "Gender Equity Movement in Schools" (GEMS) in partnership with Committee of Resource Organizations (CORO) for Literacy and Tata Institute of Social Sciences in public schools of Mumbai. Mumbai is a metro city with a population of around 12.4 million (Office of the Registrar General and Census Commissioner and India 2014). As per the latest census, 41 % of the city's population live in slums with limited facilities. GEMS project was implemented in select public schools in two wards of Mumbai, primarily catering to students from nearby slum areas, and most of the students belonging to low socioeconomic strata.

This chapter assesses the effect of the GEMS intervention on the attitude of students toward gender and violence and its association with reproductive and sexual health among young adolescents.

GEMS Project Description

GEMS draws from the social normative framework and applies it to the construction of gender and violence. It considers that the notions of dominance and power and the use of violence to resolve conflicts sets-in at very early stages through various socialization processes and that these fundamental constructs must be challenged at ages when they are being formed. Further, schools are institutions that provide an opportunity to reach a large number of students in a teaching–learning environment, and bring sustained and larger normative impact. It is here that learning, not only in terms of knowledge, but also learning of values, norms, and behaviors get reinforced.

GEMS used a combination of the cognitive-affective approaches and life skills undertaken in institutional settings to bring transformative and sustained changes toward gender equality and violence prevention. It engaged young boys and girls of grades VI and VII in collective critical self-reflection through group education activities, enabling them to recognize and challenge inequitable gender norms and the use of violence in their everyday lives. In India, grades VI and VII mean being in formal school for 6 and 7 years respectively. These students are usually 11–13 years old.

Group reflection reciprocates and reinforces the processes of individual change among students. This, coupled with school level campaign and orientation workshops with teachers, initiates institutional discourse. These mutually reinforcing processes, at the individual and systemic level, have the potential to create lasting normative changes toward gender equality and violence prevention.

A total of 25 group education activities of 45 min to 1 h were developed around gender, body, violence, emotion, communication, and conflict resolution (Achyut et al. 2011; ICRW 2011). These activities used participatory methodologies such as role plays, games, debates, and discussions to engage students in meaningful and relevant interactions and reflection. In addition, an interactive activity book named "My GEMS Diary" was developed for students with an aim to encourage them to reflect, introspect, and express their own experiences, including the incorporation of the classroom discussions into their own personal spaces and engaging parents and siblings in the discussions. The intervention also included a week long campaign in each academic year and specific orientation meetings with teachers. Trained facilitators from partner organizations led the intervention in school.

In the first academic year (2008–2009), ten classroom sessions and one round of campaign were carried out with students of grades VI and VII. The sessions focused on building perspectives and understanding of the critical concepts of gender, gender-based discrimination, and gender-based violence. Also, discussions were held on respect for their own and others' bodies and shame and blame associated with violence. In the next academic year (2009–2010), intervention focused on deepening the understanding and skills. These sessions were conducted with only those from grade VI who had passed to grade VII. The senior cohort had graduated to grade VIII and moved to different schools. These sessions were carried out once in 2 weeks by a team of trained facilitators. In addition, orientation meetings were held with teachers to inform them about the program, seek their feedback, and engage them in the campaign.

In year 1, around 2,300 students participated in group education activities and 8,000 in the campaign, while in year 2, around 1,200 students participated in group education activities and 8,000 in campaign. Thus, in the second year, classroom sessions were carried out only with a subset of students exposed in the first round. However, the campaign was open to all the students in grades V, VI, and VII.

Data and Method

In order to assess the effect of the intervention, the project used a three arm quasi-experimental design with mixed methods of data collection at multiple time points. Arm 1 included schools with group education activities and campaign (GEA+); Arm 2 included schools with only campaign; and Arm 3 included schools with no intervention (control). Each arm had 15 schools randomly allocated from the list of 45 schools selected from two wards of Mumbai. From more than 100 public schools in the selected two wards, we narrowed down to 68, which were using Hindi and Marathi as languages of instruction. From this list, 45 schools were randomly selected. These schools, then, were randomly allocated to the three study arms.

In each of the selected schools, a class of VI and VII were randomly selected for the survey. On the day of visit, students present in the class were explained about the study and consent/assent process. The students whose parents allowed them to participate were recruited after signing consent form. Same class and process were followed during subsequent surveys.

Overall, three rounds of surveys were carried out—baseline before starting the intervention, midline after the completion of first year intervention, and endline after the completion of the second year intervention. Around 2800 students of grades VI and VII participated in baseline and midline. At endline, 1,400 students participated in the survey. The surveys were carried out using structured self-administered questionnaire and included a series of questions that measure attitude toward gender norms, sexuality, and violence. Specific questions were asked about their perceptions toward SRH outcomes and self-efficacy.

For this chapter, we have taken data from baseline and endline surveys with students of grade VI, who participated in the study over a 2-year period from GEA+ and control. Thus, the analysis is based on the data gathered from 524 girls and 462 boys at the baseline and 555 girls and 433 boys at the endline.

The key outcome variables examined here are attitude toward norms related to gender, sexuality, and violence, perception on age at marriage, comfort with their growing bodies, willingness to seek information, intention to complain about sexual violence, and intention to intervene in case of violence against women and girls. Other variables used in the analysis are age, sex, and media exposure. Specific questions were asked to assess if students have TV and DVD/CD player at home, access to mobile phone for personal use, and own bicycle to facilitate mobility. Given the young age of students, limited data were gathered on their socioeconomic status.

Gender Attitude Scale

In order to measure attitude toward gender norm and violence, we constructed a scale, similar to the one developed in Brazil and adapted in India for young men (Pulerwitz and Barker 2008; Verma et al. 2008). Students were given 24 statements related to prescribed role of men and women, dominance of men over women, attributes, and justification of violence and asked to give their response on a three point scale—agree, disagree, and not sure. Considering that 11–12 years of age is challenging, children may not have formed concrete opinions toward gender norms; therefore, the "not sure" category was given.

For the construction of scale, all the statements were made unidirectional by giving a score of 0 if response supported inequality, 1 for not sure, and 2 for supporting equality. Then, using factor analysis, we constructed the scale by using 15 statements on gender roles, attributes, and violence [Cronbach's alpha value—0.69] (Achyut et al. 2011). The total score for each student was created by adding the Cronbach's alpha score on each statement. On the scale of 0–30, students who scored between 0 and 10 were categorized as having low equitable attitude; 11–20 as having moderate; and 21–30 as having high equitable attitude.

Measures Related to Sexual and Reproductive Health

In view of the young age of students [mean age 11.5 at baseline], perception-based questions related to sexual and reproductive health were asked. To assess perception on the age at marriage for girls, students were asked "What is the appropriate age at marriage for girls?" Their response was categorized as 20 years or less, and more than 20 years. Students were asked if they feel comfortable with their growing body with response categories of not at all, somewhat comfortable, and totally comfortable. Also, students were asked if they are willing to seek information on bodily changes with response categories of Yes and No.

From childhood, both girls and boys get messages about sexual violence that blame and shame. During formative research, some students particularly girls shared that often girls do not report sexual violence to their parents for fear of being blamed and getting restricted. Others shared that sometimes girls are beaten-up for bringing shame to the family.

To understand if GEMS program is able to give confidence, and create space for students to report/complain about any experience of sexual violence, the following question was asked: "If anyone touches your body or exposes himself/herself, would you complain to someone?" The response categories included: definitely complain, probably complain, and not at all. To assess their intention to intervene in case of violence against girls, students were asked about the action they would take if they saw someone beating a woman or a girl in their community. The possible response categories were: intervene, call someone to intervene, do nothing. Data on the key outcome variables are presented separately for girls and boys.

To measure the effect of the intervention on key outcomes, we have used Difference-in-Differences (DID) (Ashenfelter 1978; Ashenfelter and Card 1985). This method compares difference in average outcome in intervention arm before and after intervention with the difference in control. Thus, this model helps in detecting net effect of intervention on outcomes of interest. However, one of the key assumptions is that the factors external to the intervention that may influence outcome affect treatment and control in a similar way. It also cancels differences existing at the beginning of the program between intervention and control.

The analysis was carried out in STATA (version 12) separately for girls and boys, controlling for access to TV, DVD/CD player, mobile phone, and bicycle. For this chapter, outcome variables are either dichotomized or means are used. To assess change in the gender attitude, we have used two measures—mean score on attitudinal scale and proportion of students with high attitude [high attitude = 1; moderate and low = 0]. Other variables analyzed are: appropriate age at marriage for girls [21–36 years = 1; 20 years or less = 0]; comfort with growing body [totally comfortable = 1; not at all or somewhat comfortable = 0]; willingness to seek information about body change [Yes = 1; No = 0]; intention to complain about sexual violence [Definitely complain = 1; Probably complain or not at all = 0]; and intention to intervene in case of violence against women and girls [Intervene or ask someone to intervene = 1; do nothing = 0].

Results

Sample Characteristics

The sample characteristics at baseline and endline are similar (Table 9.1). Mean age of boys at baseline was 11.5 years [SD=0.93] in control arm, and 11.6 [SD=0.91] in intervention arm. At endline, mean age for boys was 12.7 [SD=0.94] and 12.8 [SD=0.91] in control and intervention arms respectively with no significant difference. Similarly, mean age for girls was 11.4 [SD=0.99] at baseline and 12.4 [SD=.84] at endline. More than 95 % of both girls and boys reported living with their parents with no significant difference over time and between arms.

When asked about household amenities at baseline, two-thirds of boys from control and three-fourths from intervention arm reported having TV, while a third mentioned DVD/CD player with no significant difference between arms. About a quarter of the boys reported having their own bicycles. This increased to around a third at endline in both arms. In comparison to boys, while similar proportion of girls reported owning a bicycle at baseline, a gap was observed over time in both arms indicating restriction in the use of bicycles for girls. Interestingly, at baseline, 26.1 % of boys from control arm reported having a mobile phone for personal use, compared to 35.9 % in the intervention arm [$p<0.05$]. However, no significant difference was found between the two arms at endline. Similar pattern was observed among girls. At baseline, 28.9 % of girls from control and 43.6 % from intervention

Table 9.1 Selected characteristics of 12–14 years boys and girls in GEMS project, Mumbai, India 2008–2010

	Male				Female			
	Baseline		Endline		Baseline		Endline	
	Control	GEA	Control	GEA	Control	GEA	Control	GEA
Mean age [SD]	11.5 [0.93]	11.6 [0.91]	12.7 [0.94]	12.8 [0.91]	11.4 [0.99]	11.5 [0.84]	12.4 [0.84]	12.5 [0.85]
Living with parents (%)	97.7	98.0	97.4	96.5	96.5	94.8	98.4	98.3
Having TV at home (%)	67.7	75.8	77.0	81.9	76.5	82.1	81.7	88.8**
Having CD/DVD player at home	35.7	34.8	41.1	49.5	34.1	36.8	40.5	50.8**
Having own bicycle	21.2	26.8	30.5	34.7	22.1	24.3	18.7	20.1
Having mobile phone for personal use	26.1	35.9**	34.8	36.1	28.9	43.6***	24.6	23.8
Number of students (N)	198	264	199	228	212	312	303	249

Note: **significant at $p<0.05$; ***significant at $p<0.001$

[$p < 0.001$] reported having access to a mobile phone for personal use. However, at endline, whereas 24.6 % of girls in the control reported having access to a mobile phone for personal use, 23.8 % of girls from the intervention group reported having access to a mobile phone for personal use.

Gender Attitude

Before the start of the intervention, the majority of the students, both girls and boys in each arm, scored moderately on the attitudinal scale (Table 9.2). Only 7.6 % of boys from control and 10.6 % from GEA+ were in high attitudinal category, while, 21.6 % from control arm and 11.6 from GEA+ were in low category [$p < 0.05$]. On the other hand, at baseline, girls showed positive gender attitude in both arms with about one-quarter of respondents being in high attitudinal category.

At endline, there was a 16 % net increase in the proportion of boys in the high attitudinal category among GEA+ compared to control [in control, it moved from 8 to 12 %, while in GEA+, it increased from 11 to 31 %]. Controlling for background characteristics, this increase is significant [Adjusted DID score = 0.166; $p < 0.001$]. This increase is primarily due to improvement in attitudinal change of boys from moderate to high, rather than from low to moderate. However, the mean attitude score of boys does not significantly change from baseline to endline in GEA+ compared to control [adjusted DID estimate for high equitable gender attitude category = 0.939].

For girls, the shift in attitude from baseline to endline is much more dramatic. There is net increase of almost four points in mean attitudinal score among girls in the GEA+ group. In terms of change in the proportion of girls in different attitudinal categories, there is a net increase of 35 % point in the proportion of girls with high equitable gender attitude among those exposed to the intervention [in control, it increased by 2.2 % point from 24.0 to 26.2 %, while in GEA+, it increased from 25.5 to 63.0 %]. The adjusted DID estimate for high equitable attitude category is 0.337, which is statistically significant at $p < 0.001$.

Among the 15 statements, boys showed significant positive shift on 4 statements. Among these, two statements are on gender specific attributes (statements 2 and 3), one on gender role (statement 6), and one on sexuality (statement 10). At baseline, 52.9 % of boys from control and 55.8 % from GEA+ agreed with the statement— "Boys are naturally better at math and science than girls". At endline, there is a 6.5 point decrease in the proportion of boys agreeing to this statement in control arm, while a 27.9 point drop in the GEA+ group is observed [adjusted DID mean score 0.313; p = <0.001]. For the statement "boys are naturally better than girls in sports", there is an 18.1 point net reduction in the proportion of boys in the GEA+ agreeing to the statement [76.6–55.4 %] compared to control [64.8–61.7 %] [adjusted DID mean score 0.292; $p = <0.001$]. On the statement related to gender roles (statement 6), "only men should work outside home," GEA+ arm recorded a reduction of 17.9 points among those who supported this notion compared to 5.4 in control arm.

Table 9.2 Attitudes and perceptions of students toward norms related to gender, sexuality, violence, and SRH, GEMS, Mumbai, India 2008–2010

		Boys					Girls				
		Baseline		Endline		Adjusted DID estimates	Baseline		Endline		Adjusted DID estimates
		Control	GEA	Control	GEA		Control	GEA	Control	GEA	
Attitudinal score (mean)		13.6	15	15.4	17.6	0.939	16.9	17.2	17.6	22	3.833***
Gender attitude category	High	7.6	10.6	11.8	31.2	0.166***	24	25.5	26.2	63	0.337***
	Moderate	70.8	77.8	75	59		66	66	65.1	35.6	
	Low	21.6	11.6	13.2	9.8		9.9	8.5	8.7	1.3	
Statements on gender attributes											
1. Girls cannot do well in Math and Science	Disagree	30	38.1	36.2	43.1	0.084	45.8	46.2	62.2	64.1	0.132
	Not sure	28.5	14.7	34.4	29.4		14.1	8.1	11.2	15.9	
	Agree	41.4	47.2	29.5	27.5		40.1	45.7	26.5	19.9	
2. Boys are naturally better at math and science than girls.	Disagree	21.3	29.4	23.7	42.6	0313***	47.4	58	54.3	68.6	0.01
	Not sure	25.9	14.7	29.9	29.4		22.4	21.7	27.5	21.7	
	Agree	52.9	55.8	46.4	27.9		30.1	20.3	18.2	9.7	
3. Boys are naturally better than girls in sports	Disagree	18.6	17.3	19.8	32.7	0.292***	44.5	43.4	45.1	63.9	0.337***
	Not sure	16.7	6.1	18.5	11.9		16.5	15.1	21.3	14.9	
	Agree	64.8	76.6	61.7	55.4		39	41.5	33.6	21.3	
4. A wife should always obey her husband	Disagree	11.4	18.3	25.1	35.9	0.08	20.8	24.6	26	53	0.402***
	Not sure	11	8.6	18.9	12.1		9.9	10	19.6	16.7	
	Agree	77.7	73.1	55.9	52		69.2	65.4	54.4	30.3	
Statements on gender role and privileges											
5. Men need more care as they work harder than women	Disagree	17.9	24.9	21.8	42.4	0.19	27.6	35.1	23.5	52.9	0.417***
	Not sure	13.7	14.7	24.4	19.2		17.9	14.7	21.9	18.5	
	Agree	68.4	60.4	53.8	38.4		54.5	50.2	54.7	28.6	

(continued)

Table 9.2 (continued)

| | | Boys | | | | | Girls | | | | |
| | | Baseline | | Endline | | Adjusted DID estimates | Baseline | | Endline | | Adjusted DID estimates |
		Control	GEA	Control	GEA		Control	GEA	Control	GEA	
6. Only men should work outside home	Disagree	38.2	45.7	40.5	61.3	0.261**	51.9	46	53.9	76.5	0.455***
	Not sure	14.5	9.6	17.6	11.9		15.7	9.5	23	9.5	
	Agree	47.3	44.7	41.9	26.8		32.4	44.5	23	13.9	
7. Since girls have to get married, they should not be sent for higher education	Disagree	36.1	48.7	41.3	59.5	0.005	44.2	55.7	43.9	71.1	0.162
	Not sure	22.1	17.3	33.3	17		23.1	18.6	32.1	14.4	
	Agree	41.8	34	25.3	23.5		32.7	25.7	24	14.4	
8. It's necessary to give dowry	Disagree	27.9	50.3	45.1	51.7	0.296**	41.5	39.3	41	64.4	0.367***
	Not sure	16	16.8	19.5	18.7		16.1	25.1	22.5	21.8	
	Agree	56.1	33	35.4	29.6		42.4	35.5	36.5	13.8	
9. Giving bath and feeding kids are the mother's responsibility	Disagree	14.6	25	12.4	27.6	0.003	15.4	12.7	11.3	41	0.583***
	Not sure	9.6	15.8	11.5	7		3.5	7.1	9.3	9.7	
	Agree	75.9	59.2	76.1	65.3		81	80.2	79.4	49.3	
Statements on sexuality and violence											
10. Girls provoke boys with short dresses	Disagree	32.7	23.9	30.1	34.8	0.243***	53.8	48.1	41.2	48.7	0.153
	Not sure	29.3	23.9	36.3	28.9		27.2	29.5	44.8	36.6	
	Agree	38	52.3	33.6	36.3		18.9	22.4	14	14.8	
11. It is a girl's fault if a male student or teacher sexually harasses her	Disagree	57.8	58.9	62.7	65.8	-0.066	65.1	66	61	75.6	0.034
	Not sure	28.1	33.5	29.3	23.6		15.4	25.5	32.1	19.7	
	Agree	14.1	7.6	8	10.6		19.6	8.5	6.8	4.7	

12. There are times when a boy needs to beat his girlfriend	Disagree	51.7	63.5	56.2	57.2	−0.11	55	66	41.8	64.9	0.135
	Not sure	31.2	22.3	31	27.4		29.3	17.9	49.8	30.1	
	Agree	17.1	14.2	12.8	15.4		15.8	16	8.4	5.1	
13. A woman should tolerate violence in order to keep her family together	Disagree	50.6	57.9	49.1	58.3	−0.04	54.2	52.4	51.6	70.3	0.331***
	Not sure	16.7	15.7	28.1	20.6		21.8	17.9	29.8	18.3	
	Agree	32.7	26.4	22.8	21.1		24	29.7	18.7	11.3	
14. There are times when a woman deserves to be beaten	Disagree	54.8	54.3	51.3	56.8	0.06	63.1	63.8	57	68.2	0.149
	Not sure	23.2	21.3	28.1	19.6		24	24.3	29.1	23.4	
	Agree	22.1	24.4	20.5	23.6		12.8	11.9	13.9	8.4	
15. Girls like to be teased by boys	Disagree	62.4	67.5	56.7	62.1	−0.08	76.6	72.9	70.4	77.9	0.168**
	Not sure	17.9	16.2	32.6	24.2		16	19	24.3	20.8	
	Agree	19.8	16.2	10.7	13.6		7.4	8.1	5.3	1.3	
Perception toward SRH											
Appropriate age at marriage for girls	21–36 Years	18.0 %	11.3 %	14.9 %	20.9 %	0.131***	14.0 %	19.9 %	16.4 %	21.8 %	−0.005
	less than 21 years	82.0 %	88.7 %	85.1 %	79.1 %		86.0 %	80.1 %	83.6 %	78.2 %	
Intention to intervene in case of violence against women and girls	Intervene	64.5 %	56.8 %	57.7 %	63.9 %	0.133***	72.5 %	53.7 %	69.1 %	67.2 %	0.251***
	Tell someone to intervene	20.7 %	27.2 %	22.3 %	27.8 %		17.0 %	21.5 %	14.8 %	28.0 %	
	Will do nothing	14.9 %	16.0 %	20.0 %	8.2 %		10.5 %	24.9 %	16.0 %	4.7 %	
Being comfortable with growing body	Not at all	42.1 %	53.1 %	26.0 %	31.6 %	0.02	50.9 %	50.6 %	29.5 %	29.3 %	0.003
	Somewhat	31.8 %	31.1 %	26.5 %	29.5 %		21.5 %	27.4 %	26.9 %	33.9 %	
	Totally comfortable	26.0 %	15.8 %	47.5 %	38.9 %		27.7 %	22.0 %	43.6 %	36.8 %	
Willingness to seek information about body change	Yes	62.3 %	75.8 %	51.8 %	63.1 %	−0.02	70.4 %	59.7 %	56.0 %	71.2 %	0.265***
	No	37.7 %	24.2 %	48.2 %	36.9 %		29.6 %	40.3 %	44.0 %	28.8 %	

(continued)

Table 9.2 (continued)

		Boys					Girls				
		Baseline		Endline		Adjusted DID estimates	Baseline		Endline		Adjusted DID estimates
		Control	GEA	Control	GEA		Control	GEA	Control	GEA	
Intention to complain in case of sexual violence	Definitely complain	58.3 %	54.0 %	57.8 %	66.2 %	0.203***	64.5 %	50.7 %	77.6 %	79.8 %	.227***
	Probably complain	20.5 %	22.2 %	15.6 %	15.8 %		14.2 %	28.0 %	10.3 %	11.9 %	
	Not at all complain	21.2 %	23.8 %	26.6 %	18.0 %		21.3 %	21.3 %	12.2 %	8.3 %	

Note: adjusted DID mean score is calculated controlling for TV, DVD/CD player, bicycle, and mobile phone

**Significant at $p < 0.05$; ***significant at $p < 0.001$

Similarly, GEA+ arm noted 16.0 points decline in proportion agreeing to the statement related to sexuality—"girls provoke boys with short dresses" [52.3–36.3 %] compared to 4.4 points in control [38.0–33.6 %].

Out of 15 statements, a positive shift was noted on 8 statements among girls—two on gender attributes (statement 3 and 4), four on gender role and privileges (statements 5, 6, 8 and 9), and two on violence (statements 13 and 15) (Table 9.2). Overall, these changes are more remarkable on gender role and privilege items. At baseline, around 80 % girls from both the arms agreed to the statement "Giving bath and feeding kids are the mother's responsibility". At endline, while no significant change was observed in the control arm, proportion agreeing to it declined to 49.3 % in GEA+. The net increase in adjusted mean score was 0.583 [$p<0.001$] on a scale of 0–2. For the statements "Only men should work outside home" and "men need more care as they work harder than women," net increase in adjusted mean scores were 0.455 [$p<0.001$] and 0.417 [$p<0.001$] respectively.

Compared to gender roles and privileges, overall, lesser support for violence against women and girls was noted at baseline in both the arms. The net effect of intervention was evident on two statements—"A woman should tolerate violence in order to keep her family together" [Adjusted DID mean score=0.331; $p<0.001$] and "Girls like to be teased by boys" [Adjusted DID mean score=0.168; $p<0.001$]. There are some differences in the statements on which girls and boys showed changes. For example, while boys from GEA+ showed significant net positive shift on the statements "Boys are naturally better at math and science than girls" and "girls provoke boys with short dresses," no significant net changes were noted among girls.

Perception Toward SRH

In India, legal age at marriage for girls is 18 years, however, a large proportion of women get married before the legal age. When asked about appropriate age at marriage for girls at baseline, 18.0 % of boys from control arm and 11.3 % from GEA+ reported 21 years or more (Table 9.2). After the intervention, 20.9 % of boys reported 21 years and more in GEA+, while 14.9 % in control. Thus, there was a net increase of 12.7 % points in the proportion of boys who reported 21 years or more. This increase is statistically significant. However, no such significant change was noted among girls following intervention exposure.

Students reported higher self-efficacy in terms of bystander intervention (Table 9.2). When asked about their response to violence against women and girls, 64.5 % of boys from control and 56.8 % GEA+ noted that they would intervene; 20.7 % of boys in the control arm and 27.2 % in the GEA+ arm reported that they would tell someone to intervene. At endline, there was an increase of 7.7 points in students who reported that they would intervene or tell someone to intervene in GEA+ arm [84.0–91.7 %] compared to 5.1 points decline in control arm [85.1–80.0 %]. The net positive shift in GEA+ is significant with adjusted DID estimate for intention to intervene being 0.133 [$p<0.001$]. Girls from GEA+ also reported a positive shift in intention to intervene [DID estimate=0.251; $p<0.001$].

With time, young adolescents become more comfortable with their maturing body in both study arms. However, GEMS program contributed in enhancing their confidence and interest at two fronts—their willingness to seek information on bodily changes and intention to complain about sexual violence. Following the intervention, a significantly higher proportion of girls from GEA+ expressed their willingness to seek more information on bodily changes [59.7–71.2 %], while there was a decline in control [70.4–56.0 %]. On the other hand, lesser proportion of boys from both arms expressed such willingness at endline compared to baseline.

When asked about intention to complain in case of sexual violence, both boys and girls from GEA+ showed significant positive changes. Boys and girls from GEA+ recorded net increase of 12.7 and 16.0 points respectively in the proportion reporting "definitely complain" after the intervention exposure.

Self-Reported Change in Behavior After Intervention Exposure

At endline, students from GEA+ arm were asked questions about intervention exposure and change in certain behavior following participation in the intervention (Table 9.3). Little more than half of the boys (58.5 %) and nearly two-thirds of girls (66.0 %) reported that after participating in the intervention, they have started opposing discrimination at home more than earlier, while 8–9 % mentioned that they think about it but have not tried to do anything. Furthermore, about 80 % of girls and boys reported that they are more comfortable with students of the opposite sex after attending sessions or campaign. Similar proportion of students reported that they have talked about GEMS project with someone at home or outside the home. When asked about the person they talked to, a friend was on top of the list for

Table 9.3 Self-reported changes in behavior after intervention, GEMS, Mumbai, India 2008–2010

		Boys	Girls
Started opposing discrimination at home after attending sessions or campaign	Yes, started opposing more than earlier	58.5	66.0
	I oppose as I used to	14.5	9.0
	I think about it but have not tried it	8.0	9.0
	No, I don't oppose	19.0	16.0
More comfortable with girl/boy after attending sessions or campaign		80.2	81.0
Ever talked about GEMS program with anyone		81.3	79.8
No. of students (N)		*203*	*282*
Talked about GEMS with	Mother	25.9	45.1
	Father	3.0	0.9
	Sibling	16.2	14.3
	Friends	41.0	29.5
No. of students who talk to someone about GEMS (N)		*165*	*225*

boys with 41.0 % of boys reporting talking to friends about GEMS. About half of the girls noted that they talked to their mother, while 29.5 % said they talked with their friends.

Discussion

Engaging young adolescents in discussion, critical thinking, and self-reflection on issues of gender and sexuality, at ages when these notions are forming, positively influences their attitudes about gender roles and gender relations. GEMS, a gender equality focused program, successfully challenges and changes normative and relational constructs that underlie and shape several future sexual and reproductive health (SRH) behaviors and outcomes. In addition, it addresses specific aspects of SRH that are of importance at early ages, such as knowledge and comfort with the growing body, understanding the right to bodily integrity (both of the self and others), confidence to intervene in situations of coercion and violence, perception about appropriate age at marriage, and comfort and communication with opposite sex.

An attitude that reflects support for gender equality and disapproves of force as a means to resolve conflicts is a necessary precursor to positive sexual health and future relationships. The GEMS program results in a positive shift among both boys and girls on specific measures of gender attitude—a significantly higher proportion of boys and girls report attitudes that are in the high equitable category after program exposure. While there is a movement in the positive direction across all categories of the attitude scale (low, moderate, and high), from baseline to endline in the GEA+ arm, the DID analysis with the control arm helps us discern differences that are more specifically attributable to program exposure, and are not a result of other extraneous factors, for example, increasing age.

These findings also show that the significant improvement of children, particularly among boys, is more from the moderately equitable category to the high equitable, rather than from low equitable to moderate equitable category. This could be indicative of the fact that the program is perhaps more effective with those students whose thinking already includes some notions of gender equality. Perhaps the program messages and ideas have an inherent appeal for these girls and boys, and/or the program discussions help support, reinforce, give voice, and language to their beliefs. This finding also suggests that perhaps, more intensive efforts that last longer maybe needed to shift the "rigidly held" inequitable attitudes. It must be remembered that the GEMS program reaches out to all students in a more or less similar fashion —with sessions being held in groups of both males and females.

A specific feature of the GEMS discussion in the classroom is a conscious effort to invite different voices, ensure maximum participation as it hinges on the principle of juxtaposing differences to explore alternatives. However, practical considerations, such as the number of students in a class (approximately 40) and time limit (each session lasting about 45–60 min), constraint a nuanced and exhaustive discussion. Those constraints limit the possibility of one-on-one discussions that could be so critical in reaching out to students that have sharply divergent beliefs. Such students could feel threatened in articulating or sharing their ideas, therefore, reducing their chance of acquiring new ideas. More intensive qualitative research with such program participants can help discern and understand these patterns and also recommend elements of programmatic intervention to bring about more comprehensive and sustained shifts at younger ages.

Girls start demonstrating more gender equitable attitudes and also report a greater positive shift in their gender attitudes as compared to boys, after program exposure. Among the specific items of the gender attitude scale, there is a significant shift in four statements for boys, whereas among girls this is noted in eight statements. When the specific statements are examined, we note interesting differences even though interpretation of the findings can be difficult as we understand that attitudes are influenced by a complex interplay of several determinants. In addition, the program was not designed to give specific messages about each of these issues; rather, it was built to provide a sequential understanding of various concepts of the gender construct. The assumption was that a program focused on questioning existing gender stereotypes can have potential impact on a multitude of outcomes. The discussion on specific statements of attitude does help us reflect on areas that maybe hard to change, and require additional effort. Lastly, the attitude scale itself can have limitations for precise measurement of attitudes for children in the ages of 11–13 years.

For boys, there is significant change in statements related to school specific gender attributes—that of boys being better at subjects such as science and math, and sports. For girls, there is no significant change in perceived ability on math and science. It could be that these differential sectorial abilities are very deeply ingrained in girls and more positive reinforcement is required. An encouraging area of change after program exposure is on the statement, "Girls provoke boys by wearing short dresses". This is of special significance when related to potential SRH outcomes and future relationships as it exemplifies the "sexual gaze", which also justifies sexualization or objectification of the female body while blaming them for one's own behavior.

On the other hand, for girls the statement—"girls like to be teased by boys"—shows a significant decrease among those who agreed to it. However, the more general statements such as—"there are times when a boyfriend needs to beat his girlfriend"—do not show a significant shift for boys and girls. With violence being widely prevalent, yet normalized, it is likely that attitudes that shun violence in *all* instances and believes in "zero tolerance" will take a longer engagement. From a cognitive-learning approach, these findings indicate that concrete direct statements, which are understood as directly affecting one's feelings, are the situations the girls and boys of this age find easier to relate to and change than those requiring abstraction.

Attitudes toward specific aspects of gender roles and the division of work become more egalitarian after program exposure. Support for women to "work outside the house" increased significantly for both girls and boys. Interestingly, the domain of childcare (bathing and feeding kids) proves to be more difficult to change for boys than that of household chores more generally. The positive attitudinal change toward gender role and responsibilities can be seen as support to women in alternate roles, such as employment. It may also indicate a move away from rigid masculinity, where boys are more accepting of 'caring' and 'doing domestic chores'.

The program also brings about a significant change among boys in perceived age at marriage for girls, which is beyond the legally acceptable age of 18 years. It is important to note that while this change is significant for boys who are exposed to the program, its effect on girls is positive but not significant. This could mean that as adolescent girls grow older, and into ages where discussion around marriage becomes more obvious, they could be aspiring for pushing age at marriage. But, with boys, this is not only a function of increasing age but such programs are necessary to create more egalitarian norms. The age itself, that is, not just 18 years, can indicate a more comprehensive support for girl's empowerment and self-development. It must be remembered that there is a specific statement in the attitude scale about higher education that shows no net positive shift following intervention exposure, but shifts in the positive direction in both arms. This could be influenced by the reality of seeing many girls going on to higher education in Mumbai.

Questions related to bodily integrity, for self and others, are specific domains related to SRH that show significant change after program exposure. In these specific domains, girls and boys express confidence to complain about someone in case of violations on self; and intent to intervene in case of violence against girls. We interpret this to be directly attributable to the specific program session on respecting self and others that gave clear messages about respect of the body and blame and shame about violations. The confidence to complain about sexual violence is remarkable given the stigma associated with it. Existing literature suggests that girls do not report their experience of sexual violence because of fear of being punished. One of the studies from Nepal describes girls being harassed by boys on their way to school; and if they report this harassment, they are often punished by parents and withdrawn from school (Mathur et al. 2001). This is even more acute as boys are rarely perceived as "victims" and there is silence around this issue. This also goes against the notion of hegemonic masculinity (Easton 2013). Both these findings are significant in their influence over shaping future SRH behavior. Girls and boys, who disapprove and speak out against violation and violence, are more likely to disapprove of its use in their own relations as well. The increase in comfort with the opposite sex, after program exposure, can be viewed as another possible contributor to notions of healthy, communicative, and equal relationships.

The findings demonstrate that attitudes toward gender norms, sexuality, and violence can be transformed through gender-focused interventions within the school settings. The GEMS program had several features that contributed to intense and participatory discussion. Key to the success of the group education activities was the facilitators' ability to be interactive and reach out to children. The facilitators were trained not only for a comprehensive and nuanced perspective of gender, but also for an easy presence with the girls and boys in the classrooms. The GEMS strategies and materials ensured that there were discussions not only in classrooms, but discussions in the schools, and out-reach to parents and families through the GEMS Diary, and other interactions. The finding that close to 80 % of children have discussed the program with someone, including peers, parents, and siblings, is encouraging toward the larger goal of a gender discourse.

There are limitations inherent in the program. While the GEMS project recognizes teachers as key stakeholders in taking gender discourse forward in the institutionalization process, limited activities were carried out with teachers. In the subsequent adaption and scale-up model, teachers are involved as key implementers, being supported by a team of facilitators. The school is an important site of socialization, but it is one among many other significant influencers: the family, peers, media, and other multitude exposures for young growing children in urban metropolis such as Mumbai. Several recommendations emerge; Institutionalization of such programs is necessary but strategies for longer engagement and more intensive/repeated discussions within schools are needed. On specific issues, boys and girls may need separate and/or additional sessions. Activation of forums and platforms for interface with parents and families are necessary for sustained impact. The program addresses several notions and concepts that are precursors for shaping SRH outcomes and overall sexual health. A follow-up study with children exposed to the program is critical to see if egalitarian attitudes start translating into specific behavior at older ages. Finally, this evidence must inform advocacy efforts for inclusion of such discussions within the "education" of children in schools with the aim of influencing gender norms, equal relations, and positive outcomes about sexuality and health.

References

Achyut, P., Bhatla, N., Khandekar, S., Maitra, S., & Verma, R. K. (2011). *Building support for gender equality among young adolescents in school: Findings from Mumbai, India*. New Delhi: ICRW.

Ashenfelter, O. (1978). Estimating the effect of training programs on earnings. *Review of Economics and Statistics, 60*(1), 47–57.

Ashenfelter, O., & Card, D. (1985). Using the longitudinal structure of earnings to estimate the effect of training programs. *Review of Economics and Statistics, 67*(4), 648–660.

Barker, G. (2006). Engaging boys and men to empower girls: Reflections from practice and evidence of impact. Expert Group Meeting on Elimination of all forms of discrimination and violence against the girl child. UNICEF Innocenti Research Centre, Florence, Italy, 25–28 September.

Barker, G., Contreras, J., Heilman, B., Singh, A. K., Verma, R. K., & Nascimento, M. (2011). *Evolving men: Initial results from the International Men and Gender Equality Survey (IMAGES)*. Washington, DC: International Center for Research on Women (ICRW). Rio de Janeiro: Instituto Promundo.

Barker, G., Ricardo, C., & Nascimento, M. (2007). *Engaging men and boys in changing gender-based inequity in health: Evidence from programme interventions*. Geneva: World Health Organization.

Dunne, M., Leach, F., Chilisa, B., Maundeni, T., Tabulawa, R., Kutor, et al. (2005). *Gendered school experiences: The impact on retention and achievement in Botswana and Ghana* (Education Series Research Report No. 56). London: DFID.

Easton, S. D. (2013). Masculine norms, disclosure, and childhood adversities predict long-term mental distress among men with histories of child sexual abuse. *Child Abuse & Neglect, 38*(2014), 243–251.

Go, V. F., Sethulakshmi, C. J., Bentley, M. E., Sivaram, S., Srikrishnan, A. K., Solomon, S., et al. (2003). When HIV-prevention messages and gender norms clash: The impact of domestic violence on women's HIV risk in slums of Chennai, India. *AIDS and Behavior, 7*(3), 263–272.

Haberland, N., & Rogow, D. (2007). *Sexuality and HIV education: Time for a paradigm shift* (Promoting healthy, safe, and productive transitions to adulthood brief No. 22). New York, NY: Population Council.

ICRW. (2011). *GEMS training manual for facilitators*. New Delhi: ICRW.

Karim, A. M., Magnani, R., Morgan, G., & Bond, K. (2003). Reproductive health risk and protective factors among unmarried youth in Ghana. *International Family Planning Perspective, 29*(1), 14–24.

Krishnan, S., Dunbar, M. S., Minnis, A. M., Medlin, C. A., Gerdts, C. E., & Padian, N. S. (2008). Poverty, gender inequities, and women's risk of human immunodeficiency virus/AIDS. *Annals of the New York Academy of Sciences, 1136*, 101–110. Reducing the impact of poverty on health and human development: Scientific Approaches.

Mathur, S., Malhotra, A., & Mehta, M. (2001). Adolescent girls' life aspirations and reproductive health in Nepal. *Reproductive Health Matters, 9*(17), 91–101.

Office of the Registrar General and Census Commissioner, India. (2014). Primary Census. http://www.censusindia.gov.in/2011census/population_enumeration.html. Accessed 7 July 2014.

Patel, V., & Andrew, G. (2001). Gender, sexual abuse and risk behaviours in adolescents: A cross-sectional survey in schools in Goa. *The National Medical Journal of India, 14*, 263–267.

Pinheiro, P. S. (2006). *World report on violence against children*. Geneva: United Nations.

Pulerwitz, J., & Barker, G. (2008). Measuring attitudes toward gender norms among young men in Brazil: Development and psychometric evaluation of the GEM Scale. *Men and Masculinities, 10*(3), 322–338.

Pulerwitz, J., Barker, G., Segundo, M., & Nascimento, M. (2006). *Promoting more gender-equitable norms and behaviors among young men as an HIV/AIDS prevention strategy*. Washington, DC: Population Council.

Rigby, K. (2003). Consequences of bullying in schools. *The Canadian Journal of Psychiatry, 48*, 583–590.

Santana, M. C., Raj, A., Decker, M. R., Marche, A. L., & Silverman, J. G. (2006). Masculine gender roles associated with increased sexual risk and intimate partner violence perpetration among young adult men. *Journal of Urban Health Bulletin of the New York Academy of Medicine, 83*(4), 575–585.

Sen, G., & Ostlin, P. (2007). Unequal, unfair, ineffective and inefficient. Gender inequity in health: why it exists and how we can change it. Final Report to the WHO Commission on Social Determinants of Health. http://www.who.int/social_determinants/resources/csdh_media/wgekn_final_report_07.pdf. Accessed 10 November 2014.

Sharp, S., Thompson, D., & Arora, T. (2000). How long before it hurts? An investigation into long-term bullying. *School Psychology International, 21*, 37–46.

UNAIDS. (1999). *Gender and HIV/AIDS: Taking stock of research and programs*. Geneva: UNAIDS.

Verma, R., Pulerwitz, J., Mahendra, V., Khandekar, S., Singh, A. K., Das, S., et al. (2008). *Promoting gender equity as a strategy to reduce HIV risk and gender-based violence among young men in India. Horizons final report*. Washington, DC: Population Council.

Wood, K., Maforah, F., & Jewkes, R. (1998). "He forced me to love him": Putting violence on adolescent sexual health agendas. *Social Science and Medicine, 47*(2), 233–242.

Chapter 10
Transmission of Intergenerational Spousal Violence Against Women in India

Aparna Mukherjee

Abstract Violence against women is a major human rights and public health concern. By using the large scale data of National Family Health Survey-3, this chapter attempts to find the levels and determinants of intergenerational transmission of spousal violence against women in India. The results show that childhood exposure to parental spousal violence plays an important role in shaping conformation to the set of gender role norms in India. Moreover, the findings suggest that exposure to childhood violence have a more devastating effect on building women's understanding of gender norms. Also, there is high concordance in current experience of spousal violence against women and spousal violence faced by their mothers; whereas, there is a weak association between men's involvement in spousal violence and their parents' experience of spousal violence. Given the pervasiveness of the problem of childhood exposure to parental spousal violence in India, this remains an important area for social, legal, and public policy concern.

Keywords Intergenerational transmission of violence • Childhood exposure to parental violence • India

Introduction

Violence against women is a major human rights and public health concern. The adverse health consequences that women experience due to violence are wide ranging and encompass physical, reproductive, sexual, and mental health outcomes. Unfortunately, such violence is often unnoticed and disregarded, in part, because it is considered as a forbidden topic. Moreover, violence against women is not only confined to the less developed or developing world but has remained a global challenge. As UN Secretary-General, Ban-Ki-Moon said: *"Violence against women and girls continues unabated in every continent, country and culture. It takes a devastating toll on women's lives, on their families, and on society as a whole.*

A. Mukherjee (✉)
Department of Population Policies and Programmes,
International Institute for Population Sciences, Mumbai, India
e-mail: tiya.mukherji@gmail.com

© Springer International Publishing Switzerland 2015   215
Y.K. Djamba, S.R. Kimuna (eds.), *Gender-Based Violence*,
DOI 10.1007/978-3-319-16670-4_10

Most societies prohibit such violence — yet the reality is that too often, it is covered up or tacitly condoned" (Johnson et al. 2008).

Due to its damaging repercussions to women, families, societies, and nations, violence against women has begun to draw the attention of researchers and policy makers, especially in developing countries. In these countries, women are vulnerable to many forms of violence, with domestic violence being the most common. Violence against women in the home is one of the most pervasive human rights challenges of our time. It remains a largely hidden problem that few countries, communities, or families openly confront. Violence in the home is not limited by geography, ethnicity, or status; it is a global phenomenon.

The prevalence of violence against women in India is high, especially spousal violence, which is the worst form of violence. India's National Family Health Survey-III (NFHS-3) interviewed 125,000 women in 28 states in 2005–2006; over 40 % women reported being beaten by their husbands at some point in time (Ministry of Health and Family Welfare, Government of India 2007). Over 51 % of the 75,000 men interviewed did not find anything wrong with assaulting their wives for some reason or other.

In India, cultural and social factors play an important role in developing and promoting violence against women. With the socialization process at different phases of life, men usually tend to take up the stereotyped gender roles of domination and control, whereas women grow up to follow the path of submission, dependence, and respect for authority throughout their lives. One consequence of that gendered socialization is that the home, which is supposed to be the most secure place, is where women are most exposed to violence.

The prevalence and causes of violence against women have been extensively discussed in both the social science literature and the media. The economic, social, and psychological effects of domestic (i.e., marital or spousal) violence have also received considerable attention from researchers. One focus of this attention has been the possible effects on children who witness violence within the family, including effects on their own tendency to perpetrate or experience domestic violence as adults.

The phrase "cycle of violence" is commonplace in the literature on spousal abuse. Research on effects of witnessing interparental spousal violence by children have mostly proved its association as a major risk factor with children's behavioral problems, adolescent conduct disorder, and adult intimate partner violence in their marital life. Such studies have shown that intimate partner violence between parents increased the risk for children's difficulties and can result in impulsive emotionality and aggressive personality styles in young people (Ehrensaft and Cohen 2012). Such traits get integrated before adult intimate relationships begin, increasing the likelihood that the cycle may repeat itself when conflict arises in their own marital relationships. But there are also some studies that deny any clear elevated effect or positive relationship between witnessing parental aggression and violence with their subsequent romantic partner (Kaufman and Zigler 1987; MacEwen and Barling 1988; Capaldi and Clark 1998).

Therefore, there is a need to redefine the predictive models of spousal violence that could explain the absoluteness of these phenomena of intergenerational transmission of violence.

In India, there have been many attempts to capture the causes and consequences of domestic violence, particularly spousal violence against women. However, due to lack of data and sensitivity of the pertinent issue, much of the research on that topic has been limited to socioeconomic and demographic risk factors and has failed to look into the transmission of intergenerational spousal violence at the national level (Kishor and Johnson 2004; Kaur and Garg 2008; Ghosh 2011).

The gender gap in attitudes toward violence against women is shaped by attitudes toward gender. Traditional gender-role attitudes, whether held by women or men, are associated with greater acceptance of violence against women, while egalitarian attitudes are associated with less acceptance of violence. If one can confirm that the effects of witnessing violence between parents based on the probability that children will experience violence in their own marriages, either as perpetrators or as victims, then one can conclude that the major part of gender roles accepted by women in India today are due to the transmission of gender roles from previous generations. As such, it remains important for researchers to identify the existence and extent of this inherent risk factor of spousal violence against women in India.

Therefore, the main objective of this chapter is to investigate whether the hypothesis that spousal violence against women in India depends upon the intergenerational transmission of violence within families holds true or not. A principal strand in the cycle-of-violence literature examines the effects of witnessing violence between parents on the probability that children will experience violence in their own marriages, either as perpetrators or as victims.

Review of Literature

This section contains the critical review of literature on spousal violence, the concept and theory of intergenerational transmission of violence, and a brief discussion of past research on spousal violence against women in India.

The most extensive empirical research on intimate violence has been that of Straus et al. (1980) study, which was based on over 2,000 families. The study discussed how violence becomes an inherent characteristic of family life and gets transmitted from generation to generation by simply witnessing the abuse between parents, child abuse by parents, or abuse between siblings in the childhood. In general, studies conducted in the 1990s show that spousal violence against women are indicators of the acceptance of violence, gendered attitudes, and sex role inequalities in the society (Anderson 1997; Caron and Carter 1997). Despite many attempts to reduce spousal violence against women, it continues to be widespread (Feder 1999).

Intergenerational transmission of spousal violence is often explained in terms of social transmission of behavior, where the behavior of one individual enhances the likelihood that a second individual will adopt a behavioral characteristic of the first one.

Thus, it can be said that what is actually transmitted is an "idea" about the benefits of adopting a particular behavior and that such ideas motivate particular behaviors later in life when appropriate circumstances arise (Bandura 1977). Studies have also shown that many violent men grew up in families where domestic violence was common (e.g., Rosenbaum and O'Leary 1981; Straus et al. 1980). The explanation of the intergenerational transmission of violence is often framed in terms of acquisition of aggressive behaviour (Bandura 1977). In a study by Kalmuss (1984), the exposure to interparental violence was found to be more strongly related to the enactment of violence than the experience of being abused; although this modelling of aggression was not sex specific.

Grych and Fincham (2001) found that witnessing interparental violence leads to problems in adjustment, behavior, and emotional well-being of the children and it continues to persist even when they grow up. Similarly, Johnson and O'Leary (1987) found associations between aggression and symptoms of conduct disorder, depression, and anxiety. A meta-analysis by Stith et al. (2000) found that children who have been exposed to violence in their childhood are more likely to enact or experience violence in their adult couple relations. In their studies, Miller-Perrin and Perrin (2007) concluded that witnessing interparental violence and direct experience to violence in childhood are equally dangerous.

According to studies by Johnson and Williams-Keeler (1998) and Rosenbaum and O'Leary (1981), witnessing interparental violence has comparable psychological and behavioral outcomes that hamper healthy emotional development and relational bonding in adulthood. When children are exposed to these methods of conflict resolution, they never learn prosocial alternatives to solve family problems and, therefore, lack strong alternative means for solving problems throughout life (Black et al. 2010). Another study by Owen et al. (2009) showed that children who witness family violence are more likely to enact violence with one another.

Extensive research in the past 30 years has revealed the multidimensional aspects of witnessing interparental violence in childhood (Stith et al. 2000) and its important role in quantifying its frequency and impact (Grych and Fincham 2001). Though most of the studies conclude that exposure to parental spousal violence is linked with many negative outcomes like intimate partner victimization (Feerick and Haugaard 1999), there are studies which show that there is no positive relationship between witnessing parental aggression and spousal violence in their own married life (Capaldi and Clark 1998). For example, Straus et al. (1980) found clear intergenerational effects, whereas Mihalic and Elliott (2005) found intergenerational effects that differed by sex. Similarly, other studies found a weak link or no link between aggression in the family of origin and subsequent violent behavior in adulthood (Kalmuss 1984; MacEwen 1994).

Therefore, exposure to parental spousal violence may be a risk factor for spousal violence but the relationship cannot be confirmed as absolute. Many adults who grow up in violent homes do not become violent adults, perhaps due to the effect of other factors like higher level of education, cultural difference, etc. (Kaufman and Zigler 1987). As Pollak (2002) rightly points out, witnessing domestic violence in the family of origin is not an inexorable precursor of violence, but it does increase the likelihood of violence.

Data from population-based surveys in India show that 21–48 % of women from different sociocultural settings have experienced domestic violence (Jejeebhoy 1998; Visaria 1999; International Center for Research on Women 2000; Verma and Collumbien 2003). Information from a more recent study in India called International Institute for Population Sciences (IIPS) and Population Council (2010) shows that one-fourth of young women reported that they had ever faced physical violence perpetrated by their husbands (25 %) and nearly the same fraction of young men (24 %) reported perpetrating violence on their wives.

Previous studies on domestic violence have clearly shown that spousal violence against women is pervasive and deeply rooted in sociocultural norms (Rao 1997; Visaria 1999). Kishor and Johnson (2004) indicated several socioeconomic and cultural risk factors of domestic violence in their 'multi-country' empirical study of prevalence of domestic violence, which included India.

There are some indications from previous studies that higher socioeconomic status levels, including higher levels of education among women act as protective factors against women's risk of domestic violence (Jejeebhoy 1998; Visaria 1999). Demographic factors such as age, number of living male children, and extended family residence were found to be negatively associated with the risk of spousal violence in South India (Rao 1997; Bloch and Rao 2002). Other studies in India have shown that lower level of dowry is associated with significantly higher subsequent risks of violence (Jeyaseelan et al. 2007; Singh et al. 2009). Moreover, substance abuse by men has been cited as a risk factor of spousal violence in India (Rao 1997; Kishor and Johnson 2004). Along with this, interspousal communication, ownership of property, dowry demands, and women's autonomy are important factors of spousal violence (Sahoo and Pradhan 2009; Singh et al. 2009).

The transmission of spousal violence from generation to generation in India has not received much attention from researchers though it is probably one of the most risky predictor of spousal violence. Only few studies at regional level have tried to provide some sort of picture on this phenomenon in India.

For example, studies have also revealed that male children of violent parents or men brought up in conventional patriarchal family structures are more likely to perpetrate spousal violence in their own families (Straus et al. 1980; Martin et al. 2002). Apparently, the process of gendered socialization is mainly responsible for spousal violence (Kishor and Johnson 2004). A study by Koenig et al. (2006) examined various individual and community level influences on domestic violence in Uttar Pradesh, India. Along with many other risk factors like childlessness and economic pressure, they confirmed the positive link between the intergenerational transmissions of violence and experiencing spousal violence against women in India.

Jeyaseelan et al. (2007) also confirmed that substance abuse, childhood exposure to physical violence by parents, and witnessing of parental spousal violence increase the risk of perpetrators/victims of spousal violence in adulthood. Similarly, another cross sectional study of physical spousal violence against women in Goa,

India by Kamat et al. (2010) found that women who witnessed interparental violence were more likely to accept it as a 'normal' behavior, and were more likely to be victimized.

A recent report "Youth in India: situation and needs 2006–2007" tried to capture some data on the extent of witnessing of interparental spousal violence. According to the report, one-fourth of young men and young women (24 % and 26 % respectively) reported ever witnessing their father beating their mother (Ministry of Health and Family Welfare, Government of India 2008). In contrast, just 2 % of young men and women reported that they had witnessed their mother beating their father.

In India there is deficiency of research on spousal violence against women, due to lack of data and sensitivity of the issue. Moreover, earlier research failed to consider the impact of social learning of violence and studies like that of Koenig et al. (2006) and Kamat et al. (2010) could not identify the transmission of spousal violence as an absolute and inherent factor of violence against women that is transmitted from generation to generation and has over the years made violence against women a much acceptable norm in India.

Therefore with the need to understand the gravity and extent of this level, this chapter attempts to focus on the transmission of intergeneration spousal violence in India at the national level.

Theory, Hypothesis, and Objectives

There are two basic explanations on the etiology of spousal violence—(1) feminist/patriarchal and (2) behavior learned in the family of origin, i.e., through social learning (Bandura 1977). Rising from the feminist movement of the 1970s, the feminist/patriarchal model gave the initial definition of family violence as "wife abuse" or "battering". According to the first ideology, wife abuse is viewed as being the result of an imbalance of power relations between men and women. Feminists believe that throughout history, women have been dominated by the superior patriarchal society that has limited the abilities and opportunities for women, and make women vulnerable to abuses and violent experiences within family and outside.

According to the second explanation, behaviors are learned by internalizing the observed behaviors of significant others (Burgess and Akers 1966; Bandura 1977). If we apply this to the theory of "cycle of violence", this theory postulates that children who witness or experience violence in their growing ages, learn violent behaviors from their parents and/or any other adult role models and eventually use these learned violent behaviors in their adult lives as perpetrators or as victims (Feshbach and Zagrodzka 1997).

Clearly, one of the consistent findings regarding etiological characteristics of family violence is the intergenerational transmission of violence. Unfortunately the empirical data in support of those theories are lacking.

It is assumed that men who are exposed to parental spousal violence are more likely to be violent as adults, and that women who witness parental violence as children are more likely to be tolerant with an abusive spouses. This study has three objectives:

1. To investigate the intergenerational transmission of spousal violence against women in India.
2. To understand whether the impact of childhood exposure to parental spousal violence on spousal violence is more significant on men than women.
3. To examine the differentials in this relationship in different settings of sociodemographic characteristics and cultures and also to see whether there is concordance in spousal violence against women between earlier generation and current generation.

Data Source and Methodology

This research uses data from India's Third National Family Health Survey (NFHS-3), 2005–2006, which is the first ever nationally representative survey that collected data on the dynamics of domestic violence in India. NFHS-3 was launched by the Ministry of Health and Family Welfare of Government of India, and it was conducted by the International Institute for Population Sciences and ORC Macro International. The data collected for domestic violence includes ever-married women of age 15–49. The analysis in this chapter is confined to the sample of women whose husbands were also interviewed, that is, both spouses in a couple were interviewed. The total sample size for this analysis is 28,904 couples.

Two major variables were computed to see the extent of spousal violence against women: first to determine the attitude toward spousal violence against women, and second to see the (behavioral) event of actual spousal violence against women. Exposure to parental spousal violence has been categorized into different levels depending upon the exposure in either single partner or both the partners. Based on these variables, various assessments were made with the help of different statistical tools. Binary logistic regression was also carried out with different models of background characteristics and regions in order to study the effect of childhood exposure to parental spousal violence.

To estimate spousal violence, the following questions were used to capture all types of physical spousal violence:

Does/did your husband ever do any of the following things to you?

(a) *Slap you?*
(b) *Twist your arm or pull your hair?*
(c) *Push you, shake you, or throw something at you?*
(d) *Kick you, drag you, or beat you up?*
(e) *Try to choke or burn you on purpose?*
(f) *Threaten or attack you with a knife, gun, or any other weapon?*

Conceptualization

Similar to the hypothesis, it is also conceptualized that the severity of spousal violence will considerably differ according to the exposure of men and women or both in some cases. It will help us not only to understand whether there is any association between the childhood exposures to parental spousal violence and spousal violence in adulthood but also how this process works. Possibly there could be four cases:

First, if none of them had the exposure, then if some conflict arises, the husband may not resort to violence or even if he does, then his wife will try to prevent or oppose him and eventually there will not be any future episodes of spousal violence. Therefore, among these couples there will be less or no chances of spousal violence.

Second, if only the husband had the childhood exposure to spousal violence, then if some conflict arises, he may immediately resort to violence but his wife will try to stop him and when every time this happens, the episodes of spousal violence will be reduced. Therefore, among these couples there will be moderate chances of spousal violence.

Third, the case could be where only the wife had the childhood exposure to parental spousal violence. Then, if some conflict arises between husband and wife, and the husband initiates the violence, the wife will simply accept it and it will become an approved act of solving any conflicts in the marriage and the episodes of spousal violence will continue. Therefore, among these couples there will be a high chance of spousal violence.

Fourth, it might be that both spouses had the childhood exposure to parental spousal violence. In that case, whenever there is conflict, the husband will use violence for conflict resolution and his wife will easily approve violence as a means of conflict resolution. Therefore, among these couples, there will be acute chances of spousal violence.

But obviously, the above four cases will vary with different background characteristics.

Results and Discussion

Levels of Spousal Violence According to Childhood Exposure to Parental Spousal Violence

The first part of Table 10.1 shows the difference in percentage of women who experienced spousal violence according to their own and their husband's exposure to parental spousal violence. It is quite evident that both men and women who had witnessed parental spousal violence in their childhood reported considerably higher involvement or experience of spousal violence against women than those

Table 10.1 Percent distribution of respondents by experience of spousal violence and attitude toward wife beating by exposure to parental spousal violence, India 2005–2006, NFHS-III

	Exposed to parental spousal violence	
	Yes	No
Women who experienced spousal violence according to their/husband's parental spousal violence		
Women	56.2	28.2
Men	42.7	31.4
Women and men who justify wife beating according to exposure to parental spousal violence		
Women	59.5	48.8
Men	65.7	45.3

Table 10.2 Percent distribution of spousal violence according to exposure to parental spousal violence, India 2005–2006, NFHS-III

	Percent of spousal violence	Percent of reporting couples
Spouse(s) exposure to parental spousal violence:		
None of them	25.5	58.3
Only the husband	34.8	20.3
Only the wife	53.8	12.7
Both the husband and the wife	58.5	8.7
Total	34.6	100.0

who had no such exposure. Among women, for those who witnessed parental spousal violence, 56.2 % experienced spousal violence as compared to 28.2 % of women who were not exposed to such experiences. Among male respondents, the corresponding figures are 42.7 % for "yes" and 31.4 % for "no." For both men and women, reports of wife physical abuse were much lower among those who were not exposed to parental spousal violence. These results show that exposure to parental spousal violence in childhood is associated with women's own experience of spousal violence.

The second part of Table 10.1 shows the difference in attitude of men and women who justify wife-beating, according to their childhood exposure to parental spousal violence. Both men and women who witnessed parental spousal violence justify spousal violence for any reason more than those who had no exposure. Apparently, men's exposure to parental spousal violence seems to more implicitly shape their attitudes toward their gendered behavior than women. Among those men who justify wife-beating, 65.7 % had been exposed to childhood parental spousal violence 20.4 % higher than those who had no exposure. Among those men and women who were exposed to parental spousal violence, wife-beating was justified by less than 6.2 % of women as compared to men.

Table 10.2 shows the prevalence of spousal violence according to exposure to parental spousal violence of husband and wife in their childhood. It is very clear that those couples in which both spouses witnessed spousal violence in their childhood were also more likely to report experience of spousal violence (58.5 %) than those couples who had no exposure (25.5 %). In comparative terms, couples in which both spouses were exposed to parental spousal violence reported 33 % more spousal violence than those in which no spouse had exposure. Those couples, where only the wife had childhood exposure to parental violence, reported higher prevalence of spousal violence (53.8 %) than couples, where only the husband had exposure (34.8 %).

So far, the present findings indicate that exposure to parental spousal violence does influence the transmission of violence into the second generation. It can be said that, perhaps, children witnessing fathers beating their mothers increases the risk of repeating spousal violence in their own adult marital relationships. Those women who have observed their mothers being beaten by their father tend to expect and accept the same behavior in their spousal relations as a normal behavior. Similarly, men who had the same childhood exposure experience tend to develop the attitude that beating their wives is a better way to resolve conjugal conflicts.

Figure 10.1 shows the prevalence of spousal violence in both generations. According to that figure, current spousal violence in India is 34.6 % whereas spousal violence reported for their parents by men and women are 28.7 and 20.5 % respectively.

The reported parental spousal violence by the couples is quite low, and it is even lower among women as compared to men. There could be two possibilities: either spousal violence has increased in the current generation or there is an underreporting of parental spousal violence, especially among women. It is questionable that spousal violence is lower among the respondents' parents, especially with the current change in women's position in society. Given higher female social mobility in the current generation, we expect spousal violence to be lower than in previous generations. Therefore, the lack of concordance in reporting of parental spousal violence by men and women suggests that female respondents may feel shame and guilt and hence conceal the information.

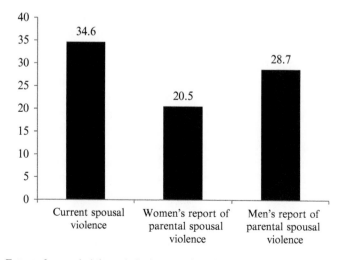

Fig. 10.1 Extent of spousal violence in both generations (%)

Patterns of Spousal Violence in Two Generations, by Selected Background Characteristics

Table 10.3 compares the differences in current prevalence and past prevalence of spousal violence by common background characteristics. In the current generation, the highest level of spousal violence is observed in the Central region of the country (42.4 %) and the lowest in the West (29.6 %). In contrast, the reported parental spousal violence by men and women was highest in the South, but the difference is considerably high. Men reported around 17 % higher prevalence of parental spousal violence in the South as compared to women. Parental spousal violence was lowest in the North as reported by women (14.8 %) and North East as reported by men (16.4 %). The lack of concordance trend in the regional variation of spousal violence between the two generations makes the picture unclear. In contrast, spousal violence is higher in rural areas as compared to urban areas in both generations. Nonetheless, in terms of the previous generation, men reported more parental spousal violence than women in both urban and rural areas.

Table 10.3 Percent distribution of respondents by spousal violence in the two generations, by selected background characteristics, India 2005–2006, NFHS-III

Background characteristics		Spousal violence	Parental spousal violence	
		Current	Women's parents	Men's parents
Region	North	30.8	14.8	17.4
	Central	42.4	16.8	22.4
	East	39.7	21.0	23.6
	North East	33.3	20.0	16.4
	West	29.6	20.5	21.4
	South	30.7	27.2	43.8
Residence	Rural	38.0	22.3	29.9
	Urban	28.9	19.5	27.2
Caste	Scheduled caste	44.9	26.9	36.2
	Scheduled tribe	38.5	26.1	32.2
	Backward caste	34.9	21.6	31.2
	General (others)	27.6	15.9	20.1
Religion	Hindu	34.5	21.2	29.3
	Muslim	39.5	20.3	25.8
	Christian	33.3	29.1	36.3
	Others	31.6	23.8	25.9
Wealth index	Poorest	47.0	24.6	32.3
	Poorer	43.4	24.0	31.0
	Middle	38.4	25.6	34.3
	Richer	31.6	21.3	30.3
	Richest	16.5	12.1	17.9
All		34.6	20.5	28.7

In both generations, the caste wise pattern in the prevalence of spousal violence is similar. In India, castes play a major role in determining one's position in society. By the constitution of India, Scheduled caste, Scheduled tribe and Other Backward castes have been given special importance, as majority of them are considered to be socially and economically disadvantaged groups. Other Backward is the term used by the Government of India to classify socioeconomically disadvantaged castes. Populations belonging to Scheduled caste had the highest prevalence and "Other castes" category had the lowest. The reports of spousal violence and parental spousal violence by religion do not show any particular consistent pattern between the two generations. In the current generation, Muslim couples reported the highest prevalence (39.5 %) followed by the Hindu couples (34.5 %), whereas the parental spousal violence rates reported by men and women were highest among the Christians.

Data on wealth index show that spousal violence decreases with increase in income. The current prevalence of spousal violence is 47.0 % among the poorest couples and 16.5 % among the richest couples. Even the parental spousal violence reported by men and women show the same trend, but the relationship is not linear.

Overall, women tend to report parental spousal violence substantially less than their male counterparts. The mass underreporting of spousal violence of women for themselves or for their mothers may be due to their social upbringing which does not allow them to speak for themselves or against any male members in their households; be it their husbands or fathers. It is important for women to understand that violence by anyone is a violation of their fundamental rights and not something to be accepted as a family norm.

Logistic Regression Analysis of Spousal Violence by Selected Background Characteristics

Table 10.4 shows the odds ratio for spousal violence by each of the background characteristics (bivariate associations). It has been separately done to clearly identify the demographic, socioeconomic, and other risk factors of spousal violence which could later help us in comparing and restricting further analysis for parental spousal violence. We have categorized various risk factors in groups like demographic, social, economic, lifestyle, and attitude related.

In terms of region of residence, compared to those who were living in the North (the reference category), residents of all other parts of India were statistically significantly more likely to have experienced spousal violence. The probability of spousal violence is highest in the Central region, followed by the East region. The Central and East regions as compared to the other regions of India are less developed and socially and economically underdeveloped hence apparently the conditions of women in these regions are worse than those of other regions. Urban areas have less likelihood of spousal violence as compared to rural areas.

Table 10.4 Odds ratio for spousal violence by selected background characteristics, India 2005–2006, NFHS-III

Predictors		Odds ratio	95 % CI
Demographic			
Region	North®	1	–
	Central	1.997***	1.796–2.220
	East	1.486***	1.312–1.684
	North East	1.301***	1.151–1.470
	West	1.225**	1.091–1.375
	South	1.171**	1.052–1.304
Residence	Rural®	1	–
	Urban	0.781***	0.728–0.839
Husband's age (in single years)		0.992	0.984–1.000
Wife's age (in single years)		1.016*	1.003–1.028
Man's age at marriage	0–19®	1	–
	20–24	0.989	0.922–1.062
	25+	0.903*	0.815–1.000
Woman's age at marriage	0–14®	1	–
	15–19	0.873**	0.809–0.943
	20+	0.723***	0.635–0.823
Marital duration	0–4®	1	–
	5–9	1.615***	1.449–1.801
	10–14	1.650***	1.430–1.905
	15–19	1.616***	1.338–1.951
	20–24	1.462**	1.148–1.863
	25–29	1.489**	1.105–2.008
	30+	1.455*	1.007–2.103
Social			
Caste	Scheduled caste®	1	–
	Scheduled tribe	0.491***	0.440–0.548
	Backward caste	0.738***	0.685–0.794
	General (others)	0.655***	0.603–0.711
Religion	Hindu®	1	–
	Muslim	1.492***	1.367–1.629
	Christian	0.754***	0.663–0.857
	Others	1.139	0.995–1.303
Husband's education	No education®	1	–
	Primary	1.112*	1.015–1.219
	Secondary	1.071	0.991–1.158
	Higher	0.977	0.886–1.078
Wife's education	No education®	1	–
	Primary	1.083	0.983–1.193
	Secondary	0.955	0.886–1.030
	Higher	0.728***	0.652–0.812

(continued)

Table 10.4 (continued)

Predictors		Odds ratio	95 % CI
Number of wives	Only 1®	1	–
	More than 1	1.694***	1.405–2.043
Economic			
Wealth index	Poorest®	1	–
	Poorer	0.928	0.844–1.021
	Middle	0.839**	0.760–0.927
	Richer	0.753***	0.673–0.843
	Richest	0.446***	0.390–0.512
Husband's occupation	Not working®	1	–
	Prof/Tech/Manager/Service	0.857	0.657–1.117
	Clerical	0.894	0.681–1.174
	Sales	0.928	0.722–1.193
	Agriculture—self employed	0.956	0.748–1.223
	Agriculture—employee	0.96	0.738–1.249
	Household domestic	1.012	0.794–1.291
Wife's occupation	Not working®	1	–
	Prof/Tech/Manager/Service	0.983	0.81–1.192
	Clerical	0.704*	0.498–0.995
	Sales	1.539***	1.315–1.801
	Agriculture—self employed	1.252***	1.160–1.352
	Agriculture—employee	1.354***	1.183–1.551
	Household domestic	1.243***	1.135–1.361
Lifestyle			
Tobacco consumption	No®	1	–
	Yes	1.098**	1.033–1.167
Alcohol consumption	No®	1	–
	Yes	2.515***	2.376–2.663
Mass media exposure men	No®	1	–
	Yes	0.920*	0.855–0.991
Mass media exposure women	No®	1	–
	Yes	1.091*	1.018–1.169
Attitude			
Those who justify beating wife	No®	1	–
	Yes	1.257***	1.187–1.331
Men justifying their right to get angry	No®	1	–
	Yes	1.123***	1.054–1.196
Marital duration 5+ and child/son preference	No child®	1	–
	No son only daughters	0.833*	0.711–0.976
	Either son/both	0.918	0.842–1.002

Notes: level of significance: ***$p<0.01$; **$p<0.05$; *$p<0.1$; ®=Reference category

Husband's age does not have any significant effect on the occurrence of spousal violence. In contrast, wife's age is positively associated with experience of spousal violence. Age at marriage is positively associated with the likelihood of spousal violence for both men and women, whereas the association between marital duration and spousal violence is positive but not linear. All couples that have been married for more than 4 years were more likely to report spousal violence than those with 0–4 years of marriage.

As compared to Scheduled caste, all other caste categories are significantly less likely to report spousal violence. The lowest odds ratio value is among members of the Scheduled Tribes. As compared to Hindu religion, couples from Muslim religion are significantly more likely to report spousal violence, whereas Christians are significantly less likely to report such behavior. Level of education plays an important role in constraining men to engage in spousal violence against their wives and women acceptance to spousal violence. Men who have only a primary level of education are significantly more likely to perpetrate spousal violence, whereas men with higher levels of education do not show any significant association, compared to uneducated men. Notably, women with the highest level of education are significantly less likely to have experienced spousal violence, which means that higher education for women can create awareness about their rights and well-being related to violence by their partners.

Men who have more than one wife are significantly more likely to indulge in spousal violence than those who have only one wife. The data in Table 10.4 also show that the probability of spousal violence decreases with income; couples from higher wealth index groups are significantly less prone to spousal violence than those in lower wealth index groups. Men's occupation is not significantly associated with spousal violence. Compared to nonworking women, women who are involved in manual labor, such as agriculture and domestic help, are significantly more likely to experience spousal violence. In contrast, women in clerical (white collar) jobs were significantly less likely to experienced spousal violence.

Consumption of alcohol and tobacco products may reduce men's cognitive abilities to control aggressive behavior. This holds true in case of spousal violence; those men who consume tobacco and alcohol are significantly more likely to perpetrate spousal violence, but the effect of alcohol is more devastating as it increases the likelihood by more than two times.

It is thought that mass media exposure creates awareness on various issues including women's rights but exposure to any form of mass media does not seem to work on women's perception toward spousal violence. Rather, it aggravates their acceptance to it. Perhaps, mass media has become very common and fails to make any further difference in educating women about spousal violence, or maybe current Indian media do not capture the attention of women through programs that could lead them to awareness. Unlike women, men with some exposure to mass media show lower likelihood to violence.

In order to understand whether attitudes or perceptions have any association with actual behavior, odds ratio was calculated for those men who justify beating women.

The results show that those men who think that wife-beating is justified for any reason were significantly more likely to perpetrate violence against their wives.

Due to India's rigid social structure, a woman's position in society is generally identified by her number of children and particularly by her sons. However, spousal violence seems not to be affected the number of sons alone. Controlling for duration of marriage (5 years and over), and comparing women by the number and sex of their children, only those who have daughter(s) and no son(s) are significantly less likely to report spousal violence versus those without children. Other sex combinations have no significant effect on spousal violence. This is, perhaps, due to longer marital duration which determines a woman's experience of spousal violence irrespective of the number of sons and daughters.

Predictive Models of Spousal Violence, by Exposure to Parental Spousal Violence and by Region of Residence

What are the net effects of these variables on spousal violence? This question is answered through the multivariate analysis in the form of logistic regression. The results are given in Table 10.5 for different models in which experience of parental spousal violence is the key explanatory variable. Other variables are added in subsequent models to measure changes in the predictive power of exposure to parental spousal violence on spousal violence.

There are five models. The first model controls for the demographic factors, whereas the second model controls for all demographics as well as social factors. The third model controls for the demographic and socioeconomic factors; the fourth model controls for all previous factors including lifestyle risk factors; and finally, the fifth model contains all the preceding risk factors, plus attitude/perception related factors. These variables have been identified as major risk factors of spousal violence in bivariate analyses (Table 10.4). They have been controlled so as to find out the true association between exposure to parental spousal violence and probability of perpetrating/experiencing spousal violence in respondents' own conjugal relationships.

All the models confirm that those couples among whom both the husband and wife had childhood exposure to parental spousal violence are significantly more likely to experience spousal violence in their own marital relationships compared to those who had no exposure, or only the husband or the wife had such experiences. This remains true for all the models.

Similarly, in all the models the chances of a woman experiencing spousal violence is quite higher in events where only the wife had exposure to childhood parental spousal violence as compared to only husband's exposure. Among different models, the pattern of likelihood remains the same. The difference in the odds ratio of exposure to parental violence of only husband and only wife is surprising. It is higher in case of women by almost two times. This repetitive trend in women's

Table 10.5 Results of different models of logistic regression analysis for spousal violence and parental spousal violence, India 2005–2006, NFHS-III

Predictors		Model I	Model II	Model III	Model IV	Model V
		Odds ratio	Odds ratio	Odds ratio	Odds ratio	Odds ratio
Controlled variables						Demographic
					Demographic	Social
				Demographic	Social	Economic
			Demographic	Social	Economic	Lifestyle
		Demographic	Social	Economic	Lifestyle	Attitude
Husband/wife exposure to parental violence	None of them®	1	1	1	1	1
	Only husband	1.823***	1.696***	1.658***	1.600***	1.562***
	Only wife	3.887***	3.692***	3.553***	3.299***	3.305***
	Both	5.456***	4.958***	4.792***	4.360***	4.291***

Notes: level of significance: ***$p < 0.01$; ® = Reference category

increased risk of spousal violence, again, suggests their greater acceptance of spousal violence. These findings remain significant even when logistic regression equations are run separately by region of residence, suggesting that witnessing parental spousal violence is positively associated with risk of spousal violence across India (Table 10.6).

To understand whether witnessing the father beating the mother influences a change in the attitude of men and women toward their gender roles and expectations, bivariate logistic regression analysis was carried out for those who experience spousal violence. The results are displayed in Fig. 10.2. It is clear that those men and women who had exposure to parental spousal violence are more likely to justify wife-beating than those who did not have any such exposure (reference category). But the likelihood is quite high for men (OR = 1.94) as compared to women (OR = 1.24). Similarly, men and women who had exposure to parental spousal violence also had higher chances of justifying husband's anger than those who did not have any such exposure. Again, men's perception toward their being justified to get angry for any reason is quite higher (OR = 1.58) than women's (OR = 1.18).

Likelihood of Help Seeking Behavior, Experience of Physical Injury, and Physical Hurt by Other Persons Among Married Women Who Witnessed Parental Spousal Violence

Lastly, Fig. 10.3 shows that women who had witnessed parental spousal violence are less likely to report or seek help (OR = 0.82) for spousal violence than women with no such childhood exposure. Similarly, women who had witnessed their father beating their mothers in childhood have higher chances of experiencing physical injury (OR = 1.40) and are almost twice (OR = 2.06) more likely to experience physical violence from others than those who had no such childhood exposure. Clearly, witnessing parental spousal violence poses a greater risk to women as they perceive violence as legitimate behavior for men to do and unabatedly continue to suffer from ongoing pattern of male domination in their homes and outside.

Therefore, growing up in a violent home tends to change the perception of men regarding their rights and justification of their deeds in the family and society as compared to their actual behavior. Whereas women seem to be more acceptable when they actually face violence, their opinion regarding men's rights to dominate and overpower women for any reason is not much influenced as in the case for men. Perhaps, women find themselves helpless when they face violence by their partners and silently prefer to subdue themselves to their husbands' rage. If true, such perception of inferiority among women may be a result of sprawling inequalities that exist in India in their access to education, health care, physical and financial resources, and opportunities in the political, economic, social, and cultural spheres.

Table 10.6 Results of regional analysis of logistic regression for spousal violence and parental spousal violence, India 2005–2006, NFHS-III

Predictors		Regions					
		North	Central	East	North-East	West	South
		Odds ratio	Odds ratio	Odds ratio	Odds ratio	Odds ratio	Odds ratio
Controlled variables		Demographic	Demographic	Demographic	Demographic	Demographic	Demographic
		Social	Social	Social	Social	Social	Social
		Economic	Economic	Economic	Economic	Economic	Economic
		Lifestyle	Lifestyle	Lifestyle	Lifestyle	Lifestyle	Life-style
		Attitude	Attitude	Attitude	Attitude	Attitude	Attitude
Husband/wife exposure to parental violence	None of them®	1	1	1	1	1	1
	Only husband	1.646***	1.540***	1.427***	1.645***	1.141	1.503***
	Only wife	3.700***	2.454***	3.910***	3.457***	5.088***	2.447***
	Both	3.270***	2.660***	4.624***	4.720***	4.237***	4.229***

Notes: level of significance: ***$p<0.01$; ® = Reference category

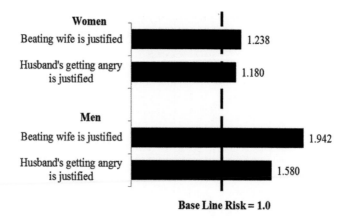

Fig. 10.2 Odds ratio for justification for violence (wife beating) and justification for husband's anger (*only for those who experienced/perpetrated spousal violence*) as reported by the husband and the wife who witnessed parental spousal violence, India 2005–2006, NFHS-III

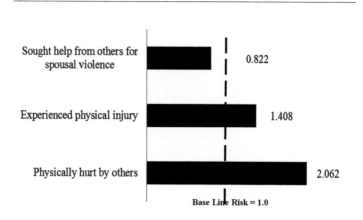

Fig. 10.3 Odds ratio for help seeking behavior, experience of physical injury, and experience of physical hurt by other persons among women who witnessed parental spousal violence, India 2005–2006, NFHS-III

Conclusion

From the analysis, it is clear that the hypothesis that was conceptualized in the beginning of this chapter is confirmed. This study reveals the impact of childhood exposure to parental spousal violence in shaping conformation to the set of gender role norms. This finding suggests that witnessing violence between one's parents while growing up is an important risk factor for the perpetration of partner violence in adulthood. Women's exposure to childhood violence seems to have more effect on building their understanding toward their gender norms. Compared to men, women are more susceptible to this phenomenon of intergenerational transmission of gender role norms.

Childhood exposure to parental spousal violence of the husband or the wife alone also have impact on spousal violence, but more so for the wife. The likelihood of experiencing or perpetrating spousal violence is higher among those spouses where both partners were exposed to childhood parental spousal violence as compared to spouses who had no such exposure or only one partner was exposed to parental spousal violence. There are similarities in current experiences of spousal violence against women and spousal violence faced by their mothers; whereas, there is a weak association between men's perpetration of spousal violence and their exposure to parental spousal violence.

Moreover, the results in the chapter show that the impact of childhood exposure to parental violence does not vary largely under different settings of sociodemographic and cultural characteristics, but remains an intrinsic risk factor to spousal violence in adulthood under all different models analyzed in this study. With differences in income quintile, lifestyle, and attitudinal related risk factors, there is a slight decline in the impact of parental spousal violence on spousal violence. Still, parental spousal violence remains a strong predictor of spousal violence even when all other covariates are added into the logistic regression equations.

The results of this study require urgent attention of policy makers to reduce spousal violence against women in India, in part, by reducing children's exposure to parental spousal violence. This will help break the intergenerational cycle of violence. Interventions are required that not only promote parental skills that strategically solve conflicts in the family, but also cultivate healthy parent-child relations, especially with girls.

Schools can play a key role in teaching children that violence of any kind and by any one is wrong. Students should be taught to avoid violence and adopt peaceful ways of conflict resolutions. Education and awareness programs on spousal violence or violence against women should focus on the impact on children and specific ways to address this hidden problem. Through some innovative programs, such as street shows and plays, teenage boys and girls should be made aware of violence at home or outside. In addition, the government and other social service organizations should take steps to reduce spousal violence. Legislative policies and laws should be passed to strengthen the message that spousal violence or violence of any type against women is a hideous crime and that perpetrators will be severely punished. These policies must focus on the protection of children and address the impact of violence on children at home.

Increasing education and training programs on spousal violence and promoting communication and referral units for women to complain and seek help at community level can help women to raise their voices and protect their children from the ill effects of spousal violence. Rising women's status in society through increase in the level of education, employment opportunities, health facilities, financing facilities, and rights to property can also bring positive changes in the reduction of violence against women in both within the family and outside.

Last, but not the least, more research should be conducted on violence against women in India, particularly domestic and spousal violence. It will help to pool information on this sensitive issue in order to allow policy makers to take action to root out this social evil from society.

Limitations

This chapter gives some insights on the phenomena and extent of transmission of intergenerational spousal violence, but there are a few limitations. Though most of the risk factors have been controlled for understanding the absoluteness of the event, we are not sure whether the exposure to childhood parental violence was also associated with victimization of children by the parents. There may be respondents who have been witnesses as well as victims of child abuse in their childhood; in that case, the effect of transmission of spousal violence may increase by many folds.

In this paper, the experience of spousal violence does not show the severity of violence nor its frequency. We have only examined those cases of spousal violence where women have ever faced physical violence in their marital relationships. If a separate analysis could be done based on a complete history of spousal aggression then it will help to substantiate whether exposure to parental spousal violence also increases the episodes and severity of violence among the couples. Perpetrators may deny or minimize their involvement while reporting spousal violence and victims may lie out of fear of reprisal if known to husband or out of feeling of shame. Therefore, the incidence of spousal violence may be much higher than what is reported here. Lastly, since some sociobiologists deny the social learning theory and emphasize that intimate violence is genetically influenced other perspectives should be considered in interpreting social behaviors, including spousal violence. That task is beyond the scope of this study.

References

Anderson, K. (1997). Gender, status, and domestic violence: An integration of feminist and family violence approaches. *Journal of Marriage and the Family, 59*, 655–669.

Bandura, A. (1977). *Social learning theory* (1st ed.). Englewood Cliffs, NJ: Prentice Hall.

Black, D., Sussman, S., & Unger, J. (2010). A further look at the intergenerational transmission of violence: Witnessing interparental violence in emerging adulthood. *Journal of Interpersonal Violence, 25*(6), 1022–1042.

Bloch, F., & Rao, V. (2002). Terror as a bargaining instrument: A case study of dowry violence in rural India. *American Economic Review, 92*, 1029–1043.

Burgess, R. L., & Akers, R. L. (1966). A differential association reinforcement theory of criminal behavior. *Social Problems, 14*, 128–147.

Capaldi, D., & Clark, S. (1998). Prospective family predictors of aggression toward female partners for at-risk young men. *Developmental Psychology, 34*(6), 1175.

Caron, S., & Carter, D. (1997). The relationships among sex role orientation, egalitarianism, attitudes toward sexuality, and attitudes toward violence against women. *The Journal of Social Psychology, 137*(5), 568–587.

Ehrensaft, M. K., & Cohen, P. (2012). Contribution of family violence to the intergenerational transmission of externalizing behavior. *Prevention Science, 13*(4), 370–383.

Feder, L. (1999). *Women and domestic violence* (1st ed.). New York: Haworth Press.

Feerick, M., & Haugaard, J. (1999). Long-term effects of witnessing marital violence for women: The contribution of childhood physical and sexual abuse. *Journal of Family Violence, 14*(4), 377–398.

Feshbach, S., & Zagrodzka, J. (1997). *Aggression: Biological, developmental, and social perspectives.* New York: Plenum Press.

Ghosh, S. (2011). Watching, blaming, silencing, intervening: Exploring the role of the community in preventing domestic violence in India. *Practicing Anthropology, 33*(3), 22–26.

Grych, J., & Fincham, F. (2001). *Interparental conflict and child development* (1st ed.). Cambridge: Cambridge University Press.

International Center for Research on Women. (2000). *Domestic violence in India: A summary report of a multi-site household survey.* Washington, DC: International Center for Research on Women.

International Institute for Population Sciences (IIPS) and Population Council. (2010). *Youth in India: Situation and needs 2006–2007.* Mumbai: IIPS.

Jejeebhoy, S. (1998). Wife-beating in rural India: A husband's right? Evidence from survey data. *Economic and Political Weekly, 33,* 855–862.

Jeyaseelan, L., Kumar, S., Neelakantan, N., Peedicayil, A., Pillai, R., & Duvvury, N. (2007). Physical spousal violence against women in India: Some risk factors. *Journal of Biosocial Science, 39*(5), 657–670.

Johnson, P., & O'Leary, K. (1987). Parental behavior patterns and conduct disorders in girls. *Journal of Abnormal Child Psychology, 15*(4), 573–581.

Johnson, H., Ollus, N., & Nevala, S. (2008). Eliminating violence against women: Forms, strategies and tools. Workshop presented at the Seventeenth Session of the United Nations Commission on Crime Prevention and Criminal Justice. Vienna: UNICRI.

Johnson, S., & Williams-Keeler, L. (1998). Creating healing relationships for couples dealing with trauma: The use of emotionally focused marital therapy. *Journal of Marital and Family Therapy, 24*(1), 25–40.

Kalmuss, D. (1984). The intergenerational transmission of marital aggression. *Journal of Marriage and the Family, 46,* 11–19.

Kamat, U., Ferreira, A., Motghare, D., Kamat, N., & Pinto, N. (2010). A cross-sectional study of physical spousal violence against women in Goa. *Healthline, 1*(1), 34–40.

Kaufman, J., & Zigler, E. (1987). Do abused children become abusive parents? *American Journal of Orthopsychiatry, 57*(2), 186–192.

Kaur, R., & Garg, S. (2008). Addressing domestic violence against women: An unfinished agenda. *Indian Journal of Community Medicine, 33*(2), 73.

Kishor, S., & Johnson, K. (2004). *Profiling domestic violence: A multi-country study.* Calverton, MA: ORC Macro.

Koenig, M., Stephenson, R., Ahmed, S., Jejeebhoy, S., & Campbell, J. (2006). Individual and contextual determinants of domestic violence in North India. *American Journal of Public Health, 96*(1), 132.

MacEwen, K. E. (1994). Refining the intergenerational transmission hypothesis. *Journal of Interpersonal Violence, 9,* 350–365.

MacEwen, K. E., & Barling, J. (1988). Multiple stressors, violence in the family of origin, and marital aggression: A longitudinal investigation. *Journal of Family Violence, 3*(1), 73–87.

Martin, S., Moracco, K., Garro, J., Tsui, A., Kupper, L., Chase, J., et al. (2002). Domestic violence across generations: Findings from northern India. *International Journal of Epidemiology, 31*(3), 560–572.

Mihalic, S. W., & Elliott, D. (2005). A social learning theory model of marital violence. In T. Chibucos & R. Leite (Eds.), *Readings in family theory* (p. 98). London, UK: Sage.

Miller-Perrin, C., & Perrin, R. (2007). *Child maltreatment* (1st ed.). Thousand Oaks, CA: Sage Publications.

Ministry of Health and Family Welfare, Government of India. (2007). *National Family Health Survey-3 (NFHS-3) (2005–2006)*. Mumbai, India: International Institute for Population Sciences.

Ministry of Health and Family Welfare, Government of India. (2008). *Youth in India: Situation and needs, 2006–2007*. Mumbai, India: International Institute for Population Sciences.

Owen, A., Thompson, M., Shaffer, A., Jackson, E., & Kaslow, N. (2009). Family variables that mediate the relation between intimate partner violence (IPV) and child adjustment. *Journal of Family Violence, 24*(7), 433–445.

Pollak, R. (2002). *An intergenerational model of domestic violence* (1st ed.). Cambridge, MA: National Bureau of Economic Research.

Rao, V. (1997). Wife-beating in rural South India: A qualitative and econometric analysis. *Social Science and Medicine, 44*(8), 1169–1180.

Rosenbaum, A., & O'Leary, K. (1981). Marital violence: Characteristics of abusive couples. *Journal of Consulting and Clinical Psychology, 49*(1), 63.

Sahoo, H., & Pradhan, M. R. (2009). Domestic violence in India: An empirical analysis. *Man in India, 89*(3), 303–322.

Singh, A., Singh, S., & Pandey, S. (2009). *Domestic violence against women in India*. Gurgaon, Haryana: Madhav Books.

Stith, S., Rosen, K., Middleton, K., Busch, A., Lundeberg, K., & Carlton, R. (2000). The intergenerational transmission of spouse abuse: A meta-analysis. *Journal of Marriage and Family, 62*(3), 640–654.

Straus, M., Gelles, R., & Steinmetz, S. (1980). *Behind closed doors*. New Brunswick, NJ: Transaction Publishers.

Verma, R., & Collumbien, M. (2003). Wife beating and the link with poor sexual health and risk behavior among men in urban slums in India. *Journal of Comparative Family Studies, 34*, 61–74.

Visaria, L. (1999). *Violence against women in India: Evidence from rural Gujarat*. Washington, DC: International Center for Research on Women.

Index

© Springer International Publishing Switzerland 2015
Y.K. Djamba, S.R. Kimuna (eds.), *Gender-Based Violence*,
DOI 10.1007/978-3-319-16670-4